Language in Psychiatry
a handbook of clinical practice

Equinox Textbooks and Surveys in Linguistics

Series Editor: Robin Fawcett, Cardiff University

Already published:

Multimodal Transcription and Text Analysis by Anthony Baldry and Paul J. Thibault

Meaning-Centered Grammar: an introductory text by Craig Hancock

Forthcoming titles in the series:

The Power of Language: how discourse influences society by Lynne Young and Brigid Fitzgerald

Genre Relations: mapping culture by J.R. Martin and David Rose

Intonation in the Grammar of English by M.A.K. Halliday and William S. Greaves

An Introduction to English Sentence Structure: clauses, markers, missing elements by Jon Jonz

The Rhetoric of Research: a guide to writing scientific literature by Beverly Lewin

Language in Psychiatry
a handbook of clinical practice

Jonathan Fine

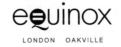

equinox

LONDON   OAKVILLE

Published by

Equinox Publishing Ltd

UK: Unit 6, The Village, 101 Amies St, London, SW11 2JW
USA: DBBC, 28 Main Street, Oakville, CT 06779

www.equinoxpub.com

Language in Psychiatry: a handbook of clinical practice by Jonathan Fine
First published 2006
© Jonathan Fine 2006

British Library Cataloguing-in-Publication Data
A catalogue record for this book is available from the British Library.

ISBN 1 904768 12 1 (hardback)

Library of Congress Cataloging-in-Publication Data
Fine, Jonathan.
  Language in psychiatry : a handbook of clinical practice / Jonathan Fine.
      p. cm. -- (Equinox textbooks and surveys in linguistics)
  Includes bibliographical references and index.
  ISBN 1-904768-12-1 (hbk.)
  1. Psychotherapy--Handbooks, manuals, etc. 2. Psycholinguistics--Handbooks, manuals, etc. 3.
Communicative disorders--Handbooks, manuals, etc. I. Title. II. Series.
  RC480.5.F465 2004
  616.89'14--dc22
                            2004008310

Typeset by Catchline, Milton Keynes (www.catchline.com)

Printed and bound in Great Britain by Antony Rowe Ltd, Chippenham

Contents

Contents

Foreword

There is a dearth of books on communication in mental illness by linguists written for non-linguists and especially for clinicians. Psychiatrists are the profession who are most likely to encounter a range of atypical speakers and they are just as puzzled as general practitioners who generally make the first clinical encounter. Developmental Paediatricians and Psychologists also meet people who are delayed or deviant in their talk. Psychiatrists have over the last century made limited stabs at explaining unusual or 'crazy talk' but it is only in the last decade that disorders such as the Pervasive Development Disorders and Schizophrenia have been subjected by Psycholinguistics to more exhaustive scrutiny. It is refreshing therefore to read a textbook which has as its opening sentence 'That the purpose of the volume is to present an approach to listening in psychiatry.' The aim of the textbook is to describe the phenomenon of psychiatric disturbances in functional linguistic terms and to enable the clinician to identify at what point the use of language or non-verbal communication becomes so atypical as to call attention to the individuals suffering from a psychiatric condition.

The clinician needs a knowledge base, which is easy to make formal and he needs ways of labelling atypical language pathological. It would not do if regional dialects or street argot were considered by the practitioner to be disturbed. Psychiatrists are currently taught the basis of classic communication deviations that people with specific syndromes show, but only extreme cases are used and the challenge is how to listen to and describe mildly deviant discourse. The topic of language and mental health has been a graveyard of research applications and funding, which is due largely to modern linguistic sophistication leaving Psychiatrists far behind. There is in Fine's book a successful aim to find linguistic characteristics of disorders by comparing affected subject's discourse and social interaction.

Fine has a high reputation for publishing across a range of clinical conditions from anxiety states to the Pervasive Developmental Disorders and is possibly the most currently highly-qualified professional to write this handbook, which does indeed cover the norms of the speech community and gives a framework to the clinician as to how functional linguistic analysis determines why the output of certain speakers is deviant.

Most attempts by linguists to communicate to clinicians deter the clinician by linguistic technology and terminology. Fine has used everyday language and clear examples of normal and deviant texts to describe and explain problems of intonation, meaning, phonology, grammar and pragmatics. The clinician and general practitioner (general practitioner or Psychiatrist) could open this book and find out forthwith why his/her patient sounds odd. The specialist may well consider the chapters on Language in Psychiatric Disorder and Pervasive Developmental Disorders the definitive works thereon. The appendices are invaluable to read with the book and to consult later in professional situations.

The clinician and the academic will see research opportunities and ways of addressing psycholinguistic questions.

Bill Fraser

Emeritus Professor of Psychiatry
University of Wales College of Medicine

Preface

This book inherently cuts across different fields and could not have been written without the help of many people and institutions.

The language data upon which the research is based have been collected in numerous settings starting in 1970 with a research project on children's language supported by the Ontario Ministry of Education and the North York Board of Education. Over the years, projects with G. Bartolucci, J.R. Martin, P. Szatmari, R. Tannock, and R. Schachar led to substantial sets of tape recordings and transcripts. I am particularly indebted to Dr. J. Pelletier for interviewing the patient at St Joseph's Hospital, Hamilton, Ontario whose language is quoted in Chapter 7. These colleagues have all permitted me to analyse and reanalyse the data. The research would not have been possible without the various speakers giving permission to be interviewed and taped. I hope that the work presented here and elsewhere justifies their confidence in research. All names have been changed or masked.

The content of this volume is developed from two key sources: Michael Halliday's *An Introduction to Functional Grammar* (second edition, London: Arnold, 1994) and *Diagnostic and Statistical Manual of Mental Disorders* (DSM 4) (fourth edition, American Psychiatric Association, 1994). An update of *An Introduction to Functional Grammar* has since been published as *An Introduction to Functional Grammar*, third edition, revised by Christian Matthiessen (London: Arnold, 2004). This third edition provides much updated material and the presentation in terms of tables and networks makes the work more accessible to the non-expert. The general lines of the analyses are similar to those of the second edition as used in the present volume. Specific references to Halliday (1994) and DSM 4 are made where appropriate. In general, though, these two works are drawn on extensively and I am pleased to acknowledge them as the starting points for the linguistic and psychiatric analyses, respectively.

Financial support has come from a number of grants and collaborations with colleagues. These include: The Ontario Mental Health Foundation (grants to Tannock and Fine; Szatmari), Medical Research Council (Canada) (grants to Bartolucci; Szatmari; Szatmari, Tuff, Bartolucci, Mahoney, Jones, Bryson and Fine), Ontario Ministry of Education (grant to Fine and Martin), Health Canada (National Health and Research Development Program (grant to Tannock & Fine number 6606–5366), and the Research and Training Committee, Hospital for Sick Children, Toronto, for support during the sabbatical years 1989–90, 1996–97.

I warmly thank Nicky Lachs, Russell Schachar, William Sledge, Peter Szatmari, Rosemary Tannock and a number of other anonymous clinical reviewers who have seen the manuscript at different stages and made detailed comments. Robin Fawcett provided me with his comments from the perspective of linguistics. They all gave me many helpful suggestions which perhaps I have not followed closely enough. These readers only can be credited with improvements. The remaining shortcomings are my own. David Graddol has contributed expert production advice that has added greatly to the ease of using the volume. On behalf of myself and my readers I thank Catchline for their dedication and care in editing, design and getting the volume into shape.

A number of institutions and the people who make them human and alive have helped me and taught me over the years. First is the English department of Glendon College, York University, Toronto, Canada where Michael Gregory introduced me to linguistics. It has remained a refreshing place to visit and share ideas, more recently with Jim Benson and Bill Greaves. The department of psychiatry of St. Joseph's Hospital, Hamilton, Ontario, Canada is where I did my first work on language and schizophrenia with Dr. Giampierro Bartolucci. He had already studied linguistics so was an excellent guide for a linguist trying to learn about psychiatric disorders. Dr. Peter Szatmari of Chedoke-McMaster Hospitals introduced me to the research and issues in pervasive developmental disorders and continues to be an inspiration to do research carefully and well. I always appreciate the human side of these collegial relations. It is much easier to do research with people you like.

The Hospital for Sick Children, Toronto, Canada, has provided me with facilities and support for my sabbatical years 1989–90, 1996–97 and a welcome mat, facilities, and plenty of stimulating conversation and collaboration during many briefer stays. The Department of Psychiatry and the Brain and Behaviour Research Programme have been encouraging, helpful and comfortable places to work. In particular, I want to thank my hosts and collaborators Russell Schachar and Rosemary Tannock for sharing their enthusiasm about research and their always willing, interested and critical ears for my ideas. They have helped shape my ideas of how to think about language and psychiatric disorders at the same time. The Department of English at Bar-Ilan University has been my academic home for over 20 years. I appreciate the collegial relations of my friends there who have encouraged my work and kept me going when the road was rough, both old timers and newcomers. My students also have prodded me endlessly to be clearer, more explicit and more detailed. Joel Walters has given much advice about how to proceed with this volume. I am so grateful. Mildred Schwartz was a constant source of academic advice and general encouragement over the years this book took its final shape. Thank you.

The manuscript and the research behind it were developed over many years that included good times and trying times. I am grateful to my family and friends who have continued with so much support. Devorah, Naomi and Ephraim: yes, it is finished. Thank you guys. The volume is dedicated to the memory of Harold Fine whose ears for the emotions and reality of language were keener with his many decades of practised listening and to the memory of Yoel Yosef Fine, who in his short years dealt deeply with the reality and dreams of the world. May their memories be for a blessing.

Jonathan Fine
August 2005

Transcription conventions
Italics: words under discussion or words that exemplify the point being discussed.
CAPITAL LETTERS: stressed pronunciation.
(Round parentheses): explanatory notes.
[Square brackets and condensed typeface]: alternative version or additional words provided by author.
Other special conventions relating to specific examples, such as bold, italics and underline, may be given in the text.

Chapter 1 contents

Why look at language in psychiatry?

Introduction

This volume presents an approach to listening in psychiatry. Much of clinical practice is dependent on information and impressions gained from interaction with patients. The clinical picture emerges from this interaction and in a holistic way leads to the diagnosis and, to some extent, suggestions for treatment. From the clinical perspective, this volume is about what goes into listening appropriately, or, put another way, what the clinician has to be aware of in language.

Speakers who are not psychiatrically normal may show their psychiatric state through the language they use. Therefore, a functional study of the language of speakers with psychiatric disorders is not the study of a side phenomenon or an epiphenomenon. It is the study of what makes the lay and clinical communities notice that something is unusual about an individual, leading ultimately to the diagnosis of a disorder. Just as the general speech community notices differences in some speakers leading eventually to clinical assessment, so the understanding of language in the clinical setting must be used to understand how that speaker will be regarded in the wider speech community where the verbal behaviour really counts.

Following from a view of language as central in psychiatric disorders, we must fit both language and the way psychiatry uses language into a concept of social reality. Language, along with non-verbal behaviour and some other signalling systems, creates interactional reality. This interactional reality includes patterns of interaction, social institutions and norms for communicating. We then use the social reality, created largely by language, as the typical background to establish what is disordered or even incomprehensible. By comparing a speaker's use of language to the typical uses of language in the speech community, we can assess how acceptable an interaction is in creating social reality. Thus we can use language, defined in a social way in the way it attains social goals, to establish the atypical and deviant uses of language that explicitly fail to accomplish social goals.

To account for how some speakers fail to be effective in the social processes that they find themselves in, we must formulate explicit tools for listening. The goal of this volume is to provide clinicians with the means for detecting the elements of language that convey psychiatric disorders and that sometimes define those disorders. To meet this goal of detecting the clinically important elements of language, we outline the elements of language that are at risk in any given disorder or speaker. By making such elements of language explicit, the practitioner can notice, arrange and probe them during clinical interaction. The hearer who is aware of the linguistic choices at risk in different disorders can more carefully listen for these particular kinds of language in context, while engaging the usual clinical listening strategies.

1.2   A linguistic model for listening in psychiatry

To construct an approach to listening, this volume presents a detailed model of communicating meaning, derived from systemic functional linguistic theory. The linguistic approach provides theoretically justified and comprehensive linguistic tools for listening to individuals with psychiatric disorders. More generally, these tools give the clinician some detailed ways to think about the problems in psychiatry that are associated with language. As well as this holistic, clinical, approach, the presentation of language and psychiatric disorders that follows is analytical in laying the groundwork for understanding the mechanisms in cognition and neuropsychology for psychiatric categories. This approach outlines how speakers are successful or not in making meaning; that is, how specific linguistic features carry those successes and failures in making meaning. The approach relates these linguistic features to psychiatric categories (from disorders to diagnostic criteria). Ultimately, the model of clinical listening and the analytical approach to the linguistic signs in psychiatry point to a way of grouping diagnostic criteria and syndromes. Specifically, the linguistic details of diagnostic criteria and syndromes can provide suggestions for what entities belong together in terms of how the speaker makes and sends meaning and the cognitive mechanisms used.

1.2.1 Language in the speech community

Language is the primary means of communication among the members of a society and in fact helps to construct and constitute that society. Language is therefore an important component in determining the individual's fit with societal norms and thus in assessing mental health. It is sensitive to how the individual follows the usual patterns of interaction. Language is also sensitive to disruptions in other areas of functioning (such as hallucinations, shyness, cognitive deterioration or developmental disorders) and so is an index of these other difficulties as well.

Language, then, is unusually sensitive to a range of disturbances. Against this tendency for variation in language, there are strong forces acting to keep the use of language as stable as possible even in the face of disruptions. This pull to keep the use of language stable is necessary for interpretable communication. As social animals, humans generally must rely on others for some of their physical and psychic needs. These needs cannot be met when language becomes far from the interpretable norms of the speech community.

What then are the 'interpretable norms of the speech community'? Interpretability in language is dependent on more or less conventional relationships between the signalling system (the vocabulary and grammar, technically, the lexicogrammar) and the meanings that are construed and are construable by the users of the signalling system. New messages and even highly original kinds of signalling as in poetry, are always possible. However, even these kinds of novel messages are based on the norms that are established and expected. The poetic value of 'screaming silence', for example, depends on the usual expectations for the use of the two words and the expectation of how an adjective modifies a noun. The effect of the new combination of words is derived from our expectation that these words are unlikely to go together in the way they are presented here. We are forced to build a new kind of meaning: the essence of the poetic process.

Although our focus is on language, the wider issue is interaction. In a society, there are activities that are part of socially defined institutions. The buying of stamps, exchanging greetings or having a cup of coffee with another person are possible activities in some societies. These possible activities derive from a 'can do' potential present in the society. Each society or community, in turn, may have similar or overlapping potentials for what can be socially 'done'. Language operates within this 'can do' potential and provides the speaker with a series of 'can mean' potentials. These terms are taken from the work of M. A. K. Halliday. That is, language use in a community offers the speaker options of the socially and linguistically 'can be meant'. For example, the existence of apology as a socially sanctioned activity, a 'can do' potential, is then expressible in language, a 'can mean' potential. This 'can mean' potential, in turn, is conveyed by the appropriate words. In some cases, the 'can do' potential of apology may be conveyed by a non-verbal means (perhaps a look of dismay or contrition). These 'can do' and 'can mean' potentials are not absolutes. Rather members of a society build up and agree on what can be done and what can be meant. In a clinical setting, individuals may have parallel verbal and non-verbal difficulties in expressing these potentials. For example, echolalia may be parallel in terms of socially defined oddness, to echopraxia. There may even be an aetiological parallel. Similarly, over talkativeness may have a relation to restlessness.

The 'can do' and 'can mean' potentials are built into the social reality that we negotiate in a community. This agreement is reflected in the social interaction of the clinical setting. A clinician builds a particular social event to reveal characteristics of a speaker. The interviewer should use the circumstances in the clinical interaction to form a variety of verbal and non-verbal contexts for the interviewee. These contexts should bring out any problems in communication and language and also should be ecologically valid in reflecting how the speaker manages in the wider speech community. There cannot be predetermined sets of rules. Rather, the clinician should be aware of the features of language and interaction at stake in a given situation. These components can then be probed in the course of clinical interaction.

Most use of language, including the language that first indicates some psychiatric pathology, is language used spontaneously in real situations. It is the family, friends and others who first recognise that a speaker is not typical in behaviour and especially in language behaviour. Such recognition is easy and reliable; the hearers may report difficulty processing and understanding the language used by someone they know well. They may notice that meanings are not typical or that meanings are not worded in a typical way. A functional linguistic approach aims to describe and formalise these intuitions of hearers in actual interaction. We wish to provide explicit tools for listening to how speakers sound different in typical contexts including the contexts that are used for the professional assessment of psychiatric state. If the differences in language that are heard in an ecologically valid clinical context can be described, then two goals will be nearer:

(1) the description will reflect the difficulties the speaker has in the
     speech community, that is, the behavioural reality apparent and the
     basis for much of diagnosis even before formal assessment;

(2) the phenomena described directly and in detail may reflect underlying mechanisms of pathology.

It is important to notice that for diagnostic criteria based on language, the language is the phenomenon itself. That is, the language is the diagnostic sign itself and is not mediated by some test or concept. The study and formulation of a linguistic approach to psychiatric disorders is an analysis of an actual element of the disorder. This kind of direct study can be compared, for example, to the study of loose associations, blocking or delusions in schizophrenia. Delusions may be studied in terms of their content as reported by the speaker. The delusions themselves are not directly accessible. However, in presenting language and communication problems within diagnostic criteria, the psychiatric community is stating that problems in communication are themselves important components of the disorders. This position is readily understandable since an individual needs adequate social interaction to be sane and within normal variation, as the society defines sanity and reasonable variation. Thus, in broader terms, the functional linguistic analysis of diagnostic criteria is the analysis of why certain speakers are not considered sane. To this extent, the study of the language of speakers with psychiatric disorders is not the study of side phenomena or epiphenomena but the study of a central characteristic of why we regard some speakers as not psychiatrically normal.

1.2.2 Language as a meaning-making resource

Primarily language is a meaning-making resource. It could be added that we are interested in meaning making in context; however, this would be redundant. The making of meaning, the sending of messages from one speaker to another, is always done in context.

Aside from the most artificial uses of language for exercise, as in textbooks for foreign language learners, all uses of language are to communicate something to someone else, or, on occasion, to oneself. Following usual systemic functional terminology:

(1) text is defined as an instance of language that is operative in   TEXT
     context;

(2) a stretch of language which is not text is one that is citational.
     Language users assume that the language they hear or read is text and
     try to make sense of it in terms of its context.

Most users of language and in particular, those using language for assessment and diagnosis, are sensitive to instances when the language is not making sense. Sometimes the language does not make sense because of some syntactic problem ('The dessert were eaten yesterday' instead of 'The dessert was eaten yesterday') and sometimes the language fails to make sense because a perfectly good, syntactically correct sentence is spoken in a context inappropriate for that sentence ('Why is he here?' in circumstances in which the 'he' is unknown to the hearer).

SYSTEMIC-
FUNCTIONAL
LINGUISTICS

This approach to language, called systemic-functional linguistics, starts from the position that language is used to convey meaning in contexts and then views the grammar, vocabulary and sounds of language as the resources speakers use to realise or encode the meaning. This is a view of language as a set of meanings that can be expressed and a set of resources that express the meanings. Speakers draw on these resources to 'word' the meanings in any particular instance of language use. Schematically, then, there are:

(1) meanings (always in context);

(2) language resources that enable those meanings to be expressed;

(3) wordings (the particular language resources that are used to express the meaning in a given instance).

1.2.3 Language as wordings

The wordings of language 'realise' the meanings by using the linguistic patterns available in the particular language. For example, in English, a speaker cannot use the personal pronoun 'you' to specifically mean either one or more than one hearer, or to specifically mean a feminine or masculine hearer. Other languages, such as French or German, make such distinctions possible and sometimes require the speaker to signal the number and sex of the hearer(s) addressed. To take another example, some languages require the speaker to specify the sex of the individual when saying 'friend'. That is, the language requires distinctions of meaning that are then expressed in the words of a particular instance of language. The English word 'you' realises certain meanings but cannot be used to carry other meanings. The English linguistic system does not have the resources for encoding meanings such as 'more than one' with the pronoun 'you'. An English speaker can, of course, send such a meaning but the wording will be more elaborate than just using the single pronoun 'you'.

It is the wordings, then, that are available for the hearer to interpret. In contrast, the meanings and the use a speaker makes of language are somewhat more abstract. The 'functional' part of a systemic-functional approach to language focuses on the meanings. The 'systemic' part of the approach refers to how the meaning distinctions are described. The basic insight is that meaning is achieved by contrast. For example, in English, 'book' means just one book whereas 'books' means two or more books. However, some languages have a form of the word 'books' that means 'a pair of', so that 'books' (a pair of) is in contrast to 'books'. In this case, 'books' means 'three or more books' since, if the speaker had intended only two books, then the speaker would have used the variant form 'books' (a pair of). Here is a contrast between 'books' (a pair of) and 'books' (three or more) which is not present in English. This contrast in forms specifies what meanings can be easily encoded in the language. Of course, meanings can be added and extended by more elaborate expressions. To take another example, the meaning of 'you', 'the person I am addressing, without specifying if there is only one or more than one addressee and without specifying the sex of the addressee' derives its meaning from there not being a term for 'the person I am addressing, who is male' or a term for 'the addressee I intend is a group of several people'. If the language has no such contrast built in, then speakers will not regularly encode such meanings about number or sex. On the other hand, 'you' does contrast with meanings for 'the speaker' ('I', 'we') and for 'neither speaker nor addressee' ('he', 'she', 'it', etc.) and it is from these contrasts that 'you' is recognised as meaning distinctively 'the person I am addressing'. In summary, there are loose connections between the meanings that can be encoded in language and the wordings of the meanings. Some meanings are easily worded by the language and others require more elaborate wordings.

MEANING AS CONTRAST

1.2.4 Language in psychological and social perspectives

Speakers thus make meaning in context by using the meaning making resources present in the language. We can conceptualise these resources as options to be chosen at various points in constructing a text. We consider the speaker to be always confronted with the question: what shall I mean in this context? The speaker then weighs what meanings are available and how they should be worded. Consider the metaphor of an intersection with a set of roads that can be taken. The language offers these options and it is up to the speaker to decide on the route. Each route means something different in the context. The 'wording' of the option can be likened to the means of travel (on foot, by car, by bicycle). Sometimes, one can get to the same place/express the same meaning by different means. If a speaker sounds rather odd, or sounds pathologically odd, then it is a matter of the meanings that have been chosen and how those meanings are worded.

As well as the meanings chosen at a certain point in a conversation, our approach to language must consider the sequence of meanings a speaker chooses. An odd remark may be unnoticed or ignored if there are not others like it. However, a pattern of unusual choices signals a strange style of meaning. Starting a sentence with 'I' or 'you' is certainly appropriate. However, in a casual conversation, if we heard ten or 20 sentences in a row (or even nine out of ten) starting with one of these words, we would at least notice the unusual style. This aspect of the use of language is referred to as DYNAMIC USE OF LANGUAGE the dynamic unfolding of language use. Since speakers usually construct their contributions to conversation in real time, they must make successive choices of meaning taking into consideration how the conversation and the interaction have developed up to that point. The clinical listener must attend especially to this dynamic aspect of language in assessing patients since an accurate impression comes from considering many successive choice points in the use of language.

This approach to language, which is centrally concerned with meaning and context, requires both a psychological, or intraorganism, perspective and a social, or interorganism, perspective. Some of the components of such a view are presented in Table 1.1.

Social dimension

SPEECH COMMUNITY The speech community (at the left of Table 1.1) is an abstraction that takes into account that many speakers interact with each other creating typical patterns of interaction and language use. These patterns may be as simple and short as how and to whom to say 'good morning' or as complicated as how to sit across a negotiating table and hammer out a collective agreement involving thousands of employees. In some sense, these patterns constitute a collective memory for how language is used to get things done in the society. Within the speech community, there will be specific generalisations about what topics are discussed in what circumstances, what kinds of formality, informality and social roles are usual, what kinds of speech events recur with special meaning (for example, does the speech community have an event called naming ships? 'I hereby name this ship the ...' or reprimanding subordinates in a hierarchy? 'It is my duty to inform you that ...'). Of course, there are many such generalisations built up in the speech community. Furthermore, as speakers interact, they constantly change these generalisations and slowly establish new norms. These norms are not dictated or imposed by some authority but, rather, emerge as people use language.

Psychological perspective			Table 1.1
Speech community	**Personal model**	**Text**	*Language in psychological and social perspectives*
Dynamically readjusting Many subtypes Register Genre	Dynamically readjusting based on previous interactions in given contexts	Text up to now: what has happened for speaker for hearer	
Collective memory of how people have communicated under specific conditions		⇓ Text at this point: what is happening for speaker for hearer	
		⇓ Text in creation: what will/can be meant for speaker: next formulation for hearer: expectation/ interpretation of 'next'	

Social perspective –

Historical register

Speech community	Personal model	Text
Generalisations from many speakers, including: • mappings from system to system • realisations • trajectories	How does it sound up to now, given how speaker wants to be heard as compared to typicalities of speech community, including: • mappings from system to system • realisations • trajectories • interactional purposes	Trajectory up to now in this context: what has happened • mappings from system to system • realisations • trajectories

Personal dimension

As well as this socially defined dimension, each individual carries a model of how language is to be used (the middle column in Table 1.1). The individual develops a personal model of language use by listening to how others use language. In terms of meaning, the individual must learn what meanings are possible and how they are typically expressed. This knowledge comes by noticing how language is used in the speech community. As with the generalisations that represent the speech community, the individual's model of how language is used is constantly in flux. As the individual is exposed to new contexts and to new speakers, the model expands. The speaker is then able to interpret and use a wider inventory of meanings and the word-ings that realise those meanings. The individual's model is therefore closely connected to the language and contexts he or she has been exposed to. As will be explored in detail later, sometimes just being exposed to a certain context is not enough. A speaker may improperly assess what is happening in the context and thus may not be 'parsing' the situation in the usual way. A fuller account of the place of possible pathology in the model is also presented later.

Text as an emerging entity

At the far right of Table 1.1 is the text itself: the stretch of language in its context. At any time, we can consider the text as it has been created up to that point; that is, what text already exists. This text may be spoken or written, but for the purposes of this discussion we will be considering spontaneously produced oral texts. For a single text, the speaker and the hearer may have somewhat different views of how the text is being formed. With the same words and in the same situation, different people may think that what is happening is either a shouting match of people who have lost their tempers or a typical family ritual that will be re-enacted according to agreed rules. In another situation, one speaker may think that there is a job offer on the table while the other speaker in the conversation may think that the prospective employee should be encouraged and complimented but is not offering employment.

As well as negotiated text, there is emerging text. In practice, we can see a text as having three parts:

(1) a part that is already constructed and open for interpretation;

(2) a point that is happening now;

(3) a part that will be created.

At any given point in the text, just as for the text up to that point, speakers must form an interpretation of what is happening. This 'happening' is in terms of what the speaker is meaning and what kind of text it is. Is it, for example, a greeting at the beginning of a conversation or an insult that is being worded carefully? The speaker and the hearer may have different interpretations of the moment-to-moment meaning of a text. Moving from the text that is being created, a text will also be created. Again, there are both the speaker's perspective and the hearer's perspective. The speaker considers two areas of choice:

(1) the possible meanings that can be presented next in the context (what things could be meant);

(2) which of those messages the speaker wishes to convey.

In a casual conversation, a speaker cannot abruptly say 'I hereby fine you a month's wages'. This possible message is not very likely in the context. As the example suggests, what is a possible message is guided by the norms of the speech community and the roles of the speakers in the community. As well as the message to be sent, the speaker can consider how that message should be worded for the hearer in the particular context. For example, if the speaker says, 'It is JOHN who took the book from the kids' (with emphasis on 'John'), the speaker implies that the hearer knows who 'John' is, that the hearer knows that someone took the book from the kids and that the hearer knows the identity of 'the kids'.

From the hearer's perspective also, a text is being created. The hearer guesses how the text will continue. That is, given the norms of the speech community and the hearer's own personal model of how interaction and language work, the hearer has expectations of what the speaker can say next. Of course, these expectations may be rather loose in some situations (e.g., after two speakers have exchanged 'Hello' at the beginning of a telephone conversation) and tighter in other situations (e.g., after 'Nice weather we're having for this time of year'). These expectations are tied to the speech community as variations in the examples show. Some speech communities have rather fixed patterns of answering a telephone such that the receiver must first say 'Hello' with the calling party then saying 'Hello'. Other speech communities require that the receiver first identify the destination of the call ('Smith family' or 'ABC Television Station') before any response from the caller. In some speech communities a typical, rather friendly and non-committal, response might be given to a comment about the weather, whereas in other speech communities the same comment would be heard as an unwelcome, too friendly and perhaps slightly suspicious overture, from a stranger. In summary, the text is interpretable as it already exists and as it is being formulated. Speakers and hearers may have different interpretation processes. Each person brings to the interpretation process and to the planning process a background of interactions in the speech community.

Building a personal model of language and interaction

The model of communicating also includes a series of generalisations developed from what may be called historical discourse registers (see Table 1.1). In a speech community, for the individual and in a text that is being formulated, there are records of what meaning choices have been taken (the roads taken, in the metaphor presented earlier) and the ways those choices were expressed in language. Each time we communicate happens after many other meaning choices. Metaphorically, there are paths of meaning choices we have taken up to the point of the current situation. In terms of the speech community, there exists a rich history of what people in the speech community have meant and how they have expressed it. We can think of a trajectory of how a communication situation usually develops from beginning to end. Activities such as buying a car or inviting a friend for dinner have a typical pattern in the speech community including verbal activity. These patterns are built up since the activities are repeated and many individuals learn the patterns.

Individuals also develop their own historical record of what has happened. The individual will consider the language used in the situation in terms of how it sounds up to that point, given that individual's model of how it should sound. The speaker matches his or her interpretation of the speech situation with his or her view of the general patterns of the speech community. For example, does this interaction sound like an insult or a joke? Since different speakers have different historical registers, accumulated by experience in specific situations, they may have different assessments of any current situation. The patterns in the individual's historical register and the objectives of the moment build a specific trajectory to achieve the speaker's goal for the interaction.

A text itself can be viewed as a historical register; that is, the set of meaning choices made in sequence. As well as the meaning choices (whether, for example, an utterance is a question or a statement), a text encodes meanings with their specific wordings or realisations. A speaker must be aware of these realisations to decide whether to say something that echoes the earlier part of the text (Mark Anthony's 'They are honourable men, they are all honourable men') or whether some variation is called for ('I want ice cream.' 'Me too'!).

Pathological interference in communicating in context 1.3

1.3.1 Possible loci of pathological interference

The model of communication suggests areas of possible difficulty for speakers with psychiatric disorders (see Table 1.2). The speech community ultimately determines typical interactions and the use of language in those interactions. Against these notions of typical, some instances stand out as atypical or even pathological.

Speech community	Personal model	Text	Table 1.2
Speech community determines the 'typical' compared to which there is 'pathological'	Problems in developing a socially appropriate model of language in context	On-line processing problems	*Sources of pathological interference in language*
	Has the speaker been exposed to contexts in the speech community?	Can/has speaker parsed the text in context appropriately up to now?	
	Can/has speaker perceived/parsed appropriately from exposures to the speech community?	Can the speaker plan an appropriate 'next' given the text in context up to 'current'?	
	Can/has speaker learnt the lexicogrammar and its mappings to functions and contexts?	Can the speaker realise the appropriate 'next'?	

Some individuals may not have developed a socially appropriate model for using language in context. Such an individual may not have developed an appropriate model for several reasons (see Table 1.3 for a summary). These reasons could be:

(1) The speaker may not have been exposed to the typical sets of contexts in the speech community.

(2) If for psychological, social or physical reasons a speaker is not familiar with the range of contexts needed to build a typical model of communication, then the speaker's contributions may not quite fit the normal patterning in the speech community.

(3) In some cases, the range of contexts was available but the speaker did not participate in them frequently enough to learn the subtle aspects of language use that other speakers did.

(4) Even if the speaker is exposed to the appropriate contexts, some speakers may have a difficulty in perceiving the significant elements of the context. For example, if a speaker does not perceive social roles clearly or does not perceive emotions well, then the personal model of communication will be incomplete or atypical.

(5) As well as problems in perception, a speaker may have a difficulty in parsing or analysing the elements of context. It is necessary to analyse social roles, meanings and even the vocabulary, grammar and sounds to fully understand and participate in interaction. If some of this analysis does not follow the typical pattern of the speech community (as, for example, in not noticing which questions are rhetorical and do not need an answer, or in not noticing that certain statements are ironic or satirical), then the speaker will construct a model for communication that does not match closely enough the models of other speakers.

(6) At the level of language, there could be problems in learning some area such as vocabulary, grammar or sounds.

(7) At more abstract levels, there could be problems in learning various genres of interaction and

(8) problems in learning various patterns in sequencing, e.g. kinds of questions, responses, statements, elliptical phrases ('Oh, yes') etc.

(9) As well as learning these structures and their orderings, speakers must appropriately map them onto meanings and contexts.

Pathology of one kind or another may interfere with any of these kinds of learning, perception or parsing, with the result that the speaker will interact atypically with language.

Table 1.3

Lack of exposure to typical contexts in the speech community

Psychological, social or physical limitations restricting exposure to the range of contexts

Speaker did not participate frequently enough in contexts to learn the subtle aspects of language use

Speaker has a difficulty in perceiving the significant elements of the context

Speaker has a difficulty in parsing or analysing the elements of context

Problems in learning some area of language such as vocabulary, grammar or sounds

Problems in learning various genres of interaction

Problems in learning various patterns in sequencing kinds of questions, responses, statements, elliptical phrases

Problems in mapping above sequences onto meanings and contexts

Factors that impair the development of an adequate model of interacting with language

As well as possible pathological interference in the development of the individual's model of communicating, some speakers may have difficulty with the on-line processing of texts. In real life interactions, individuals must comprehend and produce the speech for each activity at a rate that is typical for the community. These on-line tasks involve parsing the text in context as it has been formulated up to the present, planning an appropriate 'next' contribution given the context up to 'current' contribution and constructing the appropriate 'next' contribution. Interference with any of these tasks and the processes underlying them will result in odd language or language that may reflect some pathology.

Throughout this section, we have spoken about the interference of pathology with little exposition. In fact, it may be difficult to determine the kinds of pathology involved. There may be cognitive limitations of memory, process-ing speed, ability to integrate, generalise or to extract a pattern, etc. There may also be perceptual problems involving physical properties of speech (sounds of language or intonation, for example) or perception of social facts, emotions or other properties of situations. Difficulties may also involve psychopathology more directly in terms of attachment, reality testing, self-perception, etc. The clinician may find it difficult to determine the kind of pathology and especially the root cause. Therefore, the comments of patho-logical interference should be taken as ways of thinking about pathology or perhaps hypotheses for the kinds of difficulties that speakers may have.

1.3.2   The dynamic dimension of language in psychiatric disorders

As mentioned, language in use is built up step-by-step in context. A speaker must construct a contribution to a conversation, or construct the next part of a narrative, sequentially in relation to what has already come before. A speaker can have difficulty in building a text either sporadically or consistently. Sometimes, a sporadic difficulty can be a clear sign of a psychiatric difficulty; even one clear hallucination may change how two speakers relate to each other. In other cases, it takes a pattern of several utterances, each with a particular characteristic, to signal that something is amiss; one 'loose association' may not indicate thought-disorder, but several in a row lead to an incomprehensible stretch of talk. Similarly, we may scarcely notice one impulsive remark, but a consistent pattern of impulsive remarks in a short period will make the listener feel uncomfortable. Clinically, and in terms of research strategies, examining the rate of a particular linguistic oddity may not identify the problem in language. The approach must be to assess the effect of the linguistic structure in its context. Users of a language are usually sensitive to language in context and have a good appreciation for the meanings a speaker chooses to convey. Consequently, as hearers, they are usually aware of the cumulative effect of the choices of meaning that lead to odd sounding texts. These considerations are discussed more fully in Chapter 10.

1.3.3   Atypicality in the language of psychiatric disorders

The odd use of language by speakers with psychiatric disorders requires further clarification. As noted above, we can think of the speech community as a set of generalisations of how language is used or, in fact, how individuals interact. These generalisations cover both the language choices speakers make and the frequency of those choices in context. A pattern becomes expected or typical because speakers repeat it in certain kinds of situations and in the verbal context it unfolds. Speakers develop these typical patterns of usage by exposure, with the right frequency, to these situations. Similarly, hearers interpret language against the expected frequency of the uses of language in situation. Thus, speakers are understood against a background of meanings and their typical expressions/realisations in the community. This notion is found in standard diagnostic criteria by descriptions such as: 'limited amount of speech', 'limited range of vocabulary', 'qualitative impairment in social interaction'. The atypical frequency of some linguistic form or structure not only marks the speaker as unusual but also sends inappropriate or unintended messages. If, in a certain situation, 'Thank you' is almost always responded to with 'You're welcome', then listeners will interpret the absence of the response as unfriendliness, aloofness, or impoliteness. In other situations, we may interpret the use of 'You're welcome' as obsequiousness or cynicism. It is the degree of typicality of the utterance in the situation that affects its interpretation. The listener must therefore be familiar with the situations and the language that is used in them.

Hearers assume that others will use language with the frequency typical in the speech community. Deviations from this typicality are noticed. It is difficult to determine precise frequencies that are within the norm and frequencies that can seem just slightly atypical. Both the changing frequencies in the speech community and the difficulty of determining where a particular speaker's language falls in the speech community's range of use create this natural indeterminacy in assessing atypicality. Clinical judgement represents the clinician's assessment of issues of atypicality based on knowledge of the speech community and how speakers of different ages and social background interact.

The following section will outline some of the many aspects of language that are used to communicate in context. The next chapter covers in detail those areas of language most likely to create the effects of the language of speakers with psychiatric disorders. The approach is somewhat eclectic theoretically. That is, descriptions and parts of theory have been taken from a number of sources. Sometimes, these sources and their linguistic understanding of communication may be at odds with each other. The presentation here is in terms of the formulations that are helpful in interpreting, understanding, hypothesising about and studying psychiatric disorders. The various theoretical treatments and the descriptions are consistent in attempting to be exhaustive and theoretically coherent for each set of meanings. Textbook treatments of systemic linguistics which include the kind of detail needed for specific empirical study of the language of psychiatric disorders include: Eggins (1994) and Butt, Fahey, Spinks and Yallop (2000). Full-scale technical treatments are found in Halliday and Matthiessen (2004), Martin (1992) and Matthiessen (1995).

Linguistic factors at stake and the meanings they carry   1.4

The first part of this outline (Section 1.4.1) presents language as it fits into the context of language use and the levels of description we need when viewing language from its place in the wider communication situation. The basic kinds of meaning conveyed by language are also sketched as an introduction to the more specific analyses that follow. The next three sections deal in turn with the major kinds of meaning that language encodes: ideational (1.4.2), interpersonal (1.4.3) and textual (1.4.4).

1.4.1 The integration of meaning

REALISING MEANING

Language is a signalling system that makes concrete (that 'realises' or actualises) the meanings that are possible in a speech community. Language is one of several possible signalling systems (others include facial expressions, body movements) that convey meanings operative in the society. These meanings, however, depend on the speech situation (see Table 1.4). In some situations, only a restricted set of meanings is possible. For instance, in answering a judge's question 'How do you plead?' only a few meanings are possible. If a speaker strays from the set of possible meanings, then the speech will still be interpreted within the framework set up by the speech community. Speakers must be sensitive both to the overall pattern of meanings in the speech community and to the subsets of meanings available in particular situations (cf. Martin, 1992: 501ff.). These subsets of meaning may be delineated along the lines of the topics or issues that are the subject of conversation (technically, the field), the interpersonal relations of the speakers (the tenor) and the effect of the channel of communication (the mode). To take tenor as an example, speakers express meanings of formality, friendliness and solidarity that vary between situations. These are meanings, since language conveys in predictable and conventional ways much more than the prepositional 'content' of the sentence or clause. An important part of messages is the personal relationship expressed by one speaker to another.

Table 1.4	**Situation**	Issues that are the subject of interaction (field)
Contexts and levels of meaning		Interpersonal relations of speakers (tenor)
		Channel of communication (mode)
	Kinds of meaning in language	
	Language as message (ideational meaning)	Things of the world expressed by nominals in language
		Events of the world expressed by verbs in language
		Details of events (circumstances) expressed by adverbs, preposition phrases, etc.
	Language as exchange (interpersonal meaning)	Exchanging: information or goods and services
		Giving or demanding
	Language in context (textual meaning)	Presenting information as known or unknown to the hearer

At a most abstract level, there are recurrent situations that require typical kinds of meaning worded in typical ways. For example, when approaching a newspaper vendor there are some routine kinds of interaction such as establishing which newspaper the customer wants, determining if that newspaper is available, clarifying or confirming the price, handing over the money and handing over the newspaper. Some of these activities may be done non-verbally. This 'genre' of buying a newspaper is part of knowing how to interact appropriately in a society. At this level of interaction there are established collections of meanings that are typically combined into an overall activity, or 'social process', in the society. If a speaker does not have such a configuration of meanings available or cannot interpret such meanings when presented by another, then that speaker is restricted in interacting socially.

GENRE

SOCIAL PROCESS

As well as the subsets of meaning that relate language to situation of its use, there are three kinds of meaning encoded in language. These are:

METAFUNCTIONS OF LANGUAGE

(1) language as message (the ideational function of language) that constructs and reflects experience (Martin, 1992: 8);

(2) language as an exchange (the interpersonal function of language) that constructs the interaction and negotiation of meaning between speakers;

(3) language as it fits into a context (Table 1.4).

For this third kind of meaning, language carries meaning by forming the message to match with the expectations in the context (the textual function of language). An example of this third function is the choice between 'It is MARY that found the ball' compared to, 'It is the BALL that Mary found'.

The first kind of meaning, or 'metafunction' of language, has been seen as the 'content' of a message. However, the other kinds of meaning also express content, albeit of a different sort. As is detailed below, each of these metafunctions of language is carried by various parts of grammar and vocabulary. It is important to note that all three meanings are carried simultaneously in each utterance. An utterance is not one of ideational, interpersonal, or textual but conveys elements of all three kinds of meaning in its grammar and vocabulary. These metafunctions are a way of thinking about the different kinds of meaning that language carries and the different kinds of meaning that may be at risk in a psychiatric disorder.

1.4.2   Ideational meaning

THINGS, EVENTS,
CIRCUMSTANCES

Language reflects reality and our experience of it. In the most general way, our experience of reality is experience of things, events and circumstances. These things, events and circumstances are then expressed by language. Again in the most general way, the 'things' of the world are usually expressed or worded as nouns or groups of words centred around nouns (e.g., 'the three very large red *baskets* in the kitchen'). Such 'things' can be subcategorised in many ways to reflect the different kinds of meanings involved. For example, proper nouns (Canada, the Atlantic Ocean, King Solomon) identify a category of one, whereas common nouns (table, chair, book) identify a component of meaning that is common to a number of 'things'. Other characteristics of things that are encoded are whether they can be counted (table(s), chair(s), book(s)) or whether they are usually not counted (air, water, kindness, love) and whether they can usually be said to have volition (person, child, dog?) or not (rug, paper, reaction).

These 'things' play the role of participants in various events in the world. More than 'things', we regard the world as composed of events that happen. That is, our perception of the world is made up of various happenings. Just as with things, 'events' can be classified in various ways. There are events that happen in the material world (run, fall, destroy, move) and other events that are more intrapsychic in nature (see, love, consider, think). Events can also be expressed as happening within a certain time period (e.g., I came, I am coming, I will come). These potential meanings of time period are available to be expressed along with the event.

As well as things and events, there are meanings conveyed as 'circumstantials'. In considering events, the 'goings-on' are often described in terms of when, where or how the events take place. That is, the circumstances surrounding the events are given. In language, circumstantials can express meanings such as extent, location, manner, cause, etc. (see Halliday, 1994: 149 ff.). For example, the meanings of the circumstantials in the following sentences add different kinds of meaning to the same event:

She walked *for two hours*	temporal extent
She walked *in the meadow*	spatial location
She walked *for ten miles*	spatial extent
She walked *with determination*	manner
She walked *because of her determination*	cause

In utterances, the circumstantial element is combined with the thing and the process. The three kinds of ideational meaning come together to send a complex message encoding the reality of the external world as the speaker wishes to convey it to the hearer.

1.4.3　Interpersonal meaning

The essence of interpersonal meaning is expressing how the speaker relates to the ideational meaning of the utterance. Of course, how a speaker relates to such content is dependent on who the addressee is and how the speaker relates to the ideational meaning for that addressee. In speaking to one person, the statement may be fashioned as: 'The film was OK', but in speaking to another person the statement may be: 'You should really come to see the movie. It was the greatest'. The basic interpersonal meanings derive from two sets of contrasts:

(1) giving or demanding;

(2) exchanging information or exchanging goods and services (Halliday, 1994).

These two contrasts set up the four possibilities of: giving information ('It is sunny outside'), giving goods and services ('Here is the coffee you wanted'), demanding information ('What time is it?') and demanding goods and services ('Give me three round trip tickets to Easter Island') (see Table 1.5).

Added onto these four basic interpersonal meanings, the speaker may encode other meanings such as the degree of confidence in the truth of a statement. A speaker may express relative confidence in the statement ('It is sunny outside', 'It is definitely sunny outside') or some measure of uncertainty ('It may be sunny outside', 'It could be sunny outside', 'It is possibly sunny outside', 'It is probably sunny outside', etc.).

	Giving	Demanding	Table 1.5
Goods and services	offer *Here is the coffee you wanted*	command *Give me three round trip tickets to Easter Island*	*Basic interpersonal meanings and their combinations*
Information	statement *It is sunny outside*	question *What time is it?*	

There is an additional set of meanings that can be added onto the contrasts outlined so far: the contrast in polarity, positive or negative. An utterance may be positive or negative depending on the speaker's assessment of the truth of the statement ('It is sunny outside.' 'It isn't sunny outside'). As with most instances when speakers make 'meaning', utterances may combine different kinds of interpersonal meaning to send rather complex messages ('It *probably* isn't sunny outside', '*Could* it be that it is sunny outside my office now?'). Speakers thus build up complex interpersonal meaning by selecting options from different kinds of potential meanings. These different kinds of meaning (e.g., giving or demanding, information or goods and services, positive or negative) can be seen as organised into systems such that once in the system, a speaker must choose one option or another. For example, once a speaker is making a statement (i.e., giving information) the speaker can decide to choose from a range of options concerning how likely that event is ('They *certainly* left yesterday'. 'They *probably* left yesterday'. 'They *possibly* left yesterday'. 'They *likely* left yesterday') or leave the issue of likelihood unspecified ('They left yesterday') which is itself also an encoding of a certain meaning ('I am not going to tell you anything specific about how likely I think that the event is'). Each utterance combines interpersonal meaning with the ideational meaning.

1.4.4 Textual meaning

Ideational meanings and interpersonal meanings have to be combined and presented in a linear order in speech. In this ordering, another kind of meaning is created: the textual meaning. The textual meaning is the meaning created when fitting an utterance into its context. In determining how to word the ideational and interpersonal meanings, a speaker has a number of options. In choosing the options, the speaker must take into consideration how the utterance will fit into the context. For example, in choosing among 'Yesterday, they left', 'They left yesterday', 'It was they who left yesterday', the speaker is taking the same ideational and interpersonal meanings and shaping them differently. These different wordings are then most appropriate for different contexts. 'Yesterday, they left' is most appropriate when the speaker assumes that the hearer knows that 'they left' but wants to make sure that the hearer knows that the leaving was 'yesterday'. To take another example, a speaker can choose among 'John saw a clown', 'He saw a clown' and 'He saw the clown'. These choices depend on what information the speaker thinks is available to the hearer. At a deeper level, the speaker uses these choices to signal what information space the speaker thinks is shared with the hearer. In designing an utterance for the context, a speaker must then necessarily convey meanings about how that context is known to the hearer and meld such meanings with the ideational and interpersonal meanings of the utterance.

The approach to language in psychiatric disorders is, in summary, centrally concerned with meanings since the atypicalities in meanings are clearly a primary phenomenon in these disorders. However, there is no point considering meaning if that meaning and the process of meaning-making are not considered in real contexts. It is in such contexts that speakers are first noticed to be unusual or pathological and it is through language in other contexts that diagnosis and treatment are mainly effected.

The following chapter presents in some detail the kinds of meaning from the ideational, interpersonal and textual metafunctions that speakers use. These meanings are also presented with their typical realisations, that is, with the REALISATIONS vocabulary and grammar that are used to 'word' the meanings. Chapter 3 outlines the effects of atypicalities in the use of these language resources.

Chapter 2 contents

Chapter 2

The kinds of meanings to be heard

The structures of language and the patterns of meaning 2.1

This chapter outlines the meanings conveyed by language since hearers often take disruptions in these meanings as indicating a psychiatric disorder. To notice the unexpected, it is important to have a systematic view of the expected uses of language in context. We hear odd sounding language at two levels: odd meanings and odd wordings of meanings. Both these levels are dealt with in detail in this chapter to give the clinician tools to notice the unexpected language related to diagnosis. Outside the clinical context, the linguistic approach gives tools for thinking about the definitions and features of psychiatric disorders and how they are recognised. In discussing the role of language in psychiatry, there is a certain overlap between clinical terms and linguistic terms. This is not surprising since both fields detail the typical and atypical behaviour of individuals. For example, functional linguistics speaks of an 'ideational' metafunction for language just as a clinical description may deal with unusual ideation or, for example, specifically 'suicidal ideation'. It is important to appreciate this natural overlap of descriptive terms.

However, the linguistic terms have specific technical meanings that only partly overlap with the clinical terms. The advantage of adding a linguistic approach to the clinical approach is exactly the precision that the linguistic concepts bring. The linguistic concepts have been developed outside the clinical field in order to understand the use of language and its place in human interaction. These concepts are part of an integrated theory of human interaction. Whenever specifically linguistic concepts are used and are labelled with terms that are similar to clinical terms, the context and accompanying definitions are used to keep the linguistic and clinical terms distinct. Again, though, the overlap is natural and even helpful.

Language is not merely the words spoken but rather fits into the context and the cultural surroundings of the speakers. We need a broad view of language – from culture to the details of intonation – in order to accurately assess when a speaker is sounding odd. There may be any number of places within such a broad view that may go wrong in psychiatric disorders, from merely speaking too quickly, to sounding pedantic, to describing delusions. Each of these kinds of atypicalities may have different kinds of aetiologies and be characteristic of different disorders. In each case, though, they are relevant to clinical listening.

To consider the specifics of meaning-making in real contexts, this chapter gives an overview of how language fits into context and into the process of communication (this outline follows Ventola, 1987 and Martin, 1992 in its broad approach). To start at the most basic level, language is a signalling system to convey meaning in context. As a signalling system it has a substance, mainly sounds, in the uses being considered in psychiatric settings. These sounds are patterned in each language. For example, in English, no words can begin with the sequence of sounds [n g w]. It is not just that there are no words that start with this sequence of sounds but this combination of sounds is not possible at the beginning of English words, although possible in other languages. There are also intonations or prosodies that are used. For example, the question 'you're here?' is differentiated from the statement 'you're here' by the ups and downs of pitch.

The purpose of language is to communicate meanings from one person to another. In order to achieve this purpose, language is structured in at least three different ways (see Table 2.1). First, the sounds of a language must be spoken in specific orders. Second, the words must be combined in certain ways. We usually call this second kind of structure the 'grammar' of the language. Third, longer stretches of language, such as sentences, must be combined properly. For example, the sentences of a story cannot be uttered in random order and still produce the intended effect, no matter how well enunciated and how grammatical the sentences are.

Table 2.1	**Structure of sound**	—	sequences of sounds (Section 2.1)
Structures in language that carry meaning	**Structure of words and grammar**	—	the lexicogrammar (Section 2.1)
	Structure of discourse	—	sequences of sentences in stories, conversations, etc. (Section 2.1)

The importance of the correct sounds for a language is intuitive to us. The sounds must be recognisable and uttered in the correct order to make up words. As well as these sounds that carry the language from person to person, the language is composed of selections of words (vocabulary or lexical choice) and grammatical structures. The essence of grammatical structures (or structures of any kind for that matter) is to combine units (e.g., words or phrases) to form other units (clauses, sentences, stories) and perhaps to create dependence of one part on another (see Martin, 1992 Chapter 1, for a technical discussion). For example, a preposition like 'to' is a unit (indicated by parentheses) of one word that is combined with another word or group of words such as: '(to) (home)', '(to) (the house)', '(to) (the place over the sea and beyond the horizon)'. Together, 'to' and whatever it is placed with form a larger unit. Grammatical structures also imply the ordering of the units: it is 'to the house' and not 'the to house'. The difference between active ('The man ate the hot dog') and passive ('The hot dog was eaten by the man') is another example of a change in grammatical structure dependent on word order, a legitimate one in this case. Together, the words we select and the grammatical structures we use carry much of the meaning of language. This stratum of language is called the lexicogrammar. To communicate in a society, a speaker must have a reasonable control of the words and grammar of the language.

A third kind of structure of language, in addition to sound and the lexico-grammar, is the discourse structure of language. Knowing how words are assembled into sentences (by the lexicogrammar) is not enough to engage in a conversation or compose a letter. A language user must also arrange words and sentences into a socially acceptable pattern to send a typical kind of meaning. Some piece of language, story, conversation or anything else, that is completely and uncompromisingly in the passive would sound strange indeed. The telling of a story or the development of a conversation requires, among other things, the right amount of repetition of words, the use of conjunctions ('but', 'then', 'because', 'however', etc.) and an appropriate use of pronouns and other referring expressions ('he', 'it', 'theirs', '*the* house'). These devices help fashion a discourse structure that will be recognised by other speakers (see Eggins, 1994 for details of these devices). These discourse structures, just like the structures of sound and of lexicogrammar, carry meaning. If misused, the discourse structures send a message that is difficult to interpret. These three kinds of structuring are accessible to the hearer. There are, though, other kinds of patterning that are perhaps less evident to us. Nevertheless these patterns are relevant to recognising the odd uses of language in psychiatric disorders. We now consider these more abstract patterns that contribute to our use of language (see Table 2.2). Each of these kinds of patterning could be at risk in different psychiatric disorders.

Table 2.2

Patterns of meaning 'above' language

Culture	Patterns of behaviours of the community (Section 2.1.1)
Genre	Patterns of staged, goal-oriented, social processes (Section 2.1.2)
Situation	Patterns of specific, physical interactions (Section 2.1.3)
Register	Patterns of field – institutional focus (Section 2.1.4) Patterns of tenor – social roles Patterns of mode – channel of communication

2.1.1   Culture

At the highest level, we must recognise that culture provides the background patterns for behaviour. Culture can be understood as a community's vast series of behaviours. Some of these patterns are more frequent than others and some may be concentrated among groups of individuals. For example, people over the age of 70, or hairdressers, or lawyers may have particular kinds of interactions that are less common in other groups. The patterns of interaction include the meanings that are exchanged, the contexts those meanings are exchanged in and the language that carries the meanings.

STANDARD CONTEXTS

Standard contexts are then derived from the culture. Examples of these standard contexts can range from naming ships, swearing in members of a town council, ordering a telephone line, buying a toothbrush, making an appointment with a dentist, borrowing clothes, playing a make-believe game of mother, father and baby or trading cards of sports teams.

2.1.2   Genre

SOCIAL PROCESSES

At a lower level of abstraction, the culture generates social processes. These social processes are staged and goal-oriented. Examples of social processes in common activities are buying stamps, introducing strangers to each other, saying 'good morning' to a neighbour, or engaging in a psychiatric interview. The social processes, in turn, are structured in terms of sequences of elements and the dependencies among them. Language accomplishes or actualises many of these social processes. The way language is organised to

GENRE

achieve these social processes is in genres. Just as the genre of a mystery story has components (e.g., of introduction of characters, inciting event, search for clues and the villain, discovery of villain, denouement, etc.) so the genre that accomplishes a social process, such as a casual conversation that continues and solidifies a friendship, may have elements, or components, such as the following: greeting, approach to neutral topic like weather, approach to a substantive topic (why we are having this meeting) and leave taking. Such elements establish a schematic structure that speakers are usually familiar with. When interacting with another speaker, we have an expectation that that person will follow a predictable pattern.

Considering genres enables us to understand how social processes relate to each other. That is, some social processes seem to overlap with other social processes and result in similar genres with similar elements and structures. For example, travelling by means of public transportation is roughly similar whether it is by subway, bus, train, or ship; there is the determination of destination, determination of the fare, paying the fare, boarding the vehicle, etc. To engage smoothly in the culture, an individual must understand both the similarities and the differences among genres. The people who can give us clear examples of not knowing genres and how they are enacted through language behaviour are children, as they are progressively socialised into the culture and travellers who are moving from culture to culture. Even when the sounds, vocabulary and grammar seem familiar, there may be cultural differences that create different genres. For example, a Canadian or Briton visiting in a school classroom in the United States will not be familiar with the cultural background, the structure and the meaning of 'the pledge of allegiance to the flag', an event never performed in their home countries and cultures.

2.1.3 Situation

To bring the discussion of these abstract organisations of culture and genre to a more concrete level, we can consider the circumstances of each interaction. In any given interaction, there are physical aspects of the world that impinge on the interaction. The people in the interaction are the most obvious components that are relevant to the interaction. Other factors may be the objects in the interaction, the location of the interaction, the medium of the interaction (by face-to-face oral language, by telephone, letter, electronic mail, voice mail, etc.) and the ambient sounds. The problem in formulating an approach to situation, as this level of analysis can be called, is that there could be an endless number of relevant things. Fortunately for the speaker, hearer and the analyst of communication, only a limited set of factors impinges on the communication, or in other words, a limited set of factors are relevant to the social process at hand. The temperature at the North Pole is an external fact that is usually not relevant to interactions. However, the colour of the speaker's tie may or may not be relevant if it symbolises some concept in the society. Speakers, to the best of their ability, perceive and analyse the physical attributes of the communication event (the situation) in terms of the relevant factors.

Learning which factors are relevant is, therefore, one task in learning how to interact in a culture. To take a cross-cultural example, in some cultures, handing over an object with the left hand is taken as an insult. However, an individual who has not perceived the difference between right-handed handovers and left-handed handovers will in some situations not notice which hand offered the cup of coffee. Then the individual will not be able to act appropriately. In fact, an important meaning in the interaction may have been lost. In conclusion, situations, as the specific physical circumstances of an interaction, must be perceived and parsed in terms of what is culturally and interactionally relevant.

PURPOSE OF THE
INTERACTION

We now move from the physical attributes of the situation to a most difficult but important notion: the concept of the purpose or goal of the participants. In any given situation, there is the complicated and almost intractable problem of determining the purpose of the interaction. In part, we can work out the purpose from the standard social processes found in the culture. For example, the usual reason for buying a ticket for the next showing of a movie is to personally enter the auditorium and see the movie. The social process of buying the ticket suggests its usual purpose. However, an individual may also be buying the ticket for someone else, be doing a charitable act by giving the ticket to someone who would otherwise spend the following two hours in a cold alleyway, be exchanging a counterfeit bill for legitimate change, etc. Purpose is therefore based both on the cultural background of the community (needed for the above interpretations of the ticket buying) and on the intrapsychic reality of the individual. Since the community patterns are available to many people, we tend to base purpose or motivation on the usual expectations of the community. However, individuals may have their private and personal purposes that are much less accessible for inspection and understanding. From the perspective of the community, however, the purposes of an individual are guessed at in terms of the usual relationship between actions and purposes. If an individual is doing something, we assume it is for the usual purposes unless indicated otherwise.

2.1.4 Register

As well as social purposes that are expressed through the genres of a culture, there are differences of meaning that relate to three standard contextual variables. These three contextual variables have been referred to as field, tenor and mode.

Field

Field represents the institutional focus of what is happening. This institutional focus then leads to the 'content' of the talk. For example, a focus on the social activity of sowing grass seeds leads to the selection of certain kinds of vocabulary that is different from a focus on bicycle repairs. Institutions within the society are the focus of activity and that focus is reflected in the language.

INSTITUTIONAL FOCUS

Tenor

As well as field, a second contextual variable is the tenor. As with 'field', 'tenor' is a technical linguistic term whose meaning overlaps with some of the non-technical uses of the term. The tenor is a variable in the context that derives from the structuring of the social roles of speakers in an interaction. Speakers may have formally defined roles, such as judge and prosecutor, or less formally defined roles, such as current resident of an apartment building and incoming resident, or roles related to age, sex or family relationship. These roles, in turn, have a range in status, rules of formality and rules of interaction attached to them. The roles of speakers in an interaction are associated with certain configurations of meanings. For example, there are things that a teacher can say to a fourth grade pupil ('sit down now right away') that are not generally said by speakers in other roles in other interactions. As usual, though, a speaker may choose to go outside the bounds of the meanings commonly associated with a role. However, what is then said derives its meaning in part from the fact that it is outside the role's usual inventory of meanings. A motorist who asks a police officer for a driver's licence will be taken as making a joke, trying to insult the officer's driving habits, or being obstructive or aggressive. To take a more subtle example, if the motorist merely says 'Sir' or 'Madam' at the beginning of every sentence to the police officer, the motorist will be sending a message of how he or she understands the social roles of the interaction. The officer may either accept such signals with appreciation, since the social asymmetry is being acknowledged by the driver, or may take the comments as unnecessary or mocking obsequiousness. Speakers who misjudge the social roles of an interaction or see themselves in social roles that are not accepted by others are seen as on the fringes of the social community. Since language encodes these social roles, a close examination of language reveals how an individual is creating and fitting into social roles. Social roles are a part of all interactions and therefore there are dimensions of this linguistically defined social tenor in each interaction. The point is that these choices in tenor convey meanings of one kind or another. Chapter 3 lays out many of the atypicalities of meaning that are associated with atypicalities in the use of language. The following chapters then connect these atypicalities of meaning and their wordings to psychiatric disorders.

SOCIAL ROLES OF SPEAKERS

Mode

The third contextual variable is mode. Mode is about the role that language itself is playing in the situation; for example, is the language being spoken, written, spoken as if it were written (a newscast), or spoken as if it was not written (a play). The channel of communication (e.g., face-to-face, telephone, via windows facing each other over a roadway) can substantially affect which messages are sent and how they are formulated. As with tenor and field, though, the mode itself is an organisation of meanings. There is a meaning to interacting spontaneously that is different to the meaning of a written text. For example, in organisations one sometimes hears 'Will you put that in writing?' or 'Come say that in person'. That is, the same words with the same sender and receiver mean something different when they are in a different mode. Mode, then, takes language as itself playing a role in the situation.

Field, tenor and mode are thus sets of meanings that are typically related to specific situations. Speakers choose how the meanings of field, mode and tenor will be combined. Often, there are typical combinations of field, mode and tenor that are related to events in the society. For example, a formal speech in a legislative body will have typical fields (taxation, expenditures, services), typical tenors (a certain formality, perhaps) and typical mode (which may include reading from prepared notes, shouting out in ridicule or rebuttal, extemporising loftily and at length). Speakers are expected to combine meanings from field, tenor and mode to sound like other speakers in parallel situations. This combination of field, tenor and mode is called

REGISTER

register (see Martin, 1992). Register is thus a combination of values that represent meanings and that go together to 'achieve a text's goals' (Martin, 1992: 502-3). Some speakers may set some of these variables appropriately for the situation but use other variables inappropriately. That is, field, mode and tenor are independently variable. Thus a speaker may sound peculiar because the tenor is inappropriate for the situation even though the field (institutional focus, subject matter) and mode (channel, etc.) are appropriate. A speaker with a pervasive developmental disorder or a personality disorder who sounds too formal, or a dominating speaker who always asks questions, sets the topic of conversation and demands action, may use atypical interpersonal aspects of tenor but use field and mode typically.

In this introduction to the linguistic devices that convey information, the emphasis has been on how the use of language fits into socially defined patterns. The other side of the picture is to consider that speakers make choices of meaning as a result of interactions among the social setting, the social patterns in the community and the cognitive processes of the speaker as they have developed in social settings. Even at the abstract levels of culture, genre, situation and register, the cognitive processes of the speaker and how they may be impaired must be considered. From the point of view of pathology, impaired cognitive processes may compromise processing at these abstract levels. Looked at the other way, a skewed exposure to social settings may compromise the development of cognitive processes. There exists little data on such interactions between social and cognitive variables and these ideas are presented here as hypotheses (see Rutter, 2002). The difficulties are in both identifying cognitive impairments independently of linguistic factors and clearly describing the communication impairments that are then to be related to cognitive functioning.

Kinds of meaning in language   2.2

This section outlines the specific linguistic resources that may be affected in psychiatric disorders according to three basic types of meaning. These types of meaning will be called 'metafunctions' in order to distinguish them from the many less abstract meanings or 'functions' of language. The three metafunctions are: ideational, interpersonal and textual (see Table 2.3).

METAFUNCTIONS

Table 2.3

Overview of kinds of meanings in language: the metafunctions

Ideational meaning experience of the external world (Section 2.2.1)	Things of the external world	encoded in language as participants
	Events of the external world	encoded in language as processes
	Details of events in the external world	encoded in language as circumstances
Interpersonal meaning speaker's relation to listener (Section 2.2.2)	Speaker role in the interaction	giving, demanding
	Material being transacted in the interaction	goods and services, information
	Moves	what is speaker accomplishing in a contribution to interaction
	Speech functions	semantic roles of initiating, responding, attending, exchanging
Textual meaning fitting the language into the context (Section 2.2.3)	Thematic organisation	theme – starting point of message rheme – what is said about theme
	Given and new organisation	given – encoded for the hearer as knowable new – encoded as not known
	Cohesion	links from one clause to another such as reference, conjunction, lexis, substitution/ellipsis

These technical terms apply to specific concepts but also have similar every-day and clinical meanings that are mnemonic but potentially confusing. The metafunctions refer to the meanings in language and how language conveys those meanings. Some of these meanings are 'ideational' in that they refer to the world outside of language and, in particular, to the things, events and circumstances in the physical world. (In systemic functional linguistics textbooks, words such as Things, Events and Circumstances may be capitalised to identify them as terms meaning specific functions of language and to distinguish them as specific linguistic concepts from other everyday use of the terms.) Similarly, the interpersonal and textual metafunctions each convey certain meanings. At least in some disorders, one or another of the ideational, interpersonal or textual functions may be at risk. For example, in schizophrenia, it is the textual metafunction that shows clear atypicalities.

The following outline starts with the ideational metafunction since it is the most intuitively accessible. First we outline the metafunction, then describe with examples the linguistic devices that express the metafunction and that are then hearable and reportable by the hearer when they go wrong.

DELICACY

Before entering into the detailed analysis of meaning, we must introduce an important concept in analysing language from a functional perspective: delicacy. There are differentiations of meanings at many levels from the most basic to the most detailed and particular (see Table 2.4 for some examples).

A parallel can be made to the description of buildings. At a simple level (a level with little delicacy), buildings can be described as large or small. At a more delicate level, they may be described as one story or multi-story. At a still more delicate level of description, we can give the exact number of floors. More delicate yet, is a description in terms of the height measured in metres. After that level of delicacy, there may be a description in size based on centimetres or millimetres. So far, this description with its various levels of delicacy has treated only one dimension, literally. However, the description of a building may involve other aspects such as its use. To consider a scale of delicacy of use, the first distinction could be residential or non-residential. Then, the non-residential category could be divided into commercial or industrial. At a further level of delicacy, industrial could be divided into heavy industry or light industry. The principle is that each dimension can be described to various levels of detail, with each level dependent on distinctions made earlier in the analysis. The distinctions at each level of analysis exist because the options at that level contrast with each other. We have a distinction between residential and non-residential or between 156.8 metres and 156.9 metres because the community has established the categories and the claims they are different from each other. That is, the distinctions carry a meaning that the community regards as worth encoding.

For any given purpose or for any given analysis, only a certain level of delicacy may be useful. To return to the building example, for some property tax purposes, it may be sufficient to use a distinction between residential and non-residential. However, for purposes of urban planning, more delicate descriptions in terms of the kinds of residential (single family, multiple family) or non-residential (commercial, industrial) may be needed. Throughout the following discussion of linguistic devices, we adjust the level of delicacy to provide the tools for listening to the language of the speakers in question. In some cases, considerable delicacy is needed to outline the distinctions, whereas in other cases the level of delicacy is minimal in order to show broad and important distinctions in meaning. The guiding principle will be what kind of analysis is needed to describe the clinical phenomena and especially the phenomena that lead the lay and clinical communities to diagnose pathology. By and large, these phenomena interfere with the usual social processes in the society.

Level of delicacy	Buildings	Psychiatric categories	Linguistic categories	Table 2.4
Less delicate		axis I – axis II	participants – processes	*Delicacy of description*
	large – small			
	one story – multistory	personality disorder – communication disorder	material processes – mental processes	
	number of floors			
	height in meters	paranoid schizophrenia – schizoaffective disorder	perception mental processes – affection mental processes	
More delicate	height in centimeters			

2.2.1 Ideational metafunction

The ideational metafunction primarily carries meaning related to experience of the external world. The basic meanings of things, events and circumstances are combined into clauses (see Table 2.3). The meanings must be arranged sequentially since language is a signalling system that is overwhelmingly produced and received linearly and sequentially. The grammar of language arranges the components of meaning by structural and non-structural resources.

The most basic distinction of meaning in the world that is regularly encoded into language is of things, events and circumstances. 'Things' are the objects, people and concepts that are talked about, however abstract, fictional, or whimsical. A unicorn, Big Bang or material socialism are all things in the real world that are talked about, even though we cannot point to an instance of them. Events are the 'goings-on' that things are involved with. Again, some events are not perceptually accessible but are nevertheless much more like perceptual events than they are like things. The third category of meaning in the world (since we have not yet entered the relation between the world and how it is explicitly encoded in language) is of the surroundings of events, the circumstances that fill in details of the event. The grammar of language combines these three categories of things, events and circumstances into clauses expressing meaning about the external world.

Participants expressing the things of the external world

What is combined in the grammar are not things, events or circumstances directly, but rather the linguistic expression of them. Things are expressed in terms of a linguistic category called participants. The major kinds of participants (largely following Halliday, 1994) in terms of the meanings they express are the following (examples are given in each case):

Table 2.5a

Things of the external world encoded in language as participants

Actor	The one that does something
	The company bought the building
Goal	The one to which the process is extended
	The girl ate *the apple. The apple* was eaten
Senser	The conscious being that feels, thinks or sees
	They just know that it will snow
Phenomenon	What is being felt, thought or sensed
	They all saw *the snow*
Behaver	A conscious being who is acting physiologically or psychologically
	The children are laughing
Sayer	An entity that puts out a message
	John says it is 2:00 o'clock but *my watch* says 2:30
Receiver	One who is to receive the saying
	They told *Mary* what she needed
Verbiage	What is said
	They told Mary *what she needed*
Target	That which is targeted or the subject of saying
	Don't slander *my friends*

There is a variety of such participant roles and sometimes the roles seem to be indistinct at the borders from one category to another. This is a natural characteristic of language that we need not avoid artificially. Rather, the listener must be aware of the kinds of possible meanings that participants have in language. It is the choice and combination of these meanings that is important in noticing an atypicality in a speaker's interaction.

Processes expressing the events of the external world

To extend the notion of the ideational metafunction, just as things are expressed as participants, so events in the real world are expressed in language as processes. The terms 'participants' and 'processes' may sound rather concrete, but the terms cover a wide range of things ('the first item on the agenda', 'my concept of the universe') and events ('they *planned* to …', 'they *distinguished* those two …') that the speaker encodes as the participants and processes in discourse. The processes are often expressed in language by verbs (e.g., 'to sit', 'to draw', 'to listen') but may be expressed as nouns, as in, 'his *listening* of the music'.

Material	Doing something in the external world
Mental	Experience of the inner world
	• perception
	• affection
	• cognition
Relational	Relate one experience to another

Table 2.5b

Events of the external world encoded in language as processes

There are processes that largely express experience of the world outside of the individual. These processes are called material processes. These processes are most clearly the processes of doing (e.g., 'She *opened* the box') and typically have an actor involved as the participant. Some of these material processes are rather abstract but nevertheless express happenings in the world (e.g., 'They were *absolved* of all wrong-doing').

MATERIAL PROCESSES

In contrast to material processes, there are processes that involve experience of the individual's inner world. These are called mental processes. Mental processes include perception (e.g., 'They *heard* the music'), affection ('They *enjoyed* the music') and cognition ('They *understood* the music').

MENTAL PROCESSES

A third kind of process enables the individual to generalise by relating one kind of experience to another. This third kind of process is the relational

RELATIONAL PROCESSES

process, as in, 'John *is* short', 'The butler *is* the culprit'. These categories of processes typically are combined with certain categories of participants. For example, it is typical to say something like 'John saw the exhibition' in which 'John' has the role of 'senser' combined with 'saw', a process of mental perception. This is shown below.

John	saw	the exhibition.
participant: senser	process: mental: perception	participant: goal

Less typical but still possible in that it combines meanings in an unexpected way is, 'The stillness screamed at the room'. In this utterance, 'stillness', an inanimate and abstract thing, is presented as an actor of a material process of doing and 'the room', an inanimate, concrete thing, is presented as a receiver.

The stillness	screamed	at the room.
participant: ?actor	process: material: doing	participant: ?receiver

Such unusual combinations of meanings have a poetic sound. However, if they are sustained for a number of utterances they may be quite difficult to interpret. The point is that language conveys meaning by combining different functional components (such as participants and processes) in more or less typical and therefore expected ways. Language does thus not limit what can be said but provides a set of possible meanings that can be combined in different ways. Departing from the typical combinations of meanings expands what can be said. These departures from the usual are more or less interpretable depending on how far they depart and how they fit into context. In a book of poetry, unusual sets of meanings only reflect good or bad poetry rather than pathology. In an exchange in a grocery store, unusual sets of meanings may be heard as delusional ('Of course I don't have any money in my pocket, I am the king of France') or even criminal ('If you don't give me that, I'll punch you in the mouth').

Circumstances expressing details of events of the external world

Accompanying the participants and the processes in language are circumstances that fill in details of the events encoded in the processes. The meanings carried by circumstances are mainly of 'where' ('The exhibition was held *in the school auditorium*'), 'how' ('The exhibition was held *with great pride*'), 'when' ('The exhibition was held *on Tuesday afternoon*') and 'why' ('The exhibition was held *to satisfy the school requirement of accountability*'). Some number of circumstances can be combined if the utterance does not become too awkward ('The exhibition was held *in the school auditorium / on Tuesday afternoon / to satisfy the requirement of accountability*').

Circumstances can be further specified (according to the analysis in Halliday, 1994; see Tables 5(9) – 5(16)) into nine subcategories (with attendant further subcategories) listed as follows. Table 2.5c gives examples.

Table 2.5c

Details of events in the external world encoded in language as processes

Extent	distance:	They travelled *for three miles*
	duration:	They travelled *for three days*
Location	place:	They ate *in the lunchroom*
	time:	They ate *at noon*
Manner	means:	They built it *with scrap metal*
	quality:	They built it *carefully*
	comparison:	They built it *unlike any other*
Cause	reason:	They considered it *because it was important*
	purpose:	They considered it *in order to help the poor*
	behalf:	They considered it *for the relatives*
Contingency	condition:	She studied *in case there would be no time later*
	concession:	She studied *in spite of the noise*
	default:	She studied *in the absence of an incentive*
Accompaniment	comitative:	The couple departed *with/without the children*
	additive:	The couple departed *as well as/instead of the children*
Role	guise:	They behaved *as wild animals*
	product:	They were transformed *into angels*
Matter		She spoke *of shoes and ships and sealing wax and cabbages and kings*
Angle		Oh my papa, *to me* you are so wonderful

This outline of circumstances, as with those of participants and processes, gives the major categories of meaning and that may be compromised in psychiatric disorders. There are more detailed sets of meanings which may be relevant in specific cases; however, they are included in these general categories. Clinically, it is important to pay attention to any atypicalties in the kinds of meanings conveyed even if they are not mentioned in detail for a particular disorder. Any overabundance or scarcity of one kind of participant, process or circumstance may be a clue to a disorder and may, at least, be useful for describing the features of a case.

Language is presented here chiefly as a means of conveying meaning and therefore the different kinds of meanings of participants, processes and circumstances have been outlined first. However, these meanings are expressed by the words and structure of language. The listener hears these wordings and then forms impressions of the speaker. The next section then will deal with how participants, processes and circumstances are worded for the listener.

Wording of participants, processes and circumstances

The meanings of participants, processes and circumstances are expressed by patterns of words, or to be only slightly metaphorical, they are 'worded' or 'languaged'. To return to the metaphor of buildings, a residential building is ultimately actualised or realised by brick, wood, paint and so on. Furthermore, the paint may be white, blue, grey, etc. That is, the functions of an utterance or a building must be given structure and material substance.

Participants

Participants expressing the things in the real world (see Table 2.5a) are usually worded by nouns (table, chair, justice, mercy, unicorn) or pronouns (it, they, we, I, etc.) or by groups of words centred around a noun as in the sentence, 'my three very old black *pens* given to me by my brother.' These groups of words are called nominal groups since they are centred about a noun and usually behave as nouns when combined with other words. For example, the participants in the following three sentences are all equivalent in how they combine with the following verb and, in fact, the participants can be substituted for each other:

> I lost *my three very old black pens given to me by my brother.*
> I lost *the pens.*
> I lost *them.*

As the above example shows, various kinds of information (e.g., my, three, very old) can be associated with the participant (pens) and worded into the nominal group. This possibility is important since some speakers may express rather simple information in participants and others may be elaborate or even excessive. To start analysing the information in a nominal group, we consider the information before the noun and the information after the noun.

Table 2.6	The	three	very old	black	ballpoint	pens	given to me by my brother
Kinds of information combined with participants in the nominal group	deictic	numerative	eipthet	epithet	classifier	thing	qualifier
	pointing	how many	quality	quality	subclass		complex characterisation

Before the noun, there are four rather different kinds of information with their related wordings (the analysis follows Butt, Fahey, Feez, Spinks and Yallop, 2000, and Halliday, 1994).

In the order of the nominal group, the first kind of information is the pointing information (deictics) that helps to identify the thing to the hearer. These deictics include words that indicate which subset of the things is intended and sometimes how much of the subset. The most frequent deictics are the demonstratives (the, this, that, these, those) and possessives (my, our, his, her, their, her brother's). Such deictics signal that only a certain subset of the thing mentioned in the noun is to be considered. In the following passage, the deictics are in *italics*.

> *My* name's John. You'll be playing *this* computer game. *Every* time you see *an* X on *the* control you press *the* last button.

In this example, 'My' selects which 'name' (the thing); 'this' selects which computer game; 'every' signals the subset of the thing 'time'; 'an' signals that just one, but not any particular 'X' and 'the' signals that there is a definite 'control' and there is a definite 'last button' that the hearer knows about.

After these pointing deictics in the nominal group is information (numeratives) about how many of the thing is being considered or the order of the thing. Cardinal numbers ('*one* sister', '*four* library books', 'a *thousand* invitations') give an exact indication of how many things are meant and other words give a less exact indication of how many ('*some* pants', '*several* guests'). In conveying order, an ordinal number may be used ('the *first* winner', 'the *fifth* book') or again, as with 'how many', the order may be given less precisely ('the *subsequent* speakers'). In general then, these numeratives encode information of quantity and order about things for the hearer.

Third, after pointing and numerative information, comes information about a quality of the things. Adjectives usually fill this role of epithet and several may be combined before a particular thing ('the *old*, *dirty* and *torn* jacket'). A test of whether the information is an epithet is to see if it can be modified by the word 'very'. The epithets are in *italics* in the following passage.

> Here's the man and the horse. He ties his horse up, so he sits down and he goes to sleep. The horse goes to sleep too. Along comes the *young* boy and he is on a very *old* rocking horse. So he leaves his *little* horsy and comes and takes the man's horse and leaves his *little* horse for the man.

Epithets, then, unlike deictics and numeratives, contribute to the semantic richness and detail of the things being spoken about.

The fourth and last kind of information that can be placed before a thing in a nominal group is information about which subclass of the thing is being mentioned (hence called classifiers). As well as adjectives ('the *private* party', 'a *manual* transmission') as for epithets, classifiers can be expressed by nouns ('the *office* building', 'the *computer* table'), verbs ('a *running* dispute', 'the *shined* shoes') and even other kinds of words. Epithets can usually not be modified by 'very'. As the examples suggest, classifiers contribute much detail to the content of things.

There is one kind of information (technically called a qualifier) that is placed after the thing in the nominal group. This information (a qualifier) further characterises the thing but does so by a phrase or a clause that can itself be quite complex; for example,

the	adverse	effects	of portal caval shunting on neuropsychiatric performance in the absence of intrinsic liver disease
deictic	epithet	thing	qualifier

The information that a speaker gives about a thing may thus be relatively simple with perhaps just the thing being mentioned ('*people* bother me') or may be a combination of the five kinds of additional information ('*the first three very ripe juicy citrus* fruits *of the season*'). How much information and what kinds of information are packed into nominal groups detail the communicative and cognitive abilities of a speaker. For example, the difficulty in following a thought-disordered schizophrenic is largely attributable to problems in the deictic element of the nominal group (see Rochester and Martin, 1977; 1979). Other speakers sound atypical because they do not present other aspects of the nominal group in the usual way. Depressed patients are described clinically as having diminished interests and decreased volume and amount of speech. The decreased amount of speech may well be found in the amount of information in nominal groups. Depending what elements of the nominal group are at risk, we get different impressions of atypicality.

Processes

As well as participants that encode the things of the world, the ideational metafunction also includes processes in language that encode the goings-on in the world, the events of the world (see Table 2.5b). These processes are mainly worded by groups of words centred around a verb: verbal groups. As indicated earlier, the main kinds of meaning are material, mental and relational. These main meanings are expressed in the central lexical verb in the verbal group ('Mary *could have* **gone** home', 'George *was* **seen** in the school building', in which 'gone' and 'seen' carry the main meaning). However, there is another part of the verbal group, the finite element, that carries meaning about the time and probability of the process (see Table 2.7). This finite element may be included with the main verb as in, 'They ate lunch', for which 'ate' includes information both about the material process 'eating' and the past tense 'the action happened in a time passed'. Or the finite element may be separated from the main verb and placed before it in an auxiliary verb, as in, 'John had gone home' for which the auxiliary verb 'had' encodes the time and the main verb 'gone' encodes the lexical meaning 'to leave a place', as well as a signal that it is to be combined with an auxiliary: the use of 'gone' instead of 'go'. There may be a number of auxiliary verbs before the main lexical verb (Table 2.7), with each auxiliary adding a different kind of meaning.

In the following sentence, each auxiliary verb is labelled with the kind of meaning it is contributing. The modal 'should' indicates that the speaker is not making a positive or negative statement, but rather is casting the statement as something in-between, with a meaning of 'obligation'. 'Have' conveys the meaning that the action in the lexical verb has been completed and 'been' adds the passive meaning, that somebody should have done the emptying. At the end of the verbal group is the lexical item 'emptied' that encodes the material process in question. The verbal group thus encodes a variety of kinds of meanings in a particular order. In cases of not making sense or of making sense in unusual ways, the speaker may be using one or more of these different kinds of meaning atypically. For example, a speaker who continually uses the verbal group to refer to past time will appear to be living in the past. A speaker who very frequently uses modal verbs such as 'might', 'may', 'could', will sound excessively timid and without the commitment signalled by clear positive and negative statements.

MODAL MEANING

the boxes	should	have	been	emptied	Table 2.7
	auxilliary verb finite	auxilliary verb	auxilliary verb	lexical verb	*Kinds of information combined with processes in the verbal group*
	modal-obligation	action in past	passive	to remove the contents of	

There are two kinds of information within the verbal group that do not specifically encode information about the event. A speaker relates to the message as either positive or negative. This information is usually encoded in the verbal group with the word 'not' or its contraction 'n't' (e.g., 'The book isn't here'. 'They could *not* have seen the comets'). A speaker who is either disagreeing with another speaker, or who sounds negative in outlook or disposition may create these impressions by overusing 'not' (negative polarity) in the verbal group. As well as this positive or negative polarity,

POSITIVE OR NEGATIVE MEANINGS

the difference between active and passive voice is signalled in the verbal group. In active voice, the actor ('the one that does something') is first in the sentence and is the subject of the sentence ('*John* ate the apple'). In passive voice, a form of the verb 'be' is used, (e.g., 'is', 'are', 'was', 'were'). Also, the actor is placed later in the sentence or eliminated and some other element, often goal ('the one to which the process is extended') is placed first ('The *apple* was eaten' (by John)). The differences between active and passive are discussed later in the outline of the textual function.

Circumstances

Circumstances fill in the details of the processes. They give information about the time, location, manner, cause and so on of the process (see Table 2.5c and see Halliday, 1994 Chapter 5). Circumstances are worded by adverbs ('They swam *slowly*') and adverbial groups ('They swam *too **slowly** for my liking*') and by prepositional groups ('They swam *into the cave*'). Circumstances may be expressed by adverbs alone ('You should read *carefully*'), by adverbs connected together into a list ('You should read *slowly, carefully* and *precisely*'), or by a group of words containing an adverb that is modified ('You should read *more **carefully** than I did*'). In this last example of an adverb group, the adverb 'carefully' has the modifier 'more' before it and the modifier 'than I did' after it.

Circumstances also express information about the process through prepositional phrases. Prepositional phrases are composed of a preposition and a following nominal group. (See the examples in Table 2.8.) As with the adverb group, the more complex the prepositional phrase, the more detailed is the process and the goings-on in the world. That is, circumstances tell the hearer about the details of these happenings. The wording and frequency of circumstances provides the speaker with many options of what and how much such information to convey.

Table 2.8			
Information and structure in circumstances (details about events)	**Adverb**	they swam *slowly*	
	Adverbial group	they swam *too slowly for my liking*	
	Preposition phrase	*into*	*the red barn that was built here in the last century*
		preposition	nominal group noun *barn* with modification before it (*the, red*) and after it (*that was built here in the last century*)

The description of the wordings of participants, processes and circumstances shows how language encodes the basic meanings of participants, processes and circumstances for the hearer. In each encoding or wording, there are many options (for example, modification) that add to and colour the basic meanings. It may be difficult to categorise some wording into the underlying meaning. Language allows for this indetermination that introduces new and subtle meanings as well as various ambiguities. These ambiguities have their role in language and help the speaker to deliberately send less than completely clear messages. The ultimate constraint on the wordings and on the building of new wordings is whether members of the speech community interpret the wordings as the speaker intended them.

There are many finer grained analyses possible for each of the categories of participants, processes and circumstances. In general, it is the broader analyses of meaning that probably characterise psychiatric disorders. It is easier to imagine a speaker who over- or under- uses a category such as circumstantials or even manner circumstantials than to imagine a speaker who has an atypicality with only circumstantials specifying location: spatial: relative: near ('here', 'nearby') and not with location: spatial: relative: remote ('there'). Nevertheless, language can be used in many different ways in context and listeners should be alert to various atypicalities in ideational meanings.

Combining meanings: participants, processes and circumstances making meaning together

As mentioned, participants, processes and circumstances are usually combined in speaking or writing. It is unusual to say merely 'Mary', 'eaten' or 'in time for lunch'. However, when such things are said it is usually in a context that fills in the participants, processes or circumstances presumed to be known to the hearer. Here we must distinguish the notion of utterance from that of clause. An utterance is some stretch of language that is used in oral interaction. Most utterances are spontaneous, although they may be planned. Utterances may be relatively long or short. A clause, in contrast, is a grammatical unit that more or less conforms to the patterns of the language. There could be, therefore, several clauses in one utterance. The clause is an important unit since it is in clauses that the organisation of participants, processes and circumstances takes place. The central or defining feature of a clause is the process expressed by a verb. The participants and circumstances are dependent both semantically and structurally on the process. The nature of the process determines which kinds of participants belong with it; for example, a material process can have an actor and a goal ('Mary flew the airplane') but not a sayer, behaver or verbiage ('Mary flew the statement') participant directly associated with it. 'Mary flew the statement' sounds odd, although we might be able to interpret it metaphorically. In many languages, the process also determines grammatical order and agreement. For example, in many dialects, we can say 'They are here' but not 'They is here' since 'they' is plural and the verb encoding the process ('are') shows a sign of the grammatical connection between participant and process. There is a connection of meaning and grammatical structure among the expressions of participant, process and circumstance. These connections span the unit of the clause. Beyond the clause, there are other relationships but they are not the tight ones of structure.

When there are two or more choices in building a clause, then the difference between the choices can be interpreted as a difference of meaning. To look at it the other way round, where there are choices, they are exploited for sending different messages. To take a non-linguistic example, if two people have plain pieces of cloth as flags and pots of paint, then for each colour paint, a different message can be sent. If all the flags remain one colour, then they will all be equivalent and different messages will have to be signalled by some other system, such as the number of flags or how long they are displayed. Language uses limited resources, such as a small number of different sounds and short words, but exploits the possible variation in order, intonation, etc. to construct a large number of potential messages. Some of these different meanings may be similar ('John hit the ball', 'The ball was hit by John', 'They arrived yesterday', 'Yesterday, they arrived') but, nevertheless, the opportunity of wording something two ways opens up the possibility that the two wordings convey different meanings.

In summary, the ideational metafunction is the way language encodes the meanings from the outside world. Language is organised to provide the resources to express a vast array of meanings. For some individuals, there may be a relative increase or decrease of use of some of these meanings. If we notice a departure from a community standard, then there may be a finding of unusual 'ideation'. It is interesting that both the linguistic and psychiatric communities have used the word 'ideation' to capture the notion. The ideational metafunction in linguistics provides the details of the different kinds of meanings that are at stake and how speakers word those meanings. However, various wordings of this ideational content are influenced by the interpersonal and textual metafunctions. Sometimes, it may be necessary to both describe the ideational meanings involved (e.g., participants and processes suggesting suicide) and how those meanings are realised through the other metafunctions (e.g., active voice 'I should have died' or passive voice 'I should have been killed' within the textual metafunction). Understanding how meanings are worded is important for:

(1) developing a more specific description of the 'ideation';

(2) focusing the listener on the relevant aspects of a speaker's language;

(3) ultimately, attempting to specify how speakers diverge from the typical use of ideation.

The similarity or difference among speakers and across disorders can rest specifically in the ideational metafunction or can be in one of the other metafunctions with the attendant shaping of the ideational meanings. For example, if a speaker talks about phantoms and forces that reflect atypical choices of participants, processes and circumstances from the ideational metafunction, but the speaker frequently combines these meanings with 'hedging' choices from the interpersonal metafunction (e.g., 'possibly', 'sometimes', 'maybe', 'could be') then the effect is rather different than if the choices from the interpersonal metafunction tended to express definiteness and certainty (e.g., 'really', 'absolutely', 'always', 'certainly').

Speakers with different psychiatric disorders will have converging and diverging ideation. Presumably, speakers with the same disorder will have converging patterns of ideation. This convergence in ideation will be associated with coherent diagnostic categories. The diagnostic categories are built out of lower level diagnostic criteria or descriptive features involving ideation. The better these criteria and descriptive features are specified in terms of the ideational features of language, then the more coherent will be the diagnostic categories in terms of the ideational content.

On a micro level, specific diagnostic criteria and clinical descriptions can be made precise by providing linguistically described meanings and the wordings of those meanings. It is these clinical descriptions based on what individuals say that are the observables. The linguistic tools allow us to generalise from the individual data to the patterns of language that need to be grouped into diagnostic criteria or disorders. The generalisation is through linguistic theory. Functional linguistics provides a theory of which meanings are encodeable into language and how those meanings are typically encoded. The analysis can then go in both directions: both

(1) from the possible meanings carried by the ideational, interpersonal and textual metafunctions to the wordings;

(2) from the language used in specific cases to the meanings and combinations of meanings that are conveyed by these uses.

2.2.2 Interpersonal metafunction

As well as meanings conveyed by the ideational metafunction, there are meanings of how the speaker is interacting with the listener (see Table 2.3 for an overview). This interaction grows out of the roles of the speakers in the situation. As with the outline of the ideational function, these kinds of meanings will be developed from the basic building blocks of the interaction. Afterwards, we describe how the meanings are encoded in language. There are two main issues in outlining the meanings. The first is the role the speaker assumes in the situation. The most basic components of these roles (following Halliday, 1984, 1994) are 'giving' or 'demanding' and the commodity that is given or demanded, namely, either information or goods and services. These two dimensions are seen as kinds of meaning that derive from the roles that the speaker assumes and the corresponding roles the speaker assigns to the hearer. The dimensions combine to give four basic types of role as shown below.

	Giving	**Demanding**
Goods and services	Offer	Command
Information	Statement	Question

The essential difference between information and goods and services is that information is a linguistic function. That is, information is given by saying something, whereas goods and services are usually non-verbal commodities. A speaker who assumes the role of offerer by giving goods and services to another (e.g., a cup of coffee) then places the hearer or receiver in the complementary role of 'receiver of goods and services offered'. A hearer can decline the offer ('I'd rather not have a cup now') or even the role of being offered ('Leave me alone', 'I would never take anything from you', 'What are you trying to do?') but it is nevertheless a role defined for that speaker by the speaker of the offer.

This example points to the second issue in outlining meanings in the interpersonal function. Conversation is essentially sequential; generally, one person speaks at a time. This constraint arises naturally from the physical constraints of hearing and perceiving simultaneous messages. In some contexts, simultaneous messages are the norm (a question period in a parliament, or intentional overhearers of conversations) and speakers are assumed to monitor more than one speaker at once. However such circumstances are unusual and require learning new habits.

Turns

Since conversation is sequential and consecutive, one stretch of language is functionally dependent on another. If one speaker asks a question or makes an offer, the next speaker is heard as answering the question or reacting to that offer whatever the ideational content of the utterance. For example, after the question 'When do you think you will be home?' (a demand for information), the next utterance will be interpreted as an answer whether it be 'at eleven', 'none of your business', 'the rain in Spain falls mainly on the plain', 'I have an important meeting to get to', or anything else. That is, the sequential organisation of talk creates dependencies among utterances. Here we will have to define a new term, the turn. A turn is the talk of one speaker that is bounded by the talk of another. Turns may be very long, since in some situations other speakers do not interrupt, or they may be very short, as in an animated conversation where a simple 'yes' or 'ya' or even 'y-' may constitute a turn. Speakers are then responsible for and hold others responsible for, creating the flow of conversations with turns being dependent on each other. From this dependency one can establish adjacency pairs in conversations. These pairs, such as greeting-greeting ('Hi' – 'Hi'), invitation-acceptance or decline ('Want to come for lunch?' 'No, I'm too busy') are typically adjacent to each other in conversation and the utterance of the first partner in the pair controls the interpretation of the next turn as being the second partner in the pair. Seven adjacency pairs have been suggested (Martin, 1992: 45), with examples given:

Call	**Response to call**	John – Yes
Greeting	**Response to greeting**	Hi – Hi
Exclamation	**Response to exclamation**	Disgusting – You bet
Offer	**Acknowledge offer**	A piece of home-made pie? – Sure
Command	**Response offer to command**	Get me two painkillers – Will do
Statement	**Acknowledge statement**	Hottest day of the summer – Guess so
Question	**Response statement to question**	When will I see you? – At eleven

Although these particular pairs may not cover all examples of dependency, they illustrate the general principle that successive turns are interpreted as being tightly related to each other.

Moves

The turn is a unit defined non-functionally. It is what one person manages to say before someone else speaks. These turns, though, contain the functions that are needed to accomplish the exchange of information and goods and services. To account for what speakers have to do in conversation and how they must organise their talk, it is necessary to define a functional unit for interaction: the 'moves' that speakers make. Often, the interactions are not as straightforward as greeting – greeting, but require negotiation and clarification. Later, these moves will be seen as being combined into different kinds of exchanges and the internal make-up of the moves will be explored.

Table 2.9

Information in moves

Commodity	Orientation	
	Speaker oriented	**Hearer oriented**
Information	Primary knower	Primary knower
	Secondary knower	Secondary knower
Goods and services	Primary actor	Primary actor
	Secondary actor	Secondary actor

The systematic distinctions in meaning that are needed to analyse most moves are presented in Table 2.9 (from Martin, 1992: 49, Figure 2.10):

INFORMATION OR
ACTION?

(1) Is the interaction about information and knowledge, or is it about goods and services, that is, about action?

SPEAKER OR HEARER
AS MAIN KNOWER OR
ACTOR?

(2) Is it the speaker or the hearer that knows the information (for interactions involving information) or that does the principal action (for interactions involving goods and services)? For example, the question 'What time is it?' indicates that the speaker does not know the information. In this case, the speaker is a secondary knower. The answerer is presumed to be the primary knower, the person who knows the information. On the other hand, for the statement 'It is snowing', the speaker is the primary knower. The speaker may choose to delay displaying knowledge or may delay taking the action. In these cases, there is a 'testing' feeling about the interaction. The speaker really does know the information but is delaying the role of primary knower. A teacher asking: 'What is the capital of Greece?' is generally recognised by students as the primary knower. The teacher is delaying the display of the information for interactional and pedagogical purposes. The students are placed in the role of secondary knowers, those assumed to perhaps not know the information.

(3) Is the speaker following up on some contribution or not? For example,
there is often a third member to an adjacency pair that follows up
the second pair partner ('What's the time?' – 'Seven o'clock' – '*Still so
early*', '*Thanks*', '*Couldn't be*'. 'I've never seen you this upset before.'
– 'Just something Brian said.' – '*I thought so*'). These three distinctions can be combined with each other in various ways to generate
a considerable range of meanings. Examples follow. The meanings
chosen from these three distinctions are given in parentheses. These
choices can be seen as a list of semantic features of the interpersonal
metafunction at the level of moves.

Have some pie.	Goods and services, speaker as secondary actor, non-follow up
I'd rather not.	Goods and services, speaker as primary actor, non-follow up
Alright.	Goods and services, speaker as secondary actor, follow up
How's George doing on the new job?	Information, speaker as secondary knower, non-follow up
Could be better.	Information, speaker as primary knower, non-follow up
It's almost midnight.	Information, speaker as primary knower, non-follow up
You're kidding.	Information, speaker as secondary knower, non-follow up

The examples have been deliberately short and have demonstrated turns with
only one move. However, a number of moves may be combined in one turn.
In the following example, B's turn combines a move that asks a clarification
question with a move that gives information.

A:	What do you still find hard?	Information, speaker as secondary knower, non-follow up
B:	To do?	Information, speaker as secondary knower, non-follow up
	Oh, walking ... sometimes, if I walk too much	Information, speaker as primary knower, non-follow up

In longer turns, there may be a number of utterances that consist of the same
function. These cases point out the importance of establishing the scope of a
move as a function in conversation. It is important to know if a speaker continues with the same function or whether and under which circumstances
the speaker contributes different functions. Although not uncontroversial,
the most convenient and easily justifiable unit for establishing the scope of

the move is the 'clause selecting independently for mood' (Martin, 1992: 59 see arguments there). Such clauses are the ones that allow for the choice among the moods of interrogative, declarative, imperative, etc.

As some of the examples of moves suggest, moves often combine in typical ways that characterise certain interactions. For example, the chaining of questions often found in the talk of teachers to young children typically combines moves of (information, speaker as secondary knower, non-follow up) by the teacher, (information, speaker as primary knower, non-follow up) by the child (C) and (information, speaker as primary knower, follow up) by the teacher (T):

T:	Do you think that there's going to be guinea pigs on the farm when we get there?	Information, speaker as secondary knower, non-follow up
	What do you think that we'll find on the farm?	Information, speaker as secondary knower, non-follow up
C:	Horses	Information, speaker as primary knower, non-follow up
T:	Good	Information, speaker as primary knower, follow up

The nature of this interaction is created by the series of moves from speaker to speaker. The teacher asks information questions and follows up the answer of the child. The child provides information after the teacher's request for information. The combining of moves into typical exchanges represents patterns of meaning that recur to define how individuals typically interact in the contexts of the speech community. The systemic functional approach, then describes the interactions chiefly in terms of the meaning of the speakers.

Some speakers do not play their role in conversations since they do not provide the moves typically expected in the context of their own other moves and the moves of others. Such atypical moves may be correct in grammatical structure but just not the right thing to say in terms of the pattern of moves that creates the exchanges in interaction.

The move as a functional unit in conversation has been presented with its basic functional distinctions of information – action, identification of primary and secondary actor or knower and identification of the contribution as follow up or not. As with the basic meanings in the ideational function, these basic meanings in the interpersonal function must be worded by using the words and grammatical structures of the language. That is, the functions are realised through the lexicogrammar. We will now explore the realisations of these moves in the interpersonal function.

Speech function

The organisation of conversation into successive moves and the organisation in terms of the semantic roles speakers take become conflated. The semantic roles defined by giving – demanding and information and goods and services produce specific functions for speech (speech functions). The systematic distinctions involved in most speech functions are the following (summarised in Table 2.10, derived from Martin, 1992: 44, Figure 2.8; and Fine, 1991: 222, Table 1).

	Initiating	Responding	Table 2.10
Attending			*Meanings that combine*
Call			*into speech functions*
Greeting			
Exchanging			
Giving			
Information			
Goods and services			
Demanding			
Information			
Goods and services			

(1) All speech functions are classified as either initiating or responding.

(2) A group of speech functions deal with making sure that the speakers are attending to each other. These are then either calling or greeting. Thus a call that is initiating is typically one speaker starting the interaction (perhaps at a bit of a distance) by saying 'Joan'. A call that is responding is the second speaker's 'Ya' or 'John'. A greeting that is initiating can be 'What's up?' with a response to greeting realised by 'fine', 'the usual' or 'nothing much'.

(3) Instead of attending, speech functions may involve exchanging goods or services or exchanging information. The distinctions here are similar to those at the level of mood: information vs. goods and services; giving vs. demanding.

All these distinctions are set out systematically below:

(1)   initiating
        responding

(2)   attending
                    call
                    greeting
        exchanging
                    giving
                    demanding
        and:
                    goods and services
                    information

Each contrast or distinction can be chosen independently as long as the higher level category is chosen, for example, if [exchanging] is chosen, then either [giving] or [demanding] is chosen and either [goods and services] or [information] is also chosen. The basic meanings represented by these distinctions can then be combined to yield a dozen types of speech functions.

> initiating: attending: call
>
> initiating: attending: greeting
>
> initiating: exchange: giving: goods and services
>
> initiating: exchange: giving: information
>
> initiating: exchange: demanding: goods and services
>
> initiating: exchange: demanding: information
>
> responding: attending: call
>
> responding: attending: greeting
>
> responding: exchange: giving: goods and services
>
> responding: exchange: giving: information
>
> responding: exchange: demanding: goods and services
>
> responding: exchange: demanding: information

An important characteristic of the speech functions is that they are not always directly mapped onto moves. Consider for example the following example originally from Levinson (1983: 290) and analysed by Martin (1992: 40).

> Would you like another drink?
> Yes, I would, thank you, but make it a small one.

The first turn is a move which seems to demand information. Its speech function is a yes-no question looking for a yes or no answer. However, the move it is making is to offer goods, 'another drink' and the response 'thank you' acknowledges the offer made.

Speech functions are also related to turns in a non one-to-one way. For example, a turn may contain more than one speech function. Consider the following constructed conversation.

> A: Are you coming for dinner?
> B: Yes,
>   but not this week.
>   My brother is visiting and he is a homebody.
>   What are you doing Saturday night?

In B's turn, 'Yes' is an answer to the question of A. This stretch of conversation constitutes an adjacency pair of question (demanding information) – response statement to question (giving information). The segment 'but not this week' adds some additional or supplementary information to the answer but is not the information that was asked for directly. There is then the statement 'My brother is visiting but he is a homebody' which could be intended and taken also as supplementary information related to speaker A's question and speaker B's response or could be taken as a statement that needs a response from speaker A. The contribution 'What are you doing Saturday night?' may be an offer to get together or just a question asking for information. That is, in speaker B's turn, there are four separate speech functions combined in one turn.

SUPPLEMENTARY
INFORMATION

Speech functions and the control of interaction

In combining speech functions into turns, speakers influence the flow of conversation. The speaker of a first pair partner in an adjacency pair defines the kind of contribution that the other speaker must provide or at least be seen as rejecting. The second speaker is inevitably heard as reacting to the first pair partner as defined by the first speaker. That is, to some extent, the speaker of a first pair partner exerts local control over the interaction. This local control can be extended or reversed by the kinds of speech functions that are combined into a turn. In the following example (from Fine, 1994: 157) there is an extension of the local control over turns.

LOCAL
CONVERSATIONAL
CONTROL

> A: Do you think that there're going to be guinea pigs on the farm when we
>   get there? What do you think that we'll find on the farm?
> B: Horses
> A: Good. Have you ever been to a farm?

The first turn of speaker A has two speech functions. There first is a yes-no question that asks for information that is either 'yes' or 'no' and the second is a question that asks for specific information. Speaker B's turn provides a response to the second speech function in speaker A's turn. Speaker A's second turn combines two speech functions. The 'Good' represents an acknowledgement of speaker B's response. Within the same turn, speaker A also asks yet another question, 'Have you ever been to a farm?' That is, this second turn of speaker A continues the speaker's local control of the conversation, placing speaker B in the position of answering or declining to answer another demand for information. Such chaining of demands, whether for information or goods and services, is typical of situations in which there is an asymmetry of socially defined roles with one speaker (often teacher or clinician, assuming and/or expected to assume) the role of guiding the interaction.

As well as combining speech functions to continue the local control of conversation, there can be a turn-over of local control. These turn-overs are often accomplished by combining a second pair partner and a first pair partner in one turn. The following segment of a real conversation represents a turn-over of local conversational control from speaker A to speaker B (Fine, 1994: 157).

> A: Do you like playing? ... I mean like at recess.
> B: Yes ... what kinda game do you play at recess?

In the first turn, speaker A asks a question (a demand for 'yes' or 'no' information) that is then clarified with the statement 'I mean like at recess'. In the second turn, speaker B uses the speech function of giving information ('yes') and is thus providing the second pair partner (an answer) to the question of speaker A. However, the second speech function of speaker B's turn demands information ('what kinda game do you play at recess?'). This turn of speaker B places speaker A in the position of having to respond with a second pair partner. The local control of the conversation has moved from speaker A to speaker B. These turn-overs are typical in conversations between speakers who see each other as having equal social roles in the situation. The example here is between two children of the same age. The ordering of utterances and their functional impact produces a local organisation of talk that influences the flow of conversation.

Mood

The speech functions just explored are then worded or realised by the grammar of the language. An outline of these realisations follows. Speech functions are chiefly worded by the relationship of part of the verb to the subject in the clause. This wording of the subject and verbal element produces the mood of the clause. The part of the verb in question is the finite verb which is usually the main verb or an auxiliary verb if there is one. The essential characteristic of the finite verb is that it can show time and takes the negative 'not' or 'n't'. The function of the finite element is to make the proposition definite enough to be 'at stake' in the conversation. In 'They ate the sandwich with the melting cheese' the verb 'ate' can be negated with the addition of the auxiliary verb 'do' ('didn't eat') and the proposition can be argued about ('No, they didn't eat the sandwiches') whereas 'melting cheese' is not presented as what is at stake in the conversation.

FINITE VERB

By combining the finite verb and the subject in different ways, grammar creates a series of grammatical patterns that realise the speech functions. If there is no subject, finite verb and main verb, then the clause is called a minor clause and its role in conversation is as greetings ('Hi') or calls ('John'), as exclamations ('Wow') and sometimes as responses to questions ('Are you OK?' – 'Sure'). If there is no subject but there is a main verb, then the clause is in the imperative mood. The speaker is presenting no claim about the truth (or falsity) of the clause's ideational meaning and the subject is presumed to be the hearer ('(you) Get the book now', 'Don't (you) wait around here'). The imperative mood can thus be a realisation of the speech function of: initiating: exchanging: demanding: goods and services. Non-finite verbs ('the *melting* cheese', 'the *melted* cheese') typically are not part of clauses that have mood.

IMPERATIVE MOOD

The moods and combinations of subject and finite verbal element presented so far are incomplete in that one or more components of the clause that can occur (subject, finite element) is missing. There are three kinds of mood that have all the elements present and that often provide the wording for specific speech functions. Declarative mood structure puts the subject before the finite verbal element as in the following examples.

DECLARATIVE MOOD

Mary	came	home.
Mary	has	come home.
They	are	thinking about it.
They	should	be thinking about it.
subject	**finite element**	

There are two kinds of interrogative mood which both put something other than the subject first. In yes-no interrogatives, the information required is whether the ideational content of the clause is true; that is, the answer is either 'yes' or 'no' ('Did they arrive yet?'). The grammatical way to get this meaning is to place a finite verbal element before the subject as in the following examples.

Did	Mary	come home?
Has	Mary	come home?
Are	they	thinking about it?
Should	they	be thinking about it?
finite element	**subject**	

A second kind of interrogative is a wh- interrogative in which there is a questioning not about the truth or falsity of the statement but rather about certain information in the statement. Wh- words such as what, who, when, why, how signal that there is some part of the statement that the speaker wishes the hearer to supply. The relevant wh- word is placed at the beginning of the clause before other elements such as finite verbal element and subject that may be needed. The ordering of the key elements of wh- interrogative clauses is exemplified in the following clauses.

Where	have	all the flowers gone?
How	can	those crooks win the election?
Who	ought	to win?
Why	are	the dogs loose?
Wh- word	**finite element**	

These different moods of minor ('Hi'), non-finite ('running dogs'), imperative ('come in'), declarative ('The time is right'), yes-no interrogative ('Is the time right?') and wh- interrogative ('When will the time be right?') each have specific structural characteristics and each can be used to encode the different speech functions. The reason for analysing both speech functions and moods separately is that there is not a simple mapping between the speech functions and the grammar. That is, a single speech function may be worded in several ways using different grammatical structures. For example, an 'offer' speech function involving the features of initiating: exchange: giving: goods and services may be encoded in mood as minor ('Here'), imperative ('Take one'), declarative ('I made it myself'), yes-no interrogative ('Would you like one?'), or a wh- interrogative ('Which would you like?'). This choice in how to map from speech function to mood gives the speaker the opportunity to convey slightly different meanings. That is, the choice of the mood adds something to the meaning of the speech function.

This distinction between the speech function and how it is worded by mood is important for considering how speakers construct either typical messages or atypical messages. The question is whether the atypicality is at the level of the speech function or at the level of the mood. For example, is the speaker offering goods and services too frequently, too infrequently or in unusual contexts, or is the speaker wording those offers in unusual ways?

Degree of commitment

The analysis of the interpersonal metafunction has focused on how speakers interact with each other and express their roles in interaction. Another aspect of the interpersonal metafunction is how much the speaker is committed to the utterance presented to the hearer. This concept of the speaker's attitude can be called modality since it modulates the level of commitment (see Butt, Fahey, Feez, Spinks and Yallop, 2000). The basic meanings (following Halliday, 1994) available to the speaker are: probability ('Joan *possibly* came') and usuality ('Joan *usually* comes') for information exchanges and obligation ('Joan is *supposed* to come') and inclination ('Joan *must* come') for goods and services exchanges (see Table 2.11). There are four ways that these meanings are usually expressed: modal verbs, modal adjuncts, attitudinal epithets and adjectives in the predicate (see Table 2.12). Modal verbs (should, ought, could, would, may, might, must, can, shall, will) express the speaker's attitude to the process. These modal verbs can be used with both declarative clauses ('John *will* be here at noon') and the two kinds of interrogative clauses ('*Will* John be here at noon?' 'Who *will* be here at noon?' 'Where *could* John be?'). Each of the modal verbs conveys a different kind of commitment to the utterance. These meanings are clear to most speakers. Monitoring a speaker's modal verbs is therefore one way to focus on the commitment of the speaker to the content of utterances and how that commitment may change from addressee to addressee or from topic to topic.

	Kind of exchange	Examples	Table 2.11
Probability	information	possibly, probably	*Degree of commitment:*
Usuality	information	usually, often, rarely	*meanings*
Obligation	goods and services	supposed to	
Inclination	goods and services	want to	

Table 2.12		Kind of meaning	Examples
Degree of commitment: wordings	**Modal verbs**	attitude to process in clause	should, ought, could
	Modal adjuncts (see details in Table 2.13)	attitude to clause	probably, in fact, actually
	Attitudinal epithets	attitude to participant	disgusting, lovely
	Adjectives in predicate	objective quality of participant	unusual, record-breaking

As well as modal verbs, the speaker's attitude to an utterance can be encoded in modal adjuncts. These adjuncts express meanings mainly through various adverbs. The list in Table 2.13 (Halliday, 1994: 49, 82-3) is indicative of some of the most frequent adjuncts which express a speaker's attitude. There are more such adjuncts and some of the boundaries of the categories may not be clear. However, it is possible that for some speakers and for some disorders the atypicality language is centred around only a subset of the meanings that are then represented by a subset of adjuncts (see Table 2.13).

Table 2.13	Kind of meaning	Examples
Adjuncts expressing degree of commitment	**Polarity and modality**	
	polarity	yes, not, so, no
	probability	probably, possibly, maybe
	usuality	always, usually, sometimes, rarely, never
	readiness	willingly, readily, easily
	obligation	definitely, by all means
	Temporality	
	time	yet, still, already
	typicality	mainly, regularly, occasionally
	Mood	
	obviousness	of course, surely
	intensity	in fact, actually, merely, just
	degree	completely, totally, almost, nearly, scarcely
	Comment	
	opinion	in my opinion, personally
	admission	frankly
	persuasion	honestly, seriously
	presumption	apparently, presumably
	desirability	fortunately, hopefully
	evaluation	understandably, wisely, foolishly

Modal verbs and modal adjuncts tend to affect the whole of the meaning of the clause or the process which is the centre of the clause (e.g., '*Certainly*, I ate dinner before ten. I *could* wish for more'). That is, the speaker is conveying a sense of commitment about the major meaning in the clause. However, the speaker can also give an opinion about a specific participant by using an attitudinal epithet in the nominal group. Like other epithets, attitudinal epithets express a quality of the thing being described ('the *disgusting* weather'). Attitudinal epithets differ from other epithets by describing the speaker's opinion about the thing rather than some more objective quality. Non-attitudinal epithets (the predicate adjectives) include examples such as 'the *warm* weather', 'the *record-breaking* weather', 'the *unusual* weather', whereas attitudinal epithets convey more opinion: 'the *lovely* weather', 'the *fantastic* weather', 'the *beastly* weather'. As with the other ways of expressing opinions, some speakers may use attitudinal epithets to signal only restricted meanings. It is to capture this kind of specificity and to potentially distinguish one kind of speaker from another that it is useful to consider the separate meaning creating capacities in the interpersonal metafunction.

ATTITUDINAL
EPITHETS

The interpersonal metafunction contributes meanings of how the speaker sees the interaction between speakers. The meanings are contributed at a number of levels from move to speech function and on into the grammatical expression of attitude. A few basic points about the interpersonal metafunction should be reiterated. Firstly, every utterance has meanings that are derived from the interpersonal metafunction. That is, every utterance encodes meanings about the speaker's role in the interaction. Sometimes these roles may be emphasised and realised unambiguously ('*In my opinion*, you *certainly should* dump that *disgusting, so-called* friend') but in other cases the absence of such clear signals is still signalling the speaker's (perhaps neutral) attitude in the interaction. In terms of moves, speech functions and mood, it is clear that every utterance draws on these resources and signals interpersonal meaning. Interpersonal meanings are linked to the context of the interaction and draw meanings that are possible in the context. The presence of different interlocutors and how the speaker regards the social roles of those interlocutors influence which interpersonal meanings are drawn on and how they are expressed.

A second basic point about the interpersonal metafunction is that these meanings must be seen in the context of and as interacting with meanings from the other metafunctions. For example, the meanings of the ideational metafunction and the interpersonal metafunction must be considered together. The interpersonal meanings expressed when dealing with one kind of ideation may be different from those expressed when dealing with another kind of ideation. Any speaker will be sensitive to issues such as who can be asked about (using initiating speech functions) personal feelings or finances (a special set of ideational choices) and who probably should not be asked about them or who can be bossed around (using initiating speech functions for goods and services) concerning which road to take (ideational metafunction) and who should not.

A third point is that the unusual language may be at a number of levels of our analysis or at several specific levels at the same time. If the interpersonal metafunction is the locus of the atypicalities in language then the distinctive 'not being in touch with other speakers' will be created. The specification of exactly which parts of the interpersonal metafunction are at risk then provides information about the particular nature of the interpersonal odd-ness of the speaker.

2.2.3   Textual metafunction

The textual metafunction covers the meanings that fit an utterance into its context. Choices in grammar and vocabulary create structures up to the level of the clause and sometimes further as clauses are combined together. However, to make an utterance fit into its context, speakers must order and manipulate the material from the ideational and interpersonal metafunc-tions. The differences among 'John ate the pie yesterday', 'He ate the pie yesterday' and 'Yesterday, John ate the pie' concern how the speaker is fitting the utterance into the context; namely, is 'John' presumed to be known to the hearer, has 'John' been mentioned before in the conversation and will 'he' be interpreted as unambiguous, is the time of 'yesterday' deemed to be particularly important or unknown in this context? These choices are not merely alternate ways of saying something, but link the language in different ways to what the speaker and listener know about each other and the context. That is, the speaker can encode different meanings about the message. It is a different meaning to say 'I think that you, the hearer, do not know X but do know Y and I am telling you that X is also true' instead of 'I think that you, the hearer, do know X but do not know Y and I am telling you that Y is also true'. Since these choices are sensitive to the context (what the speaker thinks that the hearer does or does not know), these choices help fit the utterance into the context. To use an example from Halliday (1994: 335), the following stretch of language has well formed sentences on a single topic but they do not create a good text since they do not follow from one another in the context: 'The magnet is at the North Star. The earth attracts the North Star. The earth does not attract the stars which are not the North Star. The stars which are not the North Star move around.' The textual metafunction contributes coherence by fitting the language into the context. To make language coherent, there must be consistency of register, genre, etc but the language must also fit with the language that has been produced up to that point (the verbal context) and fit with the physical aspects of the speech event (the non-verbal context). From how a speaker creates this fit with context, we learn about how the speaker views and presents the context and the hearer's place in it.

The textual metafunction includes a number of structural and non-structural relations that express different kinds of meaning. The structural devices encode the meaning of the starting point of the message (thematic structure in the clause) and the speaker's encoding of information as given or new (information structure in the clause). The non-structural devices deal with the linking of participants (through reference), the linking of messages (through conjunction), the continuity of lexical meaning (through lexical patterning) and the linking of large and small structural units (by substitution and ellipsis). Each of these devices will be outlined in turn with an emphasis on the meanings that are at stake and that must be selected to create a functioning text.

Structural devices: thematic organisation

Speakers can arrange their messages into two sections:

(1) 'this is where I want to start my message'

(2) 'this is what there is to say about my starting point'.

The same message can often be stated in two ways by changing the starting point. For example, 'Three carrots is all I have' and 'All I have is three carrots' are the same in ideational function and interpersonal function. However, they differ in textual function in that they are appropriate to different contexts. Halliday interprets this first meaning, the theme, as 'the point of departure of the clause as a message' or 'what the message is about'. Martin (1992: 489) interprets the theme as tying down the text by showing how the speaker looks at things. What is not theme, what comes later in the clause, is called rheme and has the meaning of 'the development of the theme'. Speakers then have two meanings that they can use: 'the starting point of the message' and 'how the message is developed' (see Table 2.14). The following examples show groups of sentences with different choices for the starting point of the message (the theme). As the examples show, the sentences are appropriate to different contexts. Speakers who seem disconnected to the context, including being disconnected to other speakers and other utterances, may be misusing this theme-rheme structure and be sending unusual messages of what is the starting point or what is the development of a message. The atypical use of theme and rheme is of course not the cause of being disconnected from context but may be one way the clinician can recognise such disconnection.

THEME

RHEME

My aunt gave this watch to me yesterday.	What happened? What did your aunt do?
Yesterday, my aunt gave this watch to me.	When did your aunt give you this watch?
This watch, my aunt gave to me yesterday.	What did your aunt give you (yesterday)?
To me, my aunt gave this watch yesterday.	Who did your aunt give the watch to?

Table 2.14

Meanings in the thematic organisation

		Theme	**Rheme**
Meaning		the point of departure of the clause as a message what the message is about	how the message is developed what is said about the theme
Examples		My aunt	gave this watch to me yesterday.
		Yesterday,	my aunt gave this watch to me.
		This watch,	my aunt gave to me yesterday.
		To me,	my aunt gave this watch yesterday.

Choosing what is to be the theme of a message is related to the mood of the clause (is it a declarative, interrogative, imperative) as well as to the context. We will now explore this relation to mood and then return to how the message is fitted into the context. In declarative mood clauses, the subject is usually placed first and becomes the theme. The subject as theme is typical and therefore 'unmarked'. The subject is theme if there is no good reason to choose another element as theme.

Mary	saw the train leave.
The man I saw	left without a word.
subject	
theme	**rheme**

In interrogative mood clauses it is not the subject that is chosen as theme but rather a wh- word (where, when, who, etc.) or an auxiliary verb (is, were, has, do, could, etc.) that is usually chosen as theme.

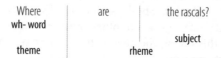

Where	are	the rascals?
wh- word		**subject**
theme	**rheme**	

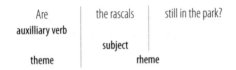

In the case of wh- questions that start with a wh- word, the theme (the wh- word) indicates that the message concerns the identity of something signalled by the wh- word (who, when, where, etc.). In the case of yes-no questions, that start with an auxiliary verb, the theme (the auxiliary verb) indicates that the polarity of positive or negative is what is at stake in the message. In summary, then, for declaratives, wh- questions and yes-no questions, the theme indicates the starting point of the message with each of these different moods having a different usual starting point: subject for declaratives ('*They* arrived'), wh-word for wh- questions ('*Who* arrived?') and auxiliary verb for yes-no questions ('*Did* they arrive?').

Focusing on the unusual: marked themes

As well as the usual starting point for a message, speakers may choose to start their message with an unusual element. In these cases, the element becomes a 'marked' theme and carries a special meaning: 'you may have thought that the message would start in some other way, but I, as speaker, have a good reason for starting the message in this unusual way'. Each different kind of message can have a marked theme:

Declarative	*Yesterday*, the backbenchers all decided to vote against the government.
Wh- question	*Around the side of the shed*, who was looking for something strange?
Yes-no question	*In spite of your misgivings*, did you really want to invite them?

The context normally determines the marked theme, since the context influences what the speaker wants to stress. For example, if the speaker wants to focus on what the backbenchers did on different days, then starting the message with 'Yesterday' ('*Yesterday*, the backbenchers all decided to vote against the government') signals that the message is centred on the time aspect of the context, rather than, perhaps, the location ('*In the Commons*, the backbenchers all decided to vote against the government') or the certainty of the statement ('*Probably*, the backbenchers all decided to vote against the government').

The following description of a task by a ten-year old keeps some themes constant from clause to clause and at other times changes the theme. The themes are in *italics*.

> Hi. *I'm* John and *I'm* telling you about the task on the computer. *This task* is very boring so *you* should come prepared. *You'll* have two letters, an X and an O and *when you see that letter pop up on the screen*, you'll have to press the button marked X or the button marked O. *If however there's a beep*, you must try to stop pressing the X or O button and press the beep button which is located on the far side of the keypad....

The first themes are mainly of the speaker ('I') or the hearer ('you') and are unmarked. The next themes that specify conditions for the rest of the message ('when you see that letter pop up on the screen', 'if however there's a beep') are marked themes. The speaker has reorganised the description from being concerned with the speaker and hearer to being concerned with what happens at different points in the task. These choices of theme then represent how the speaker wants to organise the messages in the context of neighbouring messages.

MARKED THEMES

From these examples, we see that speakers can use some marked themes to organise the message for the hearer. There is a range of meanings that marked themes can provide. Most of the following discussion pertains directly to declaratives (statements) and with certain minor changes to the other moods of interrogatives, imperatives and exclamations. Although the grammatical subject is usually the theme in declarative clauses, a complement (traditionally mainly direct or indirect objects) or adjunct may be pushed to the front of the clause and thus made the 'point of departure of the message'. In the following sentences, the complement has been made the marked theme. That is, instead of the subject and theme being the same element, they are now different, with the complement being the theme.

The sandwich,	I	fancy now.
complement	subject	
theme (marked)		rheme

The day old fish in the pantry	they	smelt.
theme (marked)		rheme

As well as a complement, an adjunct (traditionally, adverbs or phrases with prepositions) can be pushed to the front of the clause to be the theme. In the following examples, adjuncts of different kinds are pushed to the front of the clause and become marked themes. Note how the emphasis in the sentences changes compared to the unmarked versions: 'The rebirth of nature is evident in springtime'; 'They looked out the window optimistically'. The speaker has the freedom to manipulate the order of the parts of a sentence to fit the sentence into context.

In springtime,	the rebirth of nature	is evident.
adjunct	subject	
theme (marked)		rheme

Optimistically,	they	looked out of the window.
adjunct	subject	
theme (marked)		rheme

As the examples have shown, a speaker can place different kinds of information in themes. An analysis of these different kinds of information follows. A complement can be a marked theme in order to make the participant in the complement the starting point of the message. This complement can be a relatively simple nominal group ('*The sandwich*, I fancy now.') or a more elaborate structure ('*A well-organised presentation with slides, a few good jokes and a simple take-home message*, I expected'). As well as complements, adjuncts are frequently also marked themes. One category of adjuncts (conjunctive adjuncts) relates the clause to an earlier clause. A second category of adjuncts (modal adjuncts) expresses how relevant the speaker thinks the message is (Halliday, 1994: 49).

Conjunctive marked themes draw the hearer's attention to how information in two clauses is connected. This meaning then is important in evaluating how speakers develop ideas for the hearer.

There are three basic meanings available in connecting clauses: elaboration, extension and enhancement.

(1) Elaboration connects two messages by further characterising, clarifying or adding an attribute to the whole or part of the first clause (Halliday, 1994: 225). Words that express this meaning include 'that is', 'in other words', 'in any case', 'actually', as in: 'The sky is shimmering yellow. *Actually*, it looks warming and soothing to tired eyes.'   ELABORATION

(2) The second meaning is that of extension which adds something new to the first clause, worded by 'and', 'nor', 'but', 'instead', 'except', as in: 'All parties had accepted the agreement, *except* they had different interpretations of the documents.'   EXTENSION

(3) The third meaning of conjunctive marked themes (enhancement) qualifies the meaning of one clause by reference to time (as, while, when, since), place (as far as, where), manner (as if, like), cause (in order that, so that) or condition (even if, although) as in: 'He ate his supper *so that* he could go to sleep.'

These three kinds of conjunctive marked themes thus present different developments of meaning from one clause to the next.

MODAL ADJUNCTS As well as these conjunctive themes, the speaker can express opinions in a marked theme by using modal adjuncts. As mentioned, these adjuncts express how relevant the speaker thinks the message is. The expression of relevance can involve a comment on the whole proposition ('*Unfortunately*, we have not resolved the issues yet') or a signal about the time ('*Soon*, there will be no more left'), polarity ('*No*, they haven't seen the movie') or other aspect of the mood of the clause ('*Probably*, that is not the way to do it.' '*Certainly*, I'll help out.' '*In fact*, it's an ace'). The meaning expressed in the theme (the starting point of the message) can then be combined with a meaning of relating messages to each other (conjunctive adjuncts) or with the speaker's assessment of relevance (modal adjuncts). Which of these meanings are used and how frequently they are used indicate how the speaker is fitting the message into the context.

The theme-rheme structure is thus the means for signalling what is being talked about and what is said about it. At a simple but reliable level, the listener should be attuned to the beginnings of statements and other utterances. The beginnings of utterances usual signal something about the direction of the message, where it is starting and therefore where it can go. As well, the possibility of theme-marking (i.e., placing as theme some element that is usually not theme) can be used to highlight certain kinds of meaning for the hearer.

Structural devices: given and new organisation

As well as a theme-rheme structure that a speaker uses to fit language into context, there is another organisation that tailors the message to the context and to the hearer. This second textual organisation is the labelling of information as 'given' or 'new'. In clauses, there is information that the speaker can code as given or known to the hearer. This information is not necessarily known to the hearer. Rather, it is the speaker who is making an assumption that the hearer knows the information. In 'It is JOHN, who I saw coming down the stairs' (with a stress on 'John'), the speaker is assuming that the hearer knows or can pretend to know that the speaker saw someone come down the stairs. The speaker is further presenting, as new information, that it was 'John' who was coming down the stairs. The hearer may in fact know that it was John who was coming down the stairs. However, it is the speaker who is in control of how the information is presented. If the speaker has misjudged what the hearer knows, the hearer may respond with a comment such as: 'Of course I know it was John'. The distribution of information into given and new is expressed in English by word order and intonation. Since theme-rheme organisation is also expressed by word order, there will be some interaction between theme-theme organisation and given-new organisation. This interaction will be dealt with later. First, an outline of how intonation encodes the given-new distinction is given.

Intonation

The unit for expressing given and new information is the information unit. This unit consists of an obligatory new piece of information and an optional given piece of information. The new information is indicated by intonational prominence. This prominence is usually easy for hearers to detect and is produced by the pitch contour, that is, the change in direction of the pitch from low to high or high to low. The intonational prominence will be written in CAPITALS. Often, the prominence is further accentuated by a louder sound or a slower sound that makes the syllables or words easier to perceive. Each information unit has one such information prominence that marks the new information. Usually, the prominence is found at the end of the information unit, with the 'given' information coming before it. In the following example, the final word 'love' receives the intonation prominence and is marked as the new information. The information before this final word may be given or new. That is, in this case, there is indeterminacy in the boundary between given and new. The reason is that the end of the new is marked by tonic prominence but the beginning has no particular marker.

INFORMATION UNIT

All you need is   LOVE.
   given   new

To test what is given and what is new information, we can create questions to which the statement is an answer. The above statement could be an answer to the question: 'What is it that you need?' In this case, 'love' is the new information and the rest of the statement is assumed by the answerer to be known to the questioner. The statement could also be an answer to the question 'What are you telling me?' In this case, the whole statement is regarded as new information.

Having the new information fall at the end of an information unit is the typical and unmarked case. However, a speaker may choose to mark as new some piece of information other than the last one. In these cases, the intonation prominence will be again be on the new information although it is not at the end of the information unit. In the following examples, different words are given prominence and thus are signalled as new. In sentences where the information prominence is not on the usual last element, hearers interpret as 'new' just the sentence element with the intonational stress and the rest of the sentence regarded as given information.

Mary enjoyed solving	the EQUATION.
given	new

Mary enjoyed solving	THE	equation.
given	new	given

Mary enjoyed	SOLVING	the equation.
given	new	given

Mary	ENJOYED	solving the equation.
given	new	given

MARY	enjoyed solving the equation.
new	given

These sentences have identical ideational and interpersonal meanings and even have the same theme-rheme structure within the textual metafunction ('Mary' is always the theme or starting point). However, these sentences are different in terms of what is chosen as new and given information. This different distribution of given and new information would make the sentences fit into different contexts. It is rather unusual to say 'Mary solved THE equation' but the sentence is possible and appropriate when the speaker wants to mean that Mary solved the one specific, perhaps especially difficult, equation that we know about. For the sentence 'Mary ENJOYED solving the equation', the speaker is constructing a statement implying that the hearer knows that Mary solved the equation. However, with the stress on 'enjoyed', the speaker signals that the hearer does not know that Mary enjoyed the activity. Similarly, for the sentence 'MARY enjoyed solving the equation' the speaker is signalling to the hearer: 'I am assuming you know that someone enjoyed solving the equation but I want you to take note that the person was Mary since you may even think that it was someone else'. The selection of the information to be signalled as new thus involves specific assumptions about the hearer in the context.

Word order

The above examples have explored the signalling of given and new information when the theme-rheme structure was held constant; that is, the word order was kept to its typical, unmarked form. However, word order maybe varied to help realise differences in the distribution of given and new information. In the following examples, one or more elements of the sentence has been shifted to the beginning of the sentence. The element that is shifted is spoken with a separate intonation contour (indicated in written English by a comma) and is signalled as new.

They kept to their principles yesterday in the	MEETING.
given	new

YESTERDAY,	they kept to their principles in the meeting.
new	given

In the MEETING	they kept to their principles yesterday.
new	given

YESTERDAY,	in the MEETING	they kept to their principles.
new	new	given

Some of these sentences may sound rather awkward. This awkwardness is because they are rather far from the typical and unmarked uses of the given-new structure. In terms of meaning, these sentences are awkward because they are appropriate to rather special and restricted contexts. For example, the sentence 'YESTERDAY, in the MEETING, they kept to their principles' only makes sense in a context in which both the situation 'in the meeting' and the time of 'yesterday' are specifically to be brought to the attention of the hearer as new information. Thus a speaker who stresses words in unusual places in the sentence sounds odd not just in intonation but also in how the speech relates to the context. The speaker will sound less connected than expected to other speakers and to the context.

The two structural resources of theme-rheme and given-new are independent choices in the construction of a message. Theme and rheme are in terms of the starting point of the message, whereas given and new are in terms of the signalling of given and new information. Both these resources are encoded in language by structural means: theme-rheme by word order and given-new by intonation and word order. As part of the textual metafunction, these two structural resources create the texture that makes utterances fit into the verbal and non-verbal context of their use. Departures from the usual use of these resources can have the effect of disrupting the flow of the text or making the language sound out of context. Since the given-new organisation is signalled largely through intonation, any disruption in the use of intonation can have a direct effect on how the speaker seems to be presenting given and new information to the hearer. We have now outlined the structural resources of the textual metafunction. As well as these structural resources, language has a set of non-structural devices that link one piece of language to another and to the non-verbal context. These devices are collectively called cohesion.

Non-structural devices: cohesion

The grammar of language covers the structures that are assembled out of constituent elements, identifiable parts of sentences. The members of these structures are clearly related to each other by being part of the larger unit. For example, the subject of a sentence and the verb that goes with it (John eats) are part of one text by being part of the same clause. However, grammatical structures extend only as far as small clusters of dependent clauses. There are, though, links between one clause and another by non-structural links. The links that are created by cohesion are links of one clause to another, but their essence is to add meaning. These links, called cohesion, are of four types: reference, conjunction, lexis and the related pair of devices: substitution and ellipsis.

Reference

Participants in a text frequently recur as the text is developed. For example, a story about Sinbad is likely to mention Sinbad numerous times and may continue to mention relevant parts of the setting (a country, city, sea). The participants may be mentioned by using a full nominal group ('Sinbad', 'a green island with hidden treasure') or may use a device signalling that the participant was previously introduced ('he', 'it'). If the text hangs together as a whole, participants will reoccur steady as the text develops. A stretch of language with little continuity of participants or settings seems very disconnected. In the following example, there are markers of conjunction (and, so) but no continuity of the participants.

> A cat's up in a tree or a branch and a little girl's trying to tell a friend 'Go get a ladder'. So some relatives say that leaving is not possible.

Reference, then, sends signals to the hearer that the same things are being talked about. There are three basic types of reference with different kinds of meaning: personals, demonstratives and comparatives (see Table 2.15).

PERSONAL REFERENCE   Personal reference refers to a participant by specifying characteristics that help a hearer identify the participant mentioned. In English, pronouns are coded for gender (he, she, it) and for number (he, it, vs. they). These pronouns identify a participant in the verbal environment by number and gender. Demonstrative reference creates links to an earlier participant not in terms of the personal criteria of number and gender but in terms of a dimension of proximity. Demonstratives may indicate nearness ('I have never seen a machine like it.' '*This* idea is great') or remoteness ('*That* comment captures what I want to say'). The last category of reference cohesion is comparatives. Comparatives signal that the link between two participants is in terms of a similarity or difference ('The drivers started quickly – *more daring* drivers jumped ahead immediately. The *less daring* were left behind'). In each type of reference, there is an earlier participant that is presumed (or sometimes an entire concept or unit of text), a participant that is being linked back to the presumed participant and the semantic nature of the link (personal, demonstrative or comparative). Furthermore, the more often reference connects one participant to another and the longer the links are, the longer is the participant being signalled as relevant to the message. Thus texts may differ in the kind of reference that is used, what participants are linked by reference and the number and length of the links.

Type of reference	Meaning	Examples	Table 2.15
Personal	Same participant based on number and gender	Sinbad arrived. *He* was too late. The floors gleamed. *They* had been polished in the morning.	*Cohesion: reference meaning*
Demonstrative	Same participant based on proximity	I saw him immediately. *That* pilot was suspicious. You explained *those* concepts yesterday.	
Comparative	Participants are similar or different	The drivers started quickly – *more daring* drivers jumped ahead immediately. The *less daring* were left behind.	

Conjunction

As outlined in the last section, reference connects one mention of a participant to another in a text. Conjunction does not link participants but instead links clauses or other large units to each other. This type of non-structural cohesion sends a message to the hearer to 'interpret the following passage in a given way with respect to the preceding passage'. The subcategories of conjunction specify how the passages should be connected semantically. The subcategories are additive, temporal and causal (see Table 2.16). The subcategories can also be cross-categorised as linking passages within a text (internal conjunction) or linking events of the outside non-linguistic world (external conjunction). The subcategories will be outlined first and then the distinction of internal and external investigated.

Table 2.16

Cohesion: conjunction meanings

Type of conjunction	Meaning	Examples
Additive	What follows is connected to what precedes	They went into the car *and* waited for the truck to arrive.
Temporal	What follows is ordered in time to what precedes	First he inspected the tires. *Next* he checked the suspension. The rain came down in torrents. *Before that* there was thunder.
Causal	What follows is causally related to what precedes as either cause or result	They put the toys away *so* they would get a special treat. They put the toys away. *For that reason* they got a treat.

ADDITIVE
CONJUNCTION

Additive conjunction simply sends a message to the hearer that the first passage is connected to the second passage. By far the most frequent additive conjunction is 'and'. 'And' usually indicates that the speaker is connecting one stretch of language to another without any further signal of what the connection is. In the following sentences, the semantic relation between the two clauses may be clear or not. The speaker simply uses additive conjunction to indicate that the clauses should be interpreted with respect to each other: 'Just don't be ready for the beep *and* you press that button', 'You've done it already *and* maybe you can given him some help', 'They went into the car *and* they waited for the truck to arrive'. These additive links can be considered the default way of connecting information in a text. The link has limited semantic import and so is possible almost every time two clauses are linked. Young children, for example, can speak with large numbers of 'and …and …and …'.

TEMPORAL
CONJUNCTION

Temporal conjunction, on the other hand, signals that two pieces of information are linked but there is a specific kind of temporal connection between them. There is a range of temporal relations that can be encoded, including:

Following	then next	First he inspected the tires. *Next* he checked the suspension.
Preceding	before that	The rain came down in torrents. *Before that* there was thunder.
Simultaneous	at the same time	The rain came down in torrents. *At the same time* there was thunder.

These examples only illustrate a few of the many temporal relations (see Halliday, 1994: 325 and Martin, 1992: 185ff, 224ff). In all cases, it is important to stress the *relation* that is being established between two stretches of language and not merely look for a particular conjunction.

Causal conjunction, like temporal conjunction, sets up a specific semantic connection between two stretches of language. In the case of causal conjunction, the hearer is instructed to interpret the second segment of language as causally connected to the first. As with the other categories of conjunction, there are a number of different shades of meaning in the causal category, including a general meaning (so, then, therefore ...) 'They put the toys away *so* they would get a special treat' and three specific meanings: first the result (as a result ...) 'They put the toys away. *As a result* they got a treat.' Second, a specific reason (for that reason ...) 'They put the toys away. *For that reason* they got a treat.' And third, a specific purpose (for that purpose ...) 'They got a treat. *For that purpose* they had put the toys away.'

CAUSAL
CONJUNCTION

Again, the examples are not exhaustive and certain conjunctions may express more than one meaning (see Halliday, 1994: 323ff). In listening to speakers with psychiatric disorders, we must listen for unusual development of conversation by over- or under-use of these meanings expressed by conjunction. In each case, we must listen for the relation that is established between the two stretches of language and how it is realised.

As mentioned, there is a dimension of internal as opposed to external conjunction that cuts across the categories of additive, temporal and causal. External conjunctive relations signal that the hearer should connect events in the real world in a certain way. In saying '*First*, plough the field, *secondly*, plant the seeds *and finally*, harvest the crop' a speaker is using the conjunctives 'first', 'secondly', 'and finally' to signal the order in the physical world. Internal conjunctive relations, on the other hand, express relationships among stretches of language. In the following example, the conjunctives

EXTERNAL
CONJUNCTION

INTERNAL
CONJUNCTION

'first', 'secondly', 'and finally' signal how statements are sequenced rather than how events in the world are ordered:

> *First* I want to tell you, you ought to be more considerate, *secondly*, watch your language *and finally*, you should review your actions daily.

This internal-external dimension encodes the important distinction of connecting events in the real world or connecting pieces of language. In some categories of conjunction and for conjunctions, the distinction between internal and external meanings may not be clear. In these cases, the lack of clarity is itself worth noticing since it indicates that the speaker is not exploiting the possible distinction between text organisation and relations in the non-verbal 'eventful' world. It is possible and there is some evidence, that speakers with difficulty with one kind of meaning may have a lesser difficulty with the other. Conjunction, then, combines different components of meaning into a link between two stretches of language. A link may be, for example, temporal + internal or temporal + external. These links then characterise a speaker's utterances as meaning combinations that unfold as the conversation continues. Which set of meanings is used may then reflect both characteristics of the speaker and characteristics of the speech situation.

Lexical cohesion

Lexical cohesion is in some ways the weakest but most apparent link across sentences in a text. Lexical cohesion is the linking of vocabulary items one to another. By selecting vocabulary items that are connected to each other, a speaker creates a sense of a continuing text, as opposed to disjointed stretches of language (see Table 2.17). The clearest form of lexical cohesion is to repeat a vocabulary item. In the following passage, there is a repetition of the word 'pin' which contributes to the sense that the passage is one unit in context.

LEXICAL REPETITION

> Now, you got to get there... Usually five *pin* or ten *pin*. Put your fingers in the hole and try to throw down the alley to hit the *pins*.

The passage may not be completely clear, but the repetition of 'pin' helps to unify the passage in context. Sometimes the lexical item may not be repeated exactly (e.g., 'pin', 'pins') but the hearer nevertheless draws a link between the items and interprets the stretches of language as related to each other.

Type of lexical link	Meaning	Examples	Table 2.17
Repetition	Same lexical item but perhaps with different meaning	Usually five *pin* or ten *pin*. Put your fingers in the hole and try to throw down the alley to hit the *pins*.	*Cohesion: lexical meanings*
Synonyms	Some meaning is shared	It's about these two *humans* um and this old *guy* he owns a place.	
Co-occurrence	These words tend to co-occur in the same contexts	I: or did they get *arrested*? C: cause it was kinda a *sharp needle* thingy first he *shot* the boy with a *bullet* and *shoot* the other guys with a *needle* stuff	

Besides direct repetition of lexical items, synonyms also bind a text together. Synonyms share some elements of meaning but usually do not completely overlap in meaning. However, the shared elements are enough to signal that the passage has some sort of unity. Consider the following excerpt of conversation.

SYNONYMS

> I: I know it's about dinosaurs but I don't know what else it's really about
> C: it's about these two *humans* um and this old *guy* he owns a place.

The word 'guy' is presented as an approximate synonym to the word 'humans' and in contrast to 'dinosaurs'. The link between 'humans' and 'guy' helps set up the field and signal its continuity. Synonymy is not as obvious as lexical repetition and so the link may not be apparent to all speakers.

A third kind of lexical cohesion is built on the tendency of certain vocabulary items to co-occur in texts. The typical association of one content word with another can be sufficient to create a perception of textness, that the two stretches of language are part of the same text. In the following example there are a number of words from a lexical set of violence and guns that help make the language cohere.

LEXICAL CO-OCCURRENCE

> I: so he didn't *die* or anything but the *bad guys died*?
> C: mmhm
> I: or did they get *arrested*?
> C: cause it was kinda a *sharp needle* thingy first he *shot* the boy with a *bullet* and *shoot* the other guys with a *needle* stuff
> I: oh so maybe it was just a … you ever heard of a tranquillizer *gun*?

It may not be completely clear which words belong to the lexical set of violence but there are enough words that seem to fit easily to establish the textness of the passage. In fact, words that may be considered marginally related to the set may be pulled into the set (interpreted as part of the set) by the force of the clearer members of the set. Thus 'sharp' and 'needle' are less clearly part of the set with 'bad guys', 'die', 'shoot', 'bullet' and 'guns' but may be pulled into that set as the hearer interprets the passage. These clusters of vocabulary items can span several statements or turns at talk. On the other hand, shifts in the vocabulary sets may indicate that there is a shift or inconsistency in the field of discourse.

The extent and strength of lexical cohesion is hard to assess and quantify, although speakers are aware of its presence and absence. Exactly what belongs to a lexical set may depend on a speaker's knowledge of a specific field. Whether 'bug', 'install', 'launch', 'file' and 'tool' are part of the computer lexical set or more strongly associated with other lexical sets depends on a speaker's familiarity with computer software. A speaker, therefore, must construct a message taking into account how familiar the field is expected to be to the hearer and how familiar the vocabulary items are. There is no absolute, context independent construct of lexical sets. Rather, the lexical cohesion must be assessed in the context of the specific speakers and the background of the speech event.

Substitution and ellipsis

SUBSTITUTION

The fourth and last kind of cohesion, in addition to reference, conjunction and lexical cohesion, is the link set up by substitution and ellipsis. In substitution, the link is set up by using a semantically empty place marker that is interpreted in the context of some earlier more fully specified information (see Table 2.18 for meanings and examples). As the examples show, substitution involves the use of a place holder ('one', 'do' or 'so') to indicate that there is part of a grammatical unit missing. The place holder signals to the hearer that the information to fill in the full meaning is to be found elsewhere. There is then a link established between the place holder ('one', 'do', 'so') and the location of the needed information.

ELLIPSIS

Ellipsis is very similar to substitution in how it links stretches of text to each other. The difference is that in ellipsis there is no place holder at all for the information that is being linked to (see Table 2.18). As with substitution, ellipsis sets up a link across two stretches of language by making information from the first stretch of language necessary for interpretation of the second stretch. Although the link is one of meaning, the signal involves the omission of some part of the structure in the second stretch of language.

Type of link	Meaning	Examples
Substitution-nominal	Same participant	Here are some pens. I want the yellow *one*. *One* substitutes for 'pens'
Substitution-verbal	Same process	Will you eat already? Have done. *Done* substitutes for 'eat'
Substitution-clausal	Same entire clause	They think that all politicians should be rounded up and fired every three years. I think *so*. *So* substitutes for 'that all politicians should be rounded up and fired every three years'
Ellipsis-nominal	Same participant	Here are some pens. I want the yellow __. The noun 'pen' has been omitted
Ellipsis-verbal	Same process	Who is leaving? I am __. The verb 'leaving' has been omitted
Ellipsis-clausal	Same entire clause	Are you thinking of signing the documents? No __. The clause 'I am not thinking of signing the documents' has been omitted

Table 2.18

Cohesion: substitution and ellipsis

Both substitution and ellipsis are used frequently in conversation to link the speech of different speakers. In interaction, ellipsis and substitution signal that one speaker is assuming some information said by the other speaker. At this interface between two speakers, making assumptions about the other speaker's information state and linking to the other speaker's language helps mesh the meanings of one speaker with the meanings of the other speaker. In clinical and real world contexts, speakers who do not adequately use substitution and ellipsis to connect to other speakers will sound too independent of other speakers and too disconnected from the interaction.

Cohesion, in summary, is a set of non-structural devices that link one part of a text to another. These links are typically and most effective across sentences and clauses and thus have the power to link through considerable distances in the text. Cohesion, in fact, creates text, or in other words, a sense of functional unity, in rather long stretches of language. Cohesion is comprised of reference that links participants in a text, conjunction that links clauses and other larger units, lexical cohesion that sets up continuity of field (the institutional focus of what is being talked about) and substitution and ellipsis that copy meanings from one stretch of language to another. In general, the meaning of all these forms of cohesion is that the meaning of one part of the text is related to the meanings of another part of the text.

Cohesion and the structural parts of the textual metafunction (the organisation of clauses into theme-rheme and given-new) provide the devices that fit language into the verbal and non-verbal context of the speech event. The textual metafunction itself contributes the meaning of 'This is how the speaker sees his or her contribution fitting into the context'. This perspective of the speaker on the context is conveyed in every utterance along with aspects of ideational and interpersonal meanings.

2.3   Combining different kinds of meaning into a message

The ideational, interpersonal and textual metafunctions are collections of different meanings. Language, though, must express these meaning simultaneously through the vocabulary and grammar. Although each of the metafunctions tends to be expressed by specific parts of the vocabulary and grammar (e.g., interpersonal metafunction through the mood of the clause), a speaker constructs an utterance using all the metafunctions simultaneously. The choice of a verb simultaneously involves the ideational metafunction (what kind of process is involved, mental, material, etc.), the interpersonal metafunction (the verb's place in forming a question or a statement) and the textual metafunction (the possible cohesion of the verb to an earlier use of the verb or another similar verb). From the point of view of the speaker, then, meanings from the three metafunctions may be independent but the meanings are expressed simultaneously in each utterance. Certain combinations of choices from the three metafunctions express the more abstract notions in language such as register or genre. For example, the combination of yes-no questions or wh- questions (from the interpersonal metafunction), mental process verb (from the ideational metafunction) and reference to the external world (from the textual metafunction) can help to produce a certain kind of 'hospital' talk used by health care workers to patients: 'Would we like to do that now?' 'Would we like to sit down for a moment?' 'When would we like to go for a walk?'

Just as a speaker's utterances involve a combination of choices of meaning from the three metafunctions, so there may be problems or atypicalities in meaning stemming from any one metafunction. There are speakers who seem to be in touch with the interlocutor in terms of taking turns, forms of address and politeness (appropriate meanings from the interpersonal metafunction), but be difficult to follow because of infelicities in using pronouns to refer to things mentioned earlier in the conversation (problems of cohesion from the textual metafunction). At a lower level of analysis, there may be problems in one area of a metafunction but not in another. For example, there may be speakers who use conjunction appropriately to join clauses together but do not properly use another area of cohesion within the textual metafunction (pronouns to refer to things mentioned earlier, for example).

The location of atypicalities within language specifies what kinds of meaning making are at risk and what kinds of meaning making are reasonably typical in a speaker's utterances or for given disorders. There may be unusual uses of language from one or more language systems.

Individual speakers and disorders as a whole may follow the linguistic organisation of language and have problems in communication that match metafunctions or parts of metafunctions. On the other hand, a range of disturbances in meaning can co-occur that does not simply map onto how language is organised. These issues of the mapping of language onto disorders and onto diagnostic criteria are explored in Chapters 4 to 9.

2.4   Using the ideational, interpersonal and textual metafunctions in context

In using the metafunctions in context we must consider how the language is built up and sequenced in interaction. The first points have to do with the interactive and dynamic creation of conversation. A second set of points has to do with how meanings are worded. Since language is interactive and dynamic, it must be constructed in real time in relation to what the interlocutor is saying. As each contribution from the speaker or interlocutor is made, the context for the next contribution is changed. The speaker must continually up-date the record of the conversation and the immediate and more long term plans for what is to be achieved in the interaction. A change in any of the ideational, interpersonal and textual meanings can significantly alter the path of the conversation. If a speaker has ignored one of these changes, then the conversation may start sounding odd to others.

DYNAMIC CONSTRUCTION OF INTERACTION

The dynamic co-construction of the interaction by speaker and interlocutor is what is assumed by speakers in the speech community to be the standard. If there is verbal evidence that a speaker is not treating seriously the interlocutor's contributions to the conversation, then the speaker may be judged to have difficulties in either continually adjusting to the context (a dynamic on-line task) or fitting in utterances to be relevant (a cooperative co-construction task).

The construction of verbal interaction dynamically and with respect to the specific contribution of the interlocutor is also a tightly time-limited activity. Talking is an 'on-line' activity even though we tend to freeze and come back to pieces of conversation for analysis. The linguistic processing both for comprehension and production must be done within a very few seconds or parts of seconds.

As discussed earlier in this chapter, the use of language is always in terms of the expectations of others in the speech community. These expectations are built up by repeated patterns of use. An unusual pattern in the density of certain linguistic features (from the use of imperatives to the use of fixed sayings) will be reacted to as odd with the speaker judged and interacted with accordingly. To look at the build up of meanings in a slightly different way, the sequencing of different meanings from various metafunctions may itself be unusual. That is, there is a question of how often a specific linguistic pattern is used and another question of which linguistic devices are used one after another in sequence. See Chapter 10 for a discussion of this point.

In the construction of interaction on-line, the contributions must be timed appropriately. Thus, the clinical listener must consider pauses, hesitations and repetitions in the flow of speech for their effect on the interaction. If these phenomena are found in specific interpersonal or ideational contexts, then the lack of fluency for those particular meanings should be accounted for.

The use of the metafunctions in context involves not only questions of the interactive and dynamic creation of conversation but also involves questions of how the vocabulary and grammar express the ideational, interpersonal and textual meanings. As has been outlined, there is often a basic meaning that can be expressed in different ways. If a speaker uses atypical wordings, then the extra emphasis or change in meaning produced by these atypical wordings is itself part of the message. For example, if a speaker requests goods and services by the grammatical device of an exclamation (e.g., 'Crowded in here!' 'What a smell!'), then the meaning of using exclamations instead of perhaps statements ('It is crowded in here.' 'The garbage smells') or imperatives ('Leave!' 'Close the garbage can!') is added to the straightforward ideational meaning. In fact, the possibility of using a variety of ways to encode ideational meaning opens up the range of meanings we can use as speakers. Each wording somewhat adjusts the message. Some of these meanings will seem rather unusual and may be making specific points in the context (as in Winston Churchill's famous comment of 'Up with which I will not put' to indicate that avoiding a preposition at the end of a sentence can itself be odd). Such special meanings may be entirely appropriate and effective in the particular context and are achieved by deliberately using unusual or 'marked' wordings. There is thus a tension between using typical meanings and their wordings and the more atypical ones that set up special meanings by being unexpected and unusual.

'WORDING' OF MEANING

Chapter 3 contents

Chapter 3

Meaning oddly: how a speaker can sound strange

The structures of language and the patterns of meaning   3.1

Psychiatric disorders are manifested in verbal and non-verbal behaviours in many different ways. In Chapter 2 we explored how speakers may sound unusual in terms of the many kinds of meanings and wordings. This chapter starts with the different kinds of meanings and outlines how disruptions in each kind of meaning sound clinically. Succeeding chapters map specific atypicalities of meaning and wording onto disorders and diagnostic criteria.

Each kind of meaning, from culture, through the ideational, interpersonal and textual metafunctions and down to how the language words the meanings, is responsible for the atypical verbal behaviour of speakers with psychiatric disorders. In fact, the locus of the atypicality, is it ideational or interpersonal, for example, accounts for both how the speaker fails to achieve social purposes and the specific impression the speaker makes. Speakers representing different diagnostic categories and different diagnostic criteria may sound similar in some respects. It is often the cluster of diagnostic features that suggests a disorder. This clustering can be thought of more holistically as a gestalt or more molecularly as a set of specific characteristics. From the point of view of language, specific language features may typify a disorder, or there may be a number of features that together create the impression of the disorder. Furthermore, certain linguistic features – for example, speaking too quickly and pressure of speech – are found in a number of disorders. The first step in understanding this complex relationship between language

LOCUS OF
TYPICALITIES

features and psychiatric categories is to consider the phenomenological effect of linguistic atypicalities. Each of these linguistic features usually expresses specific meaning. It is these hearable parts of language that then become useful in identifying diagnostic criteria and disorders.

The purpose of this chapter is to show the effect of atypicalities in meaning and the process of meaning-making. The issue is what different meanings can be created and how others notice and react to those meanings. The chapter is organised according to the ways of expressing meaning outlined in the previous chapter. Where possible, actual examples of speech are used to illustrate the atypicalities. Some of the examples have been edited to eliminate irrelevant and distracting features found in the original. The discussion and examples are restricted to the major categories of linguistic meanings and wordings since complete coverage would require many hundreds of pages of examples and discussion. Fortunately, speakers of a language have a firm intuitive sense of changes in meaning. The task here is to outline how those atypical meanings are worded and how wording is a clue to the meanings at stake. In clinical listening, it is the meanings that are usually noticed and that are found in the diagnostic descriptions. It is then necessary to match the atypical meanings with the disorders. Listening for the specific wordings sharpens the process and makes it more objective.

Messages are created by a combination of a large number of linguistic features, drawn from the ideational, interpersonal and textual metafunctions. Any particular feature may be used in an atypical way (too many or too few pronouns or adjectives or concrete words). That is, the meaning making resource may itself be used atypically. However, in many cases, there are atypicalities scattered through various areas of language. This *pattern* of atypicalities may in fact be what characterises a speaker or a disorder. The following presentation of one atypicality at a time is intended to elucidate how language is constructed to convey meaning. That is, this chapter presents the typicalities one by one which is simpler than how individuals and disorders are found in reality.

The following chapters, which deal with disorders, view the language of disorders in a more complex way by focusing on the disorder and examining the linguistic patterns associated with them. By starting with the disorders and their diagnostic criteria, the clinical entity is preserved and the various patterns of language associated with it can be described. To understand the more detailed diagnostic criteria and features, the linguistic description starts from this clinical level. This approach then is flexible in terms of understanding both higher-level categories of disorders and lower level categories of diagnostic criteria. Such flexibility is important since disorders are reconceptualised from time to time. Although the symptoms, features and relationships among disorders change, the phenomenology remains more constant. The close study of language contributes to understanding this phenomenology.

Messages are created by a combination of linguistic means but there is also the question of how striking or unusual the atypicalities are. There are some atypicalities that immediately grab a hearer's attention and create a noticeable utterance. An ambiguous remark such as 'My father and grandfather both like basketball. He is tall' is noticed at once. Other atypicalities may not be noticeable immediately but their effect may be experienced over time. For example, continually addressing the interlocutor by first name instead of sometimes by the pronoun 'you' may not be typical and will eventually be noticed as an unusual orientation or flavour, but the use of the name will not directly draw attention and is not hard for hearers to follow. Usually the patterning in language is complex but unobtrusive. When the patterning becomes obtrusive, we notice that unusual meanings are present or perhaps that the meanings are difficult to extract or follow.

The examples presented in this chapter tend to have noticeable departures from the typical. These examples demonstrate the phenomena. However, it must be pointed out that in the effort to present clear examples of phenomena some of the examples may be more extreme than those found clinically. The different levels of analysis for language are now presented from the most abstract 'culture' to the details of each metafunction. These are the atypicalities that are potentially involved in psychiatric disorders. Each level of analysis creates different kinds of noticeable failures to accomplish social processes. Correspondingly, there are different kinds of examples for each level of analysis.

Culture and genre   3.2

3.2.1   Differences across cultures

Cultures differ in that they create different standard patterns of interaction and define different purposes for interaction. These different purposes and patterns are then reflected in the genres. To recall, genres are staged, goal-oriented social processes. There are two kinds of analysis that are important. On the one hand, different cultures may be associated with different genres. Differences in religious customs are a clear example. On the other hand, a single culture may be associated with two or more related genres that a

GENRES

speaker may not fully appreciate. For example, there are some kinds of stores and services where negotiating over price is typical and even expected and another kind where an attempt to negotiate is regarded as impudent, cheeky and completely out of place.

An example of the variation from one culture to another is how speakers greet each other and hold a casual conversation. Fine and Knizhnik (1993) outlined the differences among greetings in Russian, Hebrew and English speakers. All speakers would ask questions such as 'How are you?' or 'What's new?' However, for the Russian speakers, these questions were treated as serious inquiries that required extended and truthful answers, whereas for the English and Hebrew speakers such questions were meant and taken as routine and would be answered in a word or two 'Fine', 'Good', 'As usual'. For the Russian speakers, such short answers would be interpreted as unfriendliness or avoidance. From the other perspective, a long answer to 'How are you?' in English or Hebrew would be interpreted as meaning that things really were not normal and that the speaker wanted to explain the unusual personal situation. In this example, the different cultures are associated with slightly different genres with slightly different components. The Russian speakers expected rather full answers about well-being in even casual interactions whereas the English and Hebrew speakers regarded such interactions as requiring only the most perfunctory of information. The beginnings of a casual conversation in the different cultures are then distinct and in terms of genre are slightly different staged social processes. If a speaker does not follow the cultural pattern for whatever reason, including mood, personality disorder, psychosis, reality testing, then this cultural misalignment results.

The cross-cultural differences in genre would only be evident in disorders if a speaker from one culture is assessed or treated in another culture. The forms of such differences in culture can be as striking as the use or removal of spells or curses and the genres that are associated with them. More subtly, there can be the use of parallel genres but different components, as in the example of greeting patterns.

3.2.2   Differences across genres

A second issue involved with the distinguishing of genres is not cross-cultural but, rather, the identification of two genres within the same culture. Sometimes, a speaker may not be clear which of a number of genres is appropriate to a certain situation. In this sense, genre is similar to scripts for action. Restaurants provide ample examples. In one case, a family was sitting at a restaurant in a small village. After waiting a few minutes, they started to look around for a waiter to bring menus and take the order. No one appeared. After yet a few more minutes, one of the adults went looking for help. It was then that an employee appeared and said that the restaurant offered a buffet and that the family should take plates and help themselves. In another restaurant, in a large city's business district, customers are met by an employee who asks whether the customer has eaten in the restaurant before and if they know 'how it works here'. If the customer is new, there is an explanation of how food is paid for by weight and how certain items are included in the price of the meal without being weighed. In this second restaurant example, there is an explicit awareness that the genre is unusual and an explicit explanation of the distinctive stages in the social process of getting and paying for a meal. In both restaurant examples, individuals must identify the genre in order to act verbally and non-verbally to achieve the social objectives.

Speakers who have not, or are perhaps unable to, clearly identify genres and their place within a culture have difficulty understanding the language about them and acting so that they will be interpreted according to the patterns in the culture. If an individual chooses to pray in a therapy session, then the clinician must try to understand the source of the apparent difference in cultural expectations. Is it that the individual does not know the social processes of the therapy session? Is the individual finding a way to ignore the social processes? Is the individual involved in an obsessive behaviour that occurs in other, non-clinical, contexts where praying is also atypical for the culture? (I am indebted to Dr. R. Schachar for this example.)

As mentioned earlier, the most direct examples of difficulties in genre come from cases when a speaker is interacting within a foreign culture. Other reasonably clear examples come from situations in which speakers are likely not to know the genre and some sort of explicit 'orientation' takes place. New employees and new students often are presented with such orientations to an institution and thus to the new social processes involved. For example, an employee may be told (or gently given a suggestion) where to sit in a cafeteria, who knows answers to many simple questions, how different individuals are to be addressed (first name, last name, title) and so on. Some patients with psychiatric disorders may sound as if they are new to a culture or out of place simply because their messages do not follow cultural patterns while still following the other language patterns, such as grammar and vocabulary.

3.3   Situation

3.3.1 Language and physical context

Interactions take place in specific settings that include both relevant and irrelevant physical facts. Speakers must relate to these two kinds of facts by behaving typically and with appropriate variation for the speech community. For example, there are typical comments that are acceptable about a friend's appearance or a stranger's appearance. Compliments such as 'You look great today' or 'Is that a new X you are wearing?' have a wide range of acceptability. However, critical comments are much more restricted and are tied more closely to the relationship between the speakers. Remarks such as 'That haircut is awful', 'Isn't that shirt rather outdated now?' would not be expected between strangers. Said to a stranger, these comments indicate a misinterpretation of the situation. The speaker perhaps does not understand the social relationship of the speakers as being that of strangers or perhaps does not know what is appropriate between strangers. As well as directly commenting on elements of the situation, a speaker may not fit into the situation by talking about something usually regarded as irrelevant. Continued talk about a person's shoes or the colour of the walls may be beyond the limits of the speech community and the speaker will be heard as interacting oddly. Clinically, such talk may be interpreted as a preoccupation with certain objects or as distraction by irrelevant stimuli.

SITUATION

Language is itself part of the situation and so a speaker must react appropriately to what is said. Speakers who 'turn language in on itself' are at risk for expressing unusual meanings. For example, a speaker that attends to the phonological characteristics of language may use 'clang associations' ('They were in the room, zoom, vroom, womb') instead of the more usual semantic and syntactic ways of building utterances. Comments about language may also lead the speaker to create unusual meaning. For example, comments such as 'I always talk too much about my mother', 'They are always giving me orders', 'Why are you yelling at me?' can be entirely appropriate to the situation, or if too frequent or too densely packed, can indicate an inappropriate intrusion of talk about language.

3.3.2 Situation and genre: the language of social processes

The concepts of situation and genre (the latter specifically reflecting the social processes) interact and this interaction itself can be a source of difficulty in communicating. Speakers must be able to fit a genre into the appropriate situation. In other words, speakers must know which genres (language that creates the social process) they should use in which situations. One kind of atypicality is the insertion of one genre into a situation where it is generally not found. A subject was retelling a story as part of a neuropsychological test as follows: 'On December sixth, one week ago, ten miles from Albany, six hundred people drowned… no six hundred people caught colds and one person drowned, a man hurt his hand while saving a boy'. Until this point, the speaker is telling the story as he was instructed to. There is then an unsignalled switch into a different social process, an explanation of his performance: 'In a multiple choice sheet, I would have done quite well in a multiple choice'. Of course, such a switch in genre is not 'bad' or inappropriate in itself. The effect of the switch must be judged in terms of what is expected and how often the switch occurs. As it happens, this speaker introduced a similar switch in genre moments later after telling the story again: 'This story took place (the speaker tells the story and finishes with) they were wet, made wet by the high flood water which damaged the property'. Immediately after this statement, the speaker says: 'How is that? I, I about listen last time. Isn't that a real paradox? It's a bit like doing a mid term test and doing a final exam'. After a few follow-up questions to see if the speaker can remember more, he says 'That's all I can remember. I got a B on that. That one question'. Other speakers may insert a narrative within a dialogue or attempt to negotiate the purchase of an article of clothing in the midst of a casual conversation. What is problematic is the switch in genre, particularly when such switches are not typical in the situation. Unusual switches in genre can be made more acceptable by explicitly signalling them to the hearer. Phrases such as, 'and now I want to tell you about…' or 'wait a second I'll tell you about it…' explicitly indicate that the genre is about to change unexpectedly.

The phenomenon of a genre being atypically associated with a situation, or there being unusual shifts in genre with a situation, may relate to a number of underlying difficulties. It may be that the speaker does not appreciate how genres are associated with the situation, that the speaker has not fully analysed and identified the situation, or that the speaker does not know that what he or she said in fact expressed the inappropriate genre. Therefore, a speaker with cognitive or emotional problems affecting the learning of social processes, the apprehension of situations, or the mapping of language onto context can be expected to create atypical language involving genre.

INSERTING A GENRE

3.4   Register

Register meanings are related to the three contextual variables of field (institutional focus), tenor (social roles of speakers) and mode (role of language, channel of communication). Each of these meanings and their atypicalities are dealt with in turn and are summarised in Table 3.1.

Table 3.1
The meanings
at stake in register

Contextual variable	Kind of meaning	Atypical meanings
Field	Institutional focus 'what we talk about'	Shifting from topic to topic
Tenor	Social roles 'what is my role, what is your role' levels of formality personal solidarity friendliness goal of interaction	Inappropriate role for the speaker in the context ('I'm the judge') Shifting from one role to another
Mode	Role of language, channel of communication monologue – dialogue spontaneous – rehearsed spoken – written	Sounds like wrong channel of communication

3.4.1 Field: what we talk about

The institutional focus (the field) is largely expressed by the use of vocabulary from given sets of words. Atypicalities may include the unexpected shifting of word sets or remaining unduly in a set. The shifting of vocabulary is heard as the jumping from topic to topic. As with genre shifts, if these jumps are appropriately signalled then the speaker will not sound as disjointed as when the shifts are not signalled. Consider the following answer to the question 'Do you know any phonies?':

> No. I don't know any phonies. There's a Kincaid (name of a doctor from a television programme). He's on the loose and ah I don't think he's a phoney. He may have an operation or a factory or something. And I gotta go down and see what the college is up to too if the college wants to turn a tube on

themselves so we can see them I don't mind but ah I'm not camera shy you
know. Okay so anyways getting on the basic subject of the pill that they took
back then in was back in 1959 and ah we don't know who the ones that were
ordered to take the pills and who were the ones that haven't taken the pills.

The answer repeats a vocabulary item from the questioner ('phonies'), but
the speaker then adds the following content words: 'operation', 'factory',
'college', 'college', 'turn', 'tube', 'see', 'mind', 'camera', 'shy', 'subject', 'pill', 'took',
'know', 'ordered', 'pills', 'pills'. Within this list, 'operation' and 'factory' may
be related in terms of manufacturing, the repetition of 'college' starts to
establish an educational field and the more extensive word set of 'Kincaid',
'operation', 'pill', 'took', 'know', 'ordered', 'pills', 'pills' sets up a medical field.
The speaker shifts from one field to another without signalling the change.
At one point, 'getting on the basic subject of the pill', the speaker seems to
signal a change of field, but even here there seems insufficient warning of the
change. A comment such as 'Phonies may be phonies but I really want to tell
you about the pill they took…' would signal more clearly the change in field
for the hearer. As with all cases of interpretation, hearers may understand
word sets in different ways due to different backgrounds or outlooks. For
example, some hearers may consider that 'Kincaid' is an instance of a phoney
doctor and may associate 'factory' with 'college' or medical schools.

3.4.2   Tenor: who is speaking to whom

Register includes tenor as well as field. As field reflects the institutional
focus of the language, so tenor is a parameter in language that reflects the
social roles of speakers in interaction. Issues of formality, personal solidarity,
friendliness and the functional roles in a social process are included in tenor.
The following example illustrates a shift from a more personal tenor in which
the speakers regard each other as equals to a more formal tenor reflecting
the socially defined roles of patient (P) and clinician as interviewer (I).

1   P: do you mind if I smoke?

2   I: nope please go ahead. I smoke too these days

3   P: oh good it's a bad habit eh?

4   I: yes it is I can't shake it

5   P: I've been trying to quit you know and ummm it's ver ummm.. It's a
        very difficult thing to do. I've come down off drugs and ah.. you know
        and this is worse like I got very nauseated and. irritated like I just, you

know, I just thought I'm going to go absolutely mad you know when I when I tried quitting for three days eh I said no way I couldn't, you know, I had to smoke again. like you know

6   I: right

7   P: I just couldn't uh

8   I: those are bad days at the beginning

9   P: yea they're supposed to be if you can last seven days

10   I: right

11   P: but ah

12   I: well I quit for long periods of time but ah I seem to start again

13   P: are you a psychiatrist?

14   I: yes I am and Mrs. D is a psychologist who does the tests you have been off medication now for a while is that right?

15   P: no I still take medication

16   I: you are still taking medication?

17   P: yea I still well not I don't take it like as often as I should you know but I mean I. You know cause it like it you know I'm trying to get back to the ah working force again you know sorta like I've been dealing with the hospital and that like I've been in and out of there, mostly in there, since 19XX I believe or something like that you see. And I'm on a disability pension.

There are a number of analyses that show the personal and functional tenors of this interaction. The informal personal tenor of the beginning of the interaction is produced in part by the questions that the patient asks of the interviewer (utterances 1, 3, 13) and the words expressing emotion or personal judgement ('bad habit', 'worse', 'irritated', 'absolutely mad', 'no way'). The interviewer helps construct this informal tenor by not asking questions and by talking about himself ('I smoke too these days', 'I can't shake it', 'I quit for long periods of time but ah I seem to start again'). The more formal personal tenor starts at line 13 and is initiated by the patient's question 'Are you a psychiatrist?' The question itself directs attention to the institutionalised, formal roles of the situation. From this point on, the patient does not ask questions and the interviewer does ('You have been off medication now for a while is that right?' 'You are still taking medication?'), the patient does not express emotions and the interviewer does not speak about himself (except to acknowledge his social role 'Yes I am [a psychiatrist]'). Instead of speaking of emotions, the patient speaks of aspects of the institutions that define his role ('work force', 'hospital', 'disability pension'). The personal tenor that changes from relatively informal to relatively formal is expressed by the selection of vocabulary and the kinds of speech functions both speakers use.

The purposes of an interaction are reflected in the functional tenor. In this example, the functional tenor also changes, from discussing a mutual interest in smoking (utterances 1 to 12) to defining elements of the medical setting (utterances 13 to 17). There is clearly a correlation in the change in personal tenor (in terms of formality) and the change in functional tenor (in terms of purpose). In closing, it should be emphasised that conversation is jointly negotiated and that both speakers help to construct the tenor of the conversation, negotiating and accepting the roles each takes.

3.4.3   Mode: what channel of communication

The third contextual variable that contributes meaning related to the situation is mode. Mode is the role that language itself plays in the situation. Speakers who sound as if they are monologuing instead of engaging in conversation or speakers who sound as if they are reading prepared speeches instead of spontaneously interacting are using of an atypical mode of communication. In the following example (from Fine, 1994: 70), the patient's language sounds stilted and inappropriate due to the mode. We will now examine how this mode was created.

STILTED LANGUAGE

1   P: at the age of seven my mother by that time had remarried and we moved into a house with my adopted father and ever since then I've been trying my best to get on the so to speak usual track

2   I: yes well you seem to be ah fine person in what way do you feel you're not on the usual track?

3   P: well… it's a bit that's somewhat of a difficult question to ask.. One I suppose is never quite sure whether or not he has caught up to a so-called normal person in every respect

4   I: um hmm

5   P: cause very hard to examine the so-called normal person just exactly is normal no one can really say

6   I: right very true

7   P: it might be a state of mind it might just be a minor deviation which really doesn't make any difference

The speaker comments on the text, here and in other parts of his conversation. In utterance 1, he says 'so to speak', in utterance 3 'that's somewhat of a difficult question to answer', 'so called' and 'I suppose'. These are all com-

COMMENTING ON TEXT

ments on the language of the text or how the speaker is regarding the text. As well as directly commenting on the text, the speaker frequently hedges his comments giving the impression that the language is carefully prepared as if for a speech or written document that will be judged. The markings of this hedging include, in utterance 3: 'somewhat', 'I suppose', 'quite sure', 'every respect'; in utterance 5: 'very hard', 'exactly', 'really say'; and in utterance 7: 'might be', 'might just be', 'minor', 'really'. Although all these expressions are quite possible and useful in conversation, it is the density of them that makes the utterances sound like they are from a different kind of situation.

The variables of field, tenor and mode are sets of meanings that relate language to the situation. If there is some atypicality in these variables, it is not just a statistical property of the language, but will be heard as the speaker conveying atypical meanings for the particular situation – sounding out of place (see again Table 3.1). As some of the examples indicate, there can be a correlation among the atypical meanings in field, mode and tenor. That is, atypical meanings from one contextual variable may be associated with atypical meanings from another contextual variable. In these cases, then, the atypicality of meaning is reinforced.

3.5   Ideational metafunction

The ideational metafunction carries much of the meaning of the speaker's experience of the external world. As outlined, the basic meanings are those of things, events and circumstances. These meanings are then expressed through the choice of vocabulary and grammatical structures (the lexico-grammar). Difficulties or atypicalities in the ideational metafunction are then heard as atypicalities in what the speaker is saying about the world (see Table 3.2). Of course, an atypicality in this kind of meaning relates to the physical setting of the speech. There is not an absolute notion of making sense, but, rather, the issue is how much sense a speaker is making in a specific context.

Basic category	Kind of meaning	Atypical meanings (unusual concentration, unusual shifting)
Participant	People and objects	Unusual participants e.g. first person I, me Avoidance of certain participants Inconsistent set of participants
Process	Happenings and relations (mental, material, relational)	Concentrations, avoidance or shifting of meanings of doing, thinking, saying, classifying, identifying etc.
Circumstance	Details of happenings (extent, location, manner, cause etc.)	Unusual circumstances used Unusual concentration of given circumstances Amount of detail (too little or too much) in each circumstance

Table 3.2

The meanings at stake in the ideational metafunction

To understand the atypicalities in the ideational metafunction, we must consider the situation of the speech. In general, there are two ways that the ideational metafunction may stand out as being atypical. Firstly, there may be an unusual concentration of certain meanings. If, for example, a speaker is very concerned about a cat, parent, insect or the ozone layer, then mention of that thing will be made more frequently than expected in the speech community for given situations. Of course, there are situations in which the same frequency may be unnoticed or for which such a frequency is unusually low. Listeners naturally assess atypicality based on experience with language in the speech community. The concentration of specific ideational content is difficult to exemplify and quantitatively measure. However, members of the speech community usually notice the typical and atypical patterns of ideational meaning in specific situations.

CONCENTRATION OF MEANING

A second way that atypicalities in the ideational metafunction may stand out is by atypical switching or shifting. For example, in describing colour chips as part of a neuropsychological test, a speaker says:

> This colour is orange the colour of an orange sucker and I used to get on
> a train going to Niagara Niagara Falls on a company picnic it cost me only
> seventy cents that was in 1958 but that used to be great to Niagara Falls we
> slowly walked step by step and down the plummeting falls… with the water
> eddying and making a recession into the Dory Canyon below.. 161 feet below.'

The interviewer requested 'now describe for me that colour' while pointing to a coloured circle. The speaker starts with ideation about the task by mentioning the thing 'colour' and an exemplar of colour, 'orange'. However, there is an abrupt and unsignalled shift to usually unrelated things: 'train', 'Niagara Falls', 'picnic', 'company', 'seventy cents', 'Niagara Falls', 'we', 'falls', 'the water', 'recession', 'Dory Canyon'. Such a shift would be more typical and easier to follow if there were a signal such as 'and that colour reminds me of' or 'but what I really want to tell you about is'. Even the unsignalled shift in ideational metafunction may not be too unusual if it occurs rarely in a speaker's talk. However, repeated shifts characterise a difference between the speaker and other members of the speech community. For example, the same speaker when describing another colour chip said:

> That colour indicates amber which is caution.. caution for.. proceed with
> caution when you go through an intersection especially without so
> you won't get a ticket from the.. in August 1972 from a culvert sniper an
> unmarked police car and it just means drive carefully or stop if you can but if
> not proceed with caution.

The next chip in the sequence was described as:

> This colour is blue the colour of the swirling sea with a magnificent clear day
> and colour blue of blonds…. of beauty of Minerva the goddess of war not
> the goddess of war the goddess of of of fish and the goddess of womanhood
> of beauty of a blond like a Scandinavian blond who I'd like to have a
> proposition thirteen with.

There is thus a repeated pattern of unsignalled shifts in the ideational metafunction created by changes in the people and objects mentioned.

One way to make shifting more acceptable for most situations is to overtly signal the change in the ideational metafunction. If a speaker is describing a family event, it may sound awkward to start talking about the latest government actions or volcanic eruptions on the other side of the world. However, if the speaker can make the relation between the topics explicit and show that one is relevant to the other, then the discourse is easier to follow. As with most analyses, we must be careful not to lose sight of the higher levels of culture and genre. Cultures may differ in terms of what is clearly relevant and therefore they differ in terms of what topic seems to be connected to what other topic, even without special signalling. In some cultures, it may seem quite unremarkable to slide from a conversation about the weather into a conversation about the availability of daycare; whereas in other cultures, the weather is not a neutral topic that can easily precede any other. In this second culture, the transition from the substantive topic of weather to another substantive topic needs specific signalling. In the first mentioned culture, the sliding away from conversation about weather merely indicates that the 'real' issue at hand is beginning.

3.5.1 Participants: people and objects talked about

First person: the speaker in the situation

'Participants' in discourse are the words used for the objects of the speaker's experience. The kinds of participants are: actor, goal, senser, phenomenon, behaver, sayer, receiver verbiage and target. These are the kinds of people and objects expressed. (See Chapter 2 for the definitions and details of these subcategories.) If there is a concentration or switching of these participants in an atypical way, then we hear the messages as unusual or perhaps dysfunctional. For example, if a speaker continually speaks of himself or herself as the actor in a certain situation, then we hear the speaker as self-centred, preoccupied with the self or unable to take the perspective of others. In the following passage from a clinical interview, the speaker is mainly speaking about herself and starts several sentences with 'I' (the subjects of sentences are in *italics* with 'I' subjects in ***bold italics***).

> S: *We* had been here then for eight years so *I* took the three children and we went back and we spent two years there and *I* couldn't wait to get back again *there* were so many things *I* missed about Canada
>
> I: That's interesting what did you miss?
>
> S: *I* think *the biggest thing* was the size of everything ah *Canada* seems to be a big country even the things *you* buy in the supermarket are big like the boxes of washing powder *everything* is big
>
> I: Yea
>
> S: And then *you* go back to England and *you* feel diminished somehow

because *it's* much smaller and *it's* slower *it* took a bit of time sort of trying to get myself back into it all *I* could think of doing was saving up and coming back again but *I've* never regretted it and in a way perhaps because you know *the children* had a bit of a rocky road there for a while.

However, if this conversation is altered to introduce more uses if 'I' as the subject of sentences (retaining as far as possible other characteristics of meaning and structure), an impression of being self-centred and perhaps domineering in the conversation is created:

S: *I* had been here then for eight years so *I* took the three children and *I* went back and *I* spent two years there and *I* couldn't wait to get back again *I* missed so many things about Canada'

I: That's interesting what did you miss?

S: *I* think *the biggest thing* was the size of everything ah *Canada* seems to be a big country even the things *I* buy in the supermarket are big like the boxes of washing powder *everything* is big'

I: Yea

S: And then *I* go back to England and *I* feel diminished somehow because *it's* much smaller and *it's* slower *I* took a bit of time sort of trying to get myself back into it all *I* could think of doing was saving up and coming back again but *I've* never regretted it and in a way perhaps because you know **me** *and the children* had a bit of a rocky road there for a while.

This segment of conversation can also be altered to include more verbiage ('what is said', *in italics*) as a participant, again with changing other elements as little as possible.

S: I told you *that we had been here then for eight years* so I took the three children and we went back and we spent two years there and I said *that I couldn't wait to get back again* there were so many things I missed about Canada

I: That's interesting what did you miss?

S: I used to say *that the biggest thing was the size of everything* ah Canada seems to be a big country even the things you buy in the supermarket are big like the boxes of washing powder everything is big

I: Yea

S: And I'm saying *you go back to England and you feel diminished somehow because it's much smaller and it's slower* it took a bit of time sort of trying to get myself back into it all I said *I could do was save up and come back again* but I've never regretted it and in a way perhaps because you know the children had a bit of a rocky road there for a while.

This added verbiage as a participant distances the speaker from the statements she is making. The speaker conveys information through what has been said rather than directly asserting it for the current hearer.

The speech community defines the standards of too frequent (so as to sound like a preoccupation) and also of infrequency. If one of the semantic participants (object, person, etc.) or some combinations of participants are not used in the discourse when they would be expected, the hearer may get the impression that the speaker will not or cannot speak of those objects or people in a certain way. For example, if the speaker is never the 'actor' of action verbs or never the 'senser' of mental process verbs ('I feel like a wayfaring stranger', 'I hate potatoes') then important sets of meanings will be absent, pointing to specific cognitive or social dysfunctions.

Participants in the situation: who and what is around the interaction

So far, the examples within the ideational metafunction have dealt with the frequency of first person actors and of verbiage. Such concentrations of a particular kind of participant can occur with each of the participants. There are some other ways of considering the use of participants, however. Participants can be considered in terms of how they fit into the non-verbal context. In particular, if the major participants are not usually found in the situation, hearers may think that the speaker is having delusions or hallucinations. Statements such as 'When I met *Napoleon*, he shouted at me', 'As *Jesus*, I had the right to tell him off' or 'I saw *the Martians* eat everything I had in the refrigerator' contain a participant (in *italics*) that is now generally not recognised as possible in the speech community. In these cases, the participants do not fit with the speech community's notion of what is real for the situation. One can certainly speak of 'Napoleon', 'Jesus' and 'Martians' as verbal entities and as real entities at some other time or place. If the genre is fiction, then there are limitless possibilities. There is a continuum of how well these verbal participants fit into the situations of the speech community. For example, an expression that is interpreted as a metaphor (e.g., 'you're a prince') will be viewed one way and an expression not interpreted as a metaphor (perhaps even the same words with a non-metaphorical interpretation) will be regarded differently.

The issue of the fit of an expression can also be seen from the perspective of who belongs to the speech community, rather than from the perspective of the expression itself. That is, the definition of 'the speech community' can be changed to include only those who share a certain interpretation; for example, that Kim over there is Napoleon or a millionaire or a scoundrel or a cheater at cards. The use of language then serves to define the speech community. The speaker must mention objects, people and places in a way that is generally accepted by those addressed and taken as part of the speech community. One can exclude certain hearers from a conversation by systematically mentioning semantic 'participants' that are unknown. If I want to exclude a hearer or an overhearer from the conversation, I just have to speak about 'our friend that we saw last night' or 'that shop where we saw the bargain on shirts' and certain hearers are excluded from the conversation and the speech community for this interaction.

3.5.2   Processes: talking about events and relations in the world

As well as participants, the ideational metafunction includes the category of 'processes' that encode the actions and relations of the world. The importance of the linguistic category of processes in psychiatric syndromes is its encoding of the happenings of the world instead of the things of the world. Happenings and relations, as processes, are rather transitory in contrast to the rather more lasting perceptual quality of 'things' (see Gentner, 1982). The difference between things and events represents a dimension that is differentially perceived or manipulated by speakers. The different processes themselves encode importantly different kinds of meanings that may be selectively affected creating different kinds of impressions on the hearer. For example, the concepts of concreteness or abstractness in language may be conveyed by the use of some processes and not others. Consider the following passage from an interview with a normal control subject. The processes are in *italics*.

> Last time I *went* (to England) three years ago I *had* a British passport. Although I *had* Canadian citizenship I still *keep* my British passport and the man here *said* you know at at Toronto said ah do you *have* proof that you*'re* Canadian. And I *said* well not with me no but I *am* a citizen so he *said* well I'll *let* you *go* he said but I'm *warning* you now that you might *have* trouble *getting* back *in*. So while I *was* on the plane I *wrote* a note and *sent* it as soon as I *got* there to J. saying for heaven's sake *go* to my drawer such and such and so on and *find* the certificate and *send* it to me.

This passage has 11 material processes (processes of 'doing', including four of 'saying') and seven relational processes (processes of 'classifying' and 'identifying'). If the processes are changed (changes in **bold**) to reduce the number of material processes, the following passage results:

> Last time I **was** there (England) three years ago I *had* a British passport. Although I *had* Canadian citizenship I still **have** my British passport and the man here you know at at Toronto **wanted** me to have *have* proof that I *was* Canadian. And I **thought** well not with me no but I *am* a citizen so he was **satisfied** well I'll *let* you *go* he said but I **think** that you might *have* trouble next time. so while I *was* on the plane I *sent* a note as soon as I *got* there to J. saying for heaven's sake the certificate *is* my drawer such and such and so on and *find* the certificate and *send* it to me.

This passage has only four material processes ('sent', 'got', 'find', 'send') with the remainder of the processes being relational processes and mental processes. There is less 'doing' in this altered passage but proportionally more processes of relations and thoughts. It then sounds more abstract or less attached to the world since events are mentioned infrequently. To make the passage more concrete we can add more material processes and remove non-material processes:

> Last time I *went* (to England) three years ago I **took** a British passport. Although I **had taken out** Canadian citizenship I still *keep* my British passport and the man here *said* you know at at Toronto said ah can you **show** me proof of citizenship. And I *said* well not with me no but I *claimed* citizenship so he *said* well I'll *let* you *go* he said but I'm *warning* you now that you might **get into** trouble *coming* back *in*. So while I **was sitting** on the plane I *wrote* a note and *sent* it as soon as I *got* there to J. saying for heaven's sake *go* to my drawer such and such and so on and *find* the certificate and *send* it to me.

Processes then are the linguistic encoding of what the speaker regards as the happenings in the world. The speaker's choice of what to talk about and how much to talk about indicates the speaker's attitude and interaction with the external world. Material processes convey meanings of action, whereas mental processes convey meanings about what a speaker thinks. Processes have a central role in meaning since they relate the participants spoken about to each other. Listening for processes focuses the hearer's attention on the events that are important to the speaker and on the claims the speaker is making about them. The processes, with the accompanying participants and circumstances, encode the claims about the world that the speaker regards as relevant for the speech situation.

3.5.3 Circumstances: details of events, enriching the description

The third major category within the ideational metafunction is 'circumstance'. Circumstances encode information attendant to the process and in many cases largely fill in details of time, location and cause. Although the information in circumstances seems secondary to the more central ideational information in processes and participants, circumstances are rather frequent in utterances. Thus atypicalities in their use may be noticeable and substantially contribute to the impression a speaker makes. Circumstances situate the process as the speaker wishes to convey it to the hearer. They thus suggest the speaker's orientation to the events of the world or at least the orientation that the speaker chooses to convey. The subtypes of circumstances (extent, location, manner, cause, accompaniment, role, matter, angle) indicate the major meanings added to the information of the goings-on or happenings in the world. The issues in the atypical use of circumstances are:

(1) the kind of circumstances that are used;

(2) the frequency of circumstances;

(3) the amount of detail in each circumstance.

A speaker told the following story as a recall of a story that was told to her. Circumstances are in *italics*.

> *Once* there was a big grey fish called Albert *in an icy pond near the edge of the forest. One day, while he was swimming,* he saw this big fat juicy worm near the top of the water and Albert knew that worms were delicious, so he swam closer to the worm and bit into it cause he wanted it for his dinner. *Suddenly,* he felt a pull and the fisherman pulled Albert *into his boat* and Albert realized that he'd been caught by the fisherman and he felt sorry because he'd wished he'd been more careful.

As the circumstances indicate, the speaker is adding temporal (once, one day, while he was swimming, suddenly) and location information (in an icy pond, near the edge of the forest, into his boat) to the processes. This information is quite appropriate for the narrative being recounted. A change in circumstances changes the impression of the speaker's orientation to the information. If, for example, circumstances of cause are added to the original (indicated by **bold italics**), the speaker gives the impression of providing a further kind of detail to the story:

> *Once* there was a big grey fish called Albert *in an icy pond near the edge of the forest. One day, while he was swimming **for exercise**,* he saw this big fat juicy worm near the top of the water and Albert knew ***because of his experience***

that worms were delicious, so he swam closer to the worm *in order to take a look* and bit into it cause he wanted it for his dinner. *Suddenly*, he felt a pull and the fisherman pulled Albert *into his boat for his dinner* and Albert realized that he'd been caught by the fisherman and he felt sorry because he'd wished he'd been more careful.

If circumstances are eliminated, that is a drastic change in the frequency of circumstances, the story sounds rather detached and abstract:

There was a big grey fish called Albert. He saw this big fat juicy worm near the top of the water and Albert knew that worms were delicious, so he swam closer to the worm and bit into it cause he wanted it for his dinner. He felt a pull and the fisherman pulled Albert and Albert realized that he'd been caught by the fisherman and he felt sorry because he'd wished he'd been more careful.

A third kind of variation is to place relatively more information into the circumstances of the original story to tell the hearer that even detailed information about the events is relevant to the situation.

*Once **a long time ago** there was a big grey fish called Albert in an icy, **fresh** pond near the edge of the **green, dark** forest. One **sunny** day **towards the end of summer**, while he was swimming,* he saw this big fat juicy worm near the top of the water and Albert knew that worms were delicious, so he swam closer to the worm and bit into it cause he wanted it for his dinner. *Quite suddenly*, he felt a pull and the fisherman pulled Albert *into his **large** boat **that had many nets*** and Albert realized that he'd been caught by the fisherman and he felt sorry because he'd wished he'd been more careful.

Of course, more information, in itself, is not necessarily desirable or expected. Too much information may make the speaker seem pedantic or insecure. The kind, frequency and amount of detail in the circumstances helps make the text fit into the situation. Although this example is of a narrative that has no interruptions from another speaker, similar effects can be found in spontaneous conversation.

This section has outlined the effects that atypicalities in the ideational metafunction may have. The discussion has proceeded according to the major meanings in the metafunction. When dealing with individual speakers, of course, there may be combinations of atypicalities from each of the participant, process and circumstance areas of meaning. Such a pattern may indicate rather pervasive difficulties in encoding the outside world of experience. As with the other metafunctions, an examination of the ideational metafunction is only valid when the context of the utterance is taken into account and when the use of language is compared to how language is typically used in such contexts.

3.6   Interpersonal metafunction

The interpersonal metafunction includes those meanings between speaker and hearer that are at stake because there is interaction (see Table 3.3 for a summary of these interpersonal meanings).

Table 3.3

The meanings at stake in the interpersonal metafunction

Basic category	Kind of meaning	Atypical meanings (unusual concentration, unusual shifting)
Giving – demanding	Direction of interaction	Sounds too passive or too aggressive/too forward
Information or goods and services	Commodity being exchanged	Talk oriented (information) or activity oriented (goods and services)
Move	Configuration of: • commodity • main or secondary interactant • follow-up or not	Taking an unusual conversational stance given the roles of other speakers. Sounds out of place in the interaction but perhaps not in topic.
Speech function	Configuration of: • initiating – responding • attending – exchanging • giving – demanding commodity	Taking an unusual conversational stance given the roles of other speakers. Sounds out of place in the interaction but perhaps not in topic.
Mood	Realisations of speech function as: • declarative, imperative, • yes-no question, • wh-question	The speaker expresses the function in an unusual way
Degree of commitment	Level of commitment to truth of utterance	Sounds unduly secure/self-confident or unduly insecure and unsure

Individuals take interactional roles, such as questioner and answerer and these roles are associated with meanings. Interaction, of course, involves the exchange of ideational information. However, in exchanging this information, 'interactional' or 'interpersonal' meanings are combined with it. Speakers with difficulties in the interpersonal metafunction will seem to be 'not with' the hearer. They seem detached, not in ideation, but in the roles they are playing in the conversation and how they relate to other speakers. To repeat the basic components of the interpersonal metafunction, the following chart presents the roles of 'giving' and 'demanding' and the objects that are exchanged, 'information' and 'goods and services'.

	Giving	Demanding
Goods and services	Offer	Command
Information	Statement	Question

As with the ideational metafunction, the atypicalities in the interpersonal metafunction may be the unusual concentration of certain kinds of meaning or the atypical shifting among meanings in the metafunction.

3.6.1 Giving and demanding

The first dimension to be considered is the distinction between 'giving' and 'demanding'. This distinction is in terms of the direction of the interaction. With 'giving', the speaker has the material to be conveyed. In contrast, with 'demanding', the speaker sets up the interaction as moving goods, services or information from hearer to speaker. In terms of frequency, a speaker who more frequently than usual is in the 'giving' position or, alternatively, in the 'demanding' position would seem to be rather passive or rather aggressive, respectively. There are stages of life and even particular contexts in which either giving or demanding are expected and should be used frequently, or even exclusively. A young child may ask many questions in a row, but the behaviour is regarded as no more than 'curiosity' or 'going through a stage'. A lecturer who presents a monologue of 'giving – information' could be boring, but is using the appropriate kind of interpersonal meaning for the situation.

3.6.2 Information and goods and services

The second interactional dimension is the distinction between information and goods and services. As outlined earlier, the giving or demanding of 'information' involves language itself as the reason for the interaction. The interaction is based on the language that is demanded or given. Such texts may not seem concrete and may give the impression of being 'just talk'.

Interviews and diagnostic assessments usually involve information rather than goods and services. If, in the middle of such an interaction, either the patient or the clinician asked to open the window, then there would be a switch from interaction about information to a segment of interaction about a service (opening the window). On the other hand, an emphasis on goods and services may be heard as a focus on the external rather than the verbal world. For example, in the following conversation quoted earlier, there is a focus on goods and services that then changes to a focus on information.

1. P: do you mind if I smoke?

2. I: nope please go ahead. I smoke too these days

3. P: oh good it's a bad habit eh?

4. I: yes it is I can't shake it

5. P: I've been trying to quit you know and ummm it's ver ummm.. It's a very difficult thing to do. I've come down off drugs and ah.. you know and this is worse like I got very nauseated and. irritated like I just, you know, I just thought I'm going to go absolutely mad you know when I when I tried quitting for three days eh I said no way I couldn't, you know, I had to smoke again. like you know

6. I: right

7. P: I just couldn't uh

8. I: those are bad days at the beginning

9. P: yea they're supposed to be if you can last seven days

10. I: right

11. P: but ah

12. I: well I quit for long periods of time but ah I seem to start again

13. P: are you a psychiatrist?

14. I: yes I am and Mrs. D is a psychologist who does the tests you have been off medication now for a while is that right?

15. P: no I still take medication

16. I: you are still taking medication?

17 P: yea I still well not I don't take it like as often as I should you know but I mean I. You know cause it like it you know I'm trying to get back to the ah working force again you know sorta like I've been dealing with the hospital and that like I've been in and out of there, mostly in there, since 19XX I believe or something like that you see. And I'm on a disability pension

The first turn is a demand for service by the patient. That is, the patient wants to be able to smoke. The second turn is the interviewer's offer of the service, that is, permission to smoke. The third turn starts with an acknowledgement of the service offer ('oh good') followed by discussion about the object of the service, 'smoking', in turns 3 to 12. In turn 13 ('are you a psychiatrist?'), the patient turns the conversation from a focus on a service (permission to smoke) and the issues around it to the exchange of information. Goods and services by their nature usually refer to the physical world and the changes that speakers want to make in the world, whereas information exchanges are more centred on what can be accomplished through language.

3.6.3 Moves

The interpersonal functions of goods and services/information and demanding/giving are presented linearly in a conversation with little overlap of one speaker with another speaker. Moves are the functional units that serve to organise interpersonal functions. As outlined in Chapter 2, moves encode:

(1) whether the speaker is talking about goods and services or information;

(2) whether the speaker is the main knower (for information) or the main actor (for goods and services);

(3) whether the speaker is following up another contribution.

If there is a concentration of a single kind of move, then the speaker is taking one role in the situation. For example, if a teacher combines the 'information' and 'demanding' functions repeatedly, then the teacher is heard as the main knower who is checking if the hearers know the same information. The teacher assumes the role of a main knower who delays displaying the information. That is, the teacher does know the answer to the question but delays displaying that knowledge for pedagogical reasons. On the other hand, if a speaker seems to be demanding goods and services rather more frequently than usual, that speaker sounds dependent, demanding or perhaps like a customer who cannot be satisfied: 'Could I try one the white one now?' 'Could you please bring me a size seven?' 'Could you show me brown shoelaces to match?' 'I would like to see the lighter weight ones'. In repeating moves that give information, the speaker sounds as if there is too much information to give; for example, in response to the question 'you have been a good student haven't you?' a speaker gave the following answer:

> At times not always not always… in grade school I was an excellent student. Right up until public school I was an excellent student… When I went to

> R school I was an average student … I came out of R I graduated with my
> grade 12 diploma and I was advised to go and see about a college course but
> that kind of upset me because I really didn't want to go to college so maybe I
> should have gone and done it but oh I'm not sorry for what I did.

This speaker contributes a number of consecutive moves of giving information in the role of a main knower.

SHIFTING IN MOVES

If a speaker were to abruptly shift the kinds of moves, there would also be an
atypical construction of meaning that could be inappropriate in the situation.
Consider the above sample of conversation with the speaker adding a number of
atypical moves within the information-giving moves present in the original.

> I: you have been a good student haven't you?
>
> P: at times not always not always… in grade school I was an excellent
>   student.
>
> I: *What kind of student were you?*
>   (demanding, information)
>
> P: Right up until public school I was an excellent student… When I went to
>   R school I was an average student
>
> I: *Could you open the window for a moment?*
>   (demanding, goods and services)
>
> P: I came out of R I graduated with my grade 12 diploma and I was advised
>   to go and see about a college course but that kind of upset me because
>   I really didn't want to go to college so maybe I should have gone and
>   done it but oh I'm not sorry for what I did.
>
> I: *Have a piece of gum*
>   (giving, goods and services)

Such switching of roles in the conversation is unexpected given the context.
If a speaker juxtaposes meanings then the juxtaposition itself may be uninterpretable. A hearer may start wondering why the speaker chooses to create
such combinations of moves. The hearer will try to answer the question,
What is the point of shifting moves? The hearer may think that the speaker
is avoiding certain topics or a certain kind of interaction.

3.6.4 Speech function

Moves, then, are functional units of conversation that combine different kinds of meaning and sequence them one after another. At a more detailed level of analysis, moves are realised or expressed by speech functions. As described in Chapter 2, speech functions tell us whether the speaker is:

(1) initiating or responding;

(2) attending (checking if the speakers are communicating) or exchanging something;

(3) giving or demanding;

(4) dealing with information or goods and services.

The relevant selections from these sets of distinctions are listed in brackets and separated by colons in the following example. As with moves, uncharacteristic repetitions and shifts in speech functions send odd meanings to the hearer. In extreme cases, repetitions of calls, for example, 'Mary, Mary… Mary… John… John', would certainly mark the speaker as not following the general patterns of the speech community. In less extreme cases, repetitions of [responding:exchange:giving:information], as in the passage below, may seem to dominate the conversation.

I: you have been a good student haven't you?

(speech function [initiating:exchange:demanding:information])

P: at times not always not always **/**… in grade school I was an excellent student **/**. Right up until public school I was an excellent student…**/** When I went to R school I was an average student …**/** I came out of R **/** I graduated with my grade 12 diploma **/** and I was advised to go and see about a college course **/** but that kind of upset me **/** because I really didn't want to go to college **/** so maybe I should have gone and done it **/** but oh I'm not sorry for what I did.

The repeated speech functions of [responding:exchange:giving:information] are separated by **/**. Speech functions are often directly correlated with moves so that long explanation and exemplification of the difference is not necessary. The set of speech functions given in Chapter 2 and repeated in Table 3.4 indicates the selection of speech functions that are used to create moves in interaction. The speech functions are composed of meanings on a number of dimensions: initiating/responding; attending/exchanging; etc. see Tables 3.3 and 3.4.

Table 3.4

Speech functions and the meanings that compose them

Initiating/ responding	Attending/ exchanging	Giving/ demanding	Commodity	Example
Initiating	Attending – call			Mary
Initiating	Attending – greeting			Hi
Initiating	Exchange	Giving	Goods and services	Have a drink
Initiating	Exchange	Giving	Information	I'm hungry
Initiating	Exchange	Demanding	Goods and services	Open the window
Initiating	Exchange	Demanding	Information	When are you leaving?
Responding	Attending – call			(Mary) Yes?
Responding	Attending – greeting			(hi) hi
Responding	Exchange	Giving	Goods and services	(Could I have a drink?) Here's your tea
Responding	Exchange	Giving	Information	(When are you leaving?) I'll leave at three
Responding	Exchange	Demanding	Goods and services	(Try this on) No, I want the yellow one
Responding	Exchange	Demanding	Information	(I'm hungry) What did you have for lunch?

3.6.5   Mood: how to express the speech functions through language

In order to express the functions of moves and speech functions, speakers use various grammatical structures. As with the relation between moves and speech functions, there is not a direct one-to-one relation between speech functions and the grammatical structures that word them. In the clause, the mood is the combination of finite verb and subject that determines whether the clause will be a declarative ('They are thinking about it'), imperative ('Leave it alone'), yes-no question ('Are they thinking about it?') or wh-question ('Why are they thinking about it?') (see Table 3.3).

If a given speech function is worded by an unusual grammatical mood, then the hearer will wonder why the speaker said it that way. For example, an offer of [initiating: exchange: giving: goods and services] may be encoded as an imperative ('Take one'), a declarative ('These are really delicious'), a yes-no question ('Do you want one?') or a wh- question ('Why not have one?'). If a speaker uses a less appropriate mood in a certain context (such as a shop keeper saying 'Buy these, they're the latest style' instead of 'Would you like to buy these? They're the latest style'), the speaker conveys atypical and even counterproductive interpersonal meanings. Similar effects, perhaps disastrous for the speaker and his intentions, could be produced by saying to a new acquaintance 'Marry me' as an imperative realising the speech function of [initiating:exchange: demanding: goods and services]. The same speech function would perhaps be more appropriately worded as a statement ('I would like to marry you'), yes-no question ('Do you want to marry me?') or a wh- question ('When do you want to get married?' 'What would it take to convince you to marry me?'). CHOICE OF MOOD

As well as choosing an inappropriate mood for the context, a speaker can also give an unusual impression by the pattern of moods. If all questions are answered by minor clauses, clauses without subject and verb, then the speaker may seem minimally communicative, minimally interested in interaction. That is, a series of one-word answers such as 'yes', 'no', 'maybe', 'sure' will quickly establish the speaker as unwilling or unable to give the fuller answers expected. Even an answer such as 'I agree' or 'I am sure' in place of merely 'yes' builds somewhat more interpersonal connection with the questioner. That is, speakers have a number of ways to express the same speech function. Using these different ways, a speaker can produce variety in manner of speaking and can make the language fit the context precisely. PATTERN OF MOODS

3.6.6 Degree of commitment

Aside from the mood choices outlined, the interpersonal metafunction conveys the degree of commitment that a speaker has to the utterance. A speaker who inappropriately or consistently uses some specific level of commitment may sound unduly insecure or, at the other extreme, sure and self-confident. The following passage is extracted as it was spoken in a conversation.

> I don't know Australia at all. I don't think I'd like to be there ah. I have this basic gut feeling for two reasons. First of all the location of Australia. It's too far away from here… that is familiar to me anyway… and the other thing that I believe and I don't know whether it's correct, is that it's ah there are compartments socially for instance. I speak to Italians that come here from Australia and they have remained very much within their own communities, in part out of choice, in part because I think it's more difficult for the non-English speaking…

This passage can be rewritten to introduce more commitment to the utterances by using modal adjuncts ('definitely', 'seriously', etc.) and attitudinal epithets ('terrible', 'miserable', 'lovely', etc.) and by removing the verb 'think' that operates to modulate the level of commitment.

> I don't know Australia at all. I *definitely* don't like to be there ah. *Seriously*, I have this basic gut feeling for two reasons. First of all the *terrible* location of Australia. It's too far away from here… that is familiar to me anyway… and the other *miserable* thing that I believe and I don't know whether it's correct, is that it's ah there are compartments socially for instance. I speak to *lovely* Italians that come here from Australia and they have remained very much within their own *wonderful* communities, in part out of choice, in part because it's more difficult for the non-English speaking…

To reduce the level of commitment, the original passage can be taken and changed by adding other modal adjuncts ('sometimes', 'maybe', 'almost') and by adding modal verbs ('seems', 'could', 'may').

> I don't know Australia at all. *Sometimes,* I don't think I'd like to be there ah. *Maybe* I have this basic gut feeling for two reasons. First of all the location of Australia. It *seems* too far away from here… that is familiar to me anyway… and the other thing that I *almost* believe and I don't know whether it's

correct, is that it's ah there are compartments socially for instance. I speak to Italians that come here from Australia and they *could* have remained very much within their own communities, in part out of choice, in part because I think it *may* be more difficult for the non-English speaking….

The manipulation of level of commitment and the wording of speech function through grammatical mood (imperative, yes-no question, etc.) help a speaker build an interpersonal relationship with the hearer. If this relationship is odd, despite the ideational meaning, the speaker will be out of contact with others. The nature of the unusual relation will depend on the specific options chosen from the interpersonal metafunction.

This discussion of level of commitment and speech function completes the discussion of the kinds of meaning that can go astray within the interpersonal metafunction. The meanings at stake range from the basic meanings of giving or demanding information or goods and services at the level of move to initiating or responding, attending or exchanging at the level of speech function, to many choices of mood and commitment in the grammar. These meanings are largely chosen independently of ideational meaning. The third metafunction is the textual metafunction. Again, the meanings from the textual metafunction can be largely independent of the meanings of the ideational and interpersonal metafunctions. Like the ideational and interpersonal metafunctions, the textual metafunction contributes to the meaning and effect of an utterance in context. Therefore, disturbances in the textual metafunction result in atypicalities in meaning and in how the speaker is interpreted in context.

Textual metafunction: links to language and links to the world   3.7

The textual function creates the meaning of 'how this piece of language fits into the context'. Such a fit may seem obvious and is usually hardly noticed. It is when there is something wrong with the fit of language to its context that the language becomes difficult to interpret or sound awkward. The components of the textual metafunction have been outlined in Chapter 2 and are briefly summarised here (see Table 3.5 for the components, meanings and examples).

FITTING LANGUAGE TO CONTEXT

Table 3.5	Basic category	Kind of meaning	Atypical meanings (unusual concentration, unusual shifting)
The meanings at stake in the textual metafunction	Thematic structure theme – rheme	Point of departure of message	Compromised continuity and development of messages
	Given and new organisation	Coding information as if known or as if unknown to hearer	Sentence rhythm or stress unusual Seems to misjudge what hearer knows or does not know –misinterpretation of the hearer's perspective
	Cohesion – reference	Sustains identity of objects and people	Lack of continuity of objects and people, under-identified objects and people
	Cohesion – conjunction	Links one message to another by addition, cause, time, etc.	Incomplete trains of thought, insecurity in context, inability to develop full message
	Cohesion – lexical	Same general area of ideational meaning	Unusual shift in ideational meaning, over concentration on an ideational meaning

3.7.1   Thematic organisation: points of departure

The 'point of departure of the message' (the theme) is placed first in a clause. The development of the message is placed next in the clause. This ordering of information in the clause is the thematic structure. In conversation, the thematic structure creates the flow of the conversation. If the thematic structure is misaligned, then the contribution to the conversation may seem out of place or awkward. The following piece of conversation is presented as it occurred.

A: have you always lived in H (name of city) or you?

B: yes yes

A: ever since you've come here?

B: yep.. I like it. I'm not much for social life and my youngest daughter, she's nineteen and she thinks T (name of city) is the greatest city

A: hmm hmm

B: so she's going to H College in September

A: oh is she

B: it's just for one term one year but she'd love to live there but I don't think I'd want to I wouldn't want to go to a big big city

A: I don't like T well I like T but I don't think I'd like to live the way I would have to live there. If I could live downtown, I think I may enjoy it better, but I don't like their suburbia they're flat and uninteresting.

In the following version of the conversation, the ideational and interpersonal meanings are identical but the thematic structure has been altered to create different 'starting points' for clauses and therefore also different developments for those clauses (the newly created themes or starting points are in *italics*).

A: have you always lived in H (name of city) or you?

B: yes yes

A: ever since you've come here?

B: yep.. I like it. *social life* is not much for me and my youngest daughter, *nineteen* she is and *T* (name of city) *is the greatest city* she thinks

A: hmm hmm

B: so she's going to H College in September

A: oh is she

B: it's just for one term one year but *it* is she who would love to live there but I don't think I'd want to I wouldn't want to go to a big big city

A: *T,* I don't like, well… I like T but I don't think I'd like to live the way I would have to live there. If I could live downtown, I think I may enjoy it better, but *their suburbia,* I don't like…*flat and uninteresting* they are.

The changed version has created a number of different themes and in doing so reduced the number of times that 'I' is the theme. There is also a break in the series of themes with 'she' meaning the daughter. The effect has been to reduce the amount of continuity in the themes. This second passage sounds more like a list of separate statements compared to the original version. In terms of the textual function, the statements in the altered version sound as if they are out of context with the flow of the conversation. The meaning of 'I am speaking from one perspective' is lost.

3.7.2   Given and new organisation: what do you think I know?

As well as the distribution of information into themes, there is also a distribution of information into given and new information. The speaker can take information and decide which parts to present as new for the hearer and which parts to present as if the hearer knows them (given information). Information that is moved to the beginning of clauses is specifically marked as new information. For example, in the above conversation, '*their suburbia*, I don't like' has 'their suburbia' moved to the beginning of the clause. The effect of this change is to code 'their suburbia' as new information for the hearer. Information can also be coded as new by stressing the word. For example, if the speaker said 'I don't like THEIR suburbia', the message would be that perhaps the speaker does like some suburbias but that the speaker's dislike of 'their' suburbia is presented as unknown to the hearer.

SENTENCE STRESS

Clinically, we may hear sentence rhythm or sentence stress as unusual because of an unexpected distribution of given and new information. The segment of conversation quoted above can be altered to show the effect of an unusual distribution of given and new information. The words in CAPITALS receive stress in the following version. Some of these words are in their usual place and others have been moved to the beginnings of clauses (indicated by *ITALICISED CAPITALS*).

A: have you ALWAYS lived in H (name of city) or you?

B: yes yes

A: EVER since you've come here?

B: yep.. I like it. I'm not much for social life and MY youngest daughter, SHE's nineteen and she thinks T (name of city) is THE greatest city

A: hmm hmm

B: so *IN SEPTEMBER* she's going to H College

A: oh is she

B: it's just for one term one year but she'd love to live THERE but I don't THINK I'd want to I wouldn't WANT to go to a big big city

A: I don't like T well I like T but I don't think I'd like to live the way I would have to live there. If I could live downtown, I think I may enjoy it better, but *THEIR suburbia* I don't like they're flat and uninteresting.

In the first utterance, for example, the stress on 'always' means that the speaker thinks that the hearer would not expect the question to be about the hearer's whole life. In the fourth utterance, the emphasis on 'my', treating it as new information, means that the speaker thinks that the hearer may be thinking of someone else's daughter rather than the speaker's daughter. In the next clause, the emphasis on 'she' implies that the speaker thinks that the hearer is thinking of someone else, probably a male, since 'she' often contrasts with 'he'. If given and new information repeatedly do not seem to fit with the context, then the speaker gives the impression of not taking the hearer's perspective into account.

3.7.3   Cohesion across clauses: how does this connect to that?

The structural systems of thematic structure (the starting point of messages) and the distribution of given and new information are two ways language is fitted into context. Cohesion, made up of reference, conjunction, vocabulary choice and ellipsis, is another way to build links to context. In general, cohesion signals that one stretch of language is dependent on another.

Reference: connecting up people and objects

For reference, some information from elsewhere is needed to interpret the current stretch of language. Consider the following stretch of conversation from a florid schizophrenic (courtesy Drs. G. Bartolucci, J. Pelletier).

I: ….did someone bring you [here]?

P: did someone bring me … no nobody brought me … I flew in my very own plane … I wouldn't trust anybody down at the airport to bring me anywhere

I: why not?

P: why not … why not … for the very simple fact that I don't think that they can really handle a plane … unless they are going to lay me down as a little rose and put me back in *the box* and *they* can fly me around because there's a million people out there that can meet *the same world* … it's just world after world after a world right

I: yea

P: and there's no need to be worried about *that* and if you want *them you* can go down and get *them* and if you figure you need plastic *ones* or *other ones* if *they* figure *they* need *those things* and *they* want *those things* it's entirely up to *them*

The italicised nominals are not clear because the reference link to another part of the text cannot be followed. The hearer does not have the information to identify 'the box', 'they', 'the same world', 'other ones', 'those things', etc. Such unclear references can be very disruptive since they make the utterances quite uninterpretable. Utterances may be unusual in a less disruptive way by using relatively more or less than would be expected of some kind of reference. The following excerpt of a story is a recall given by a normal subject.

> Well there was once a lady and *her* husband was sick and to make him better *she* wanted a tiger's whisker to make medicine… now *she* was afraid of tigers so *she* thought *she* would play a trick and get the tiger's whisker. So *she* decided to take some food…

Notice the use of 'her' and 'she' to refer to the lady. If these references are systematically removed and replaced with nominals that are clear but do not refer to earlier language, the passage sounds somewhat too explicit and awkward because it does not make the usual cohesive links.

> Well there was once a lady and *a lady's* husband was sick and to make him better *a lady* wanted a tiger's whisker to make medicine… now *a lady* was afraid of tigers so *a lady* thought *she* would play a trick and get the tiger's whisker. So *a lady* decided to take some food…

If 'a lady' is replaced by 'the lady' the passage sounds better since the nominal 'the lady' makes the hearer presume that the same person is spoken about.

> Well there was once a lady and *the lady's* husband was sick and to make him better *the lady* wanted a tiger's whisker to make medicine… now *the lady* was afraid of tigers so *the lady* thought *she* would play a trick and get the tiger's whisker. So *the lady* decided to take some food…

Nevertheless, this last version is awkward because it relies only on the reference word 'the' to indicate presumed information and on the repetition of the word 'lady'. Even if the utterance is interpretable, the linking can be atypical and therefore not fit the context.

Conjunction: connecting up messages

Conjunction, the next kind of cohesion after reference, links the interpretation of one stretch of language to another. These additive, temporal and causal links may be disrupted if a speaker starts to create a link and then does not finish:

> A: enjoy the radio? do you like going to movies?
> B: no yeah but …

In this example, the speaker started a clause with the conjunction 'but'; however, the clause was not completed. Frequent incomplete conjunctive links create an impression of the speaker's insecurity in the context or inability to finish a train of thought. The speaker seems to know what is to be said next and starts the next part of the message only to leave it incomplete. If the difficulty is in one kind of link, then there may be relatively more incomplete conjunctive links with one kind of conjunction compared to another. For example, a speaker may regularly complete temporal links but leave causal links unfinished sounding incapable of explaining.

As well as the break down of conjunctive links there is possibility of the misuse, over use or under use of links. If a speaker rarely uses one kind of conjunctive link, such as temporal or causal, then the speaker will seem to ignore a semantic dimension for organising material. The following story, used earlier to illustrate referential links, has a few temporal links (in *italics*) and a few causal links (in **bold**) as well as a large number of explicitly additive links (worded by 'and').

> Well there was once a lady and her husband was sick and to make him better she wanted a tiger's whisker to make medicine... now she was afraid of tigers **so** she thought she would play a trick and get the tiger's whisker. **So** she decided to take some food and take it to this lonely tiger's cave... and *when* she got there she put the food down to entice the tiger out of his cage and she sang him some songs and the tiger came out of the cave and ate the food and listened to the lady singing and *then* the woman went up to him and cut his whisker off and *then* she ran away and the tiger felt sad and lonely **because** she'd gone

If the explicit temporal and causal links are removed, the story seems flatter or less interesting because there is less content in the links between different pieces of information:

> Well there was once a lady and her husband was sick and to make him better she wanted a tiger's whisker to make medicine... now she was afraid of tigers... she thought she would play a trick and get the tiger's whisker. She decided to take some food and take it to this lonely tiger's cave... and she got there and she put the food down to entice the tiger out of his cage and she sang him some songs and the tiger came out of the cave and ate the food and listened to the lady singing and the woman went up to him and cut his whisker off and she ran away and the tiger felt sad and lonely... she'd gone

Although this example is of a story, similar effects can also be found in conversations.

Lexical cohesion: connecting up words

In addition to reference and conjunction, the third frequent type of cohesion is lexical cohesion, i.e., the choice of vocabulary to signal that the same general area of meaning is continuing. When other parts of the textual metafunction are not sending clear meanings, lexical cohesion can signal that there is some overall coherence to the message. In the following segment from a conversation with a speaker with schizophrenia (courtesy Drs. G. Bartolucci, J. Pelletier) there are a number of problems in the textual metafunction (unclear reference, for example) and in the ideational metafunction, yet the lexical cohesion of some word sets ('kids', 'school', 'girls', 'boys', 'young', 'understand') helps build some coherence.

> It was back in fifteen hundred when they took the pill actually and it created some kind or organism and diabetes and things like this you know… the kids they're all actually fine you just gotta know how to talk to the kids and how to associate things with the kids right? Like you separate a school building and keep the girls on this half you keep the boys on this half and if you ever criss-cross a school then you run into all kinds of problems but this happened way back in fifty-nine when the kids were young and still yet you know very vigorous and enjoying themselves and it was something that the ladies thought would help the kids to understand…. we didn't use the kids really but we did help the kids to understand that the thing to wear their tupperware and things like this.

The different kinds of cohesion build up the connection of one stretch of language to another. If there is some difficulty in using cohesion, then the speaker will be heard as either not making sense or making some sense but not quite the right sense. In each case, though, it is not the linguistic characteristics of the utterances that are immediately noticeable or important. Rather, it is the failure to communicate meaning in an expected way that is disruptive to social interaction and that draws the focus of clinical attention.

3.7.4   Textual metafunction as meaning

The components of the textual metafunction are not just wordings of ideational and interpersonal meanings. Rather, meaning is added by the textual metafunction: the meaning of how the speaker is relating to the specific context of the speaking event. If these meanings are compromised, then the speaker will be as difficult to interpret and sound as inappropriate as if the ideational or interpersonal metafunctions are adversely affected. The range of possible difficulties in making meaning must be considered for each individual who is not socially appropriate. For expository purposes, the discussion of the meaning-making has been in terms of the linguistic systems and meanings. However, in terms of individuals and even psychiatric categories, there are many possible combinations of compromised meanings. It is rare that there is a spectacular and isolated difficulty in one area of meaning. Listening must involve the careful consideration of what kinds of meaning seem out of place or not clear and what kinds of meaning seem appropriate. For example, a speaker with schizophrenia may be quite cooperative and use appropriate speech functions in waiting turns, asking and answering questions and providing information. At the same time, the speaker may be using the textual or ideational metafunctions in ways that make much of the interaction uninterpretable.

The categories of psychiatric disorder or diagnostic criteria require the listener to integrate information from many linguistic components. The overall impression shapes and defines the psychiatric categories. Linguistic analysis and linguistic categories sharpen the focus the clinician and lay listener on the difficulties the speaker is having in social settings. They also direct the listeners' attention to aspects of interaction that account for the speaker's difficulties.

Chapter 4 contents

Chapter 4

Communication Disorders

Overview of Communication Disorders 4.1

Communication Disorders are disorders in communication itself rather than unusual language or communication indicating some other disorder. For example, in mood disorders, psychotic disorders or autism, the speaker communicates rather atypically but the disorders centre on constructs that are not directly communication, namely, mood, reality testing and social isolation respectively. However, impairments in communication overlap across disorders. The language behaviour of Communication Disorders, which implies no further concepts, overlaps with the language behaviour of other disorders. In these other disorders, though, the language behaviour is a sign of other concepts. Unlike other disorders, Communication Disorders as a formal psychiatric category will be capitalised to distinguish it from the informal use of the phrase. The field of Communication Disorders is a substantial field unto itself (see, for example, extended treatments in Hamaguchi, 2001; Leonard, 1998; Owens, Metz & Haas, 2002; Shames & Anderson, 2002).

In this chapter, we deal with Communication Disorders in terms of its use in psychiatry and how it relates to other psychiatric disorders. Since the language features of Communication Disorders may overlap with other disorders, it is important to separate the disorders from each other. If individuals with dissimilar substrates are combined in one disorder because the communication issues are similar, it will be very difficult to treat individuals effectively or to search for underlying factors. By separating the disorders, it is possible and perhaps even easier, to search for coherent cognitive, biological or other accounts of the disorders.

There is an inherent developmental dimension in Communication Disorders. As children, speakers with Communication Disorders apparently lag behind in the use of several aspects of language. It is not clear if the language of these children is merely delayed or whether there is a different trajectory of development. Of course, the issue has to be considered separately for each realm of language; what is true for the sounds of language may not be true for vocabulary, grammar or meanings, etc. To study these questions of delayed or different development, we need a specific understanding of the kinds of impairments in Communication Disorders. In particular this chapter details the communication features that are clinically noticed in the disorders. These features thus are a description of the phenomena that cause the social impairment in Communication Disorders.

EXPRESSIVE AND
RECEPTIVE

Communication Disorders are divided into expressive and receptive disorders. The evidence for the two kinds of disorders is different. Expressive disorders involve the production of language and so the evidence is simply what the speakers say. As we will show, the production impairment involves a number of different levels of language: meanings, wordings and even the sounds of the language. Receptive disorders, in contrast, implicate how a speaker understands language spoken by others. In this case, the evidence is more indirect since we must consider verbal and non-verbal behaviour from both speakers. Even with this evidence, though, we are inferring the receptive disorder; it is not directly accessible. For this reason, relatively more evidence is needed to firmly diagnose a receptive disorder. The evidence is both positive in indicating the disorder and negative in eliminating other kinds of disorders. If we find lack of verbal and non-verbal response, it may arise from impaired hearing, shyness, lethargy and a number of other disorders essentially quite different from a receptive Communication Disorder. For a receptive disorder, we must find evidence that the speaker can produce language appropriate to the situation and at the same time evidence that the speaker does not know what is happening verbally in the context.

Communication disorders involve impairments at a number of levels of language. The impairments in language range from meaning to lower levels of grammar, vocabulary and finally to the characteristics of sound and stuttering. We describe these levels in detail later. The lower levels, such as vocabulary, sounds (phonology) and stuttering (an impairment in the delivery of the intended sounds and words) do not directly disrupt meaning even though they may interfere with the smooth interaction.

Expressive language disorder   4.2

4.2.1 Clinical features

Expressive language disorder is defined as an impairment in language expression in the presence of less impaired or unimpaired non-verbal intellectual ability and receptive language ability. That is, there is a specific impairment only in expression. Often standardised tests are used to measure this impairment. Fundamentally, the impairment is in the spontaneous use of language covering a wide range of language phenomena. One set of impairments is a limitation of: amount of speech, range of vocabulary, variety of grammatical structures and sentence types. A second set of impairments is the way grammatical structures are expressed: simplified grammatical structure, omission of important parts of sentences, shortened sentences, unusual word order. A third set concerns vocabulary: difficulty acquiring new words and word finding and vocabulary errors. In addition, for all of these areas of language, there may be slow language development. The first set of impairments is restriction in the amount and variety of language. These restrictions narrow the speaker's range of meanings. Each restriction narrows in a particular kind of meaning. The second set of impairments (grammatical processing) seriously compromises interpretability. We hear the speaker as giving us incomplete information or just not making sense, since the utterances do not sound like expected structures. The third set of impairments concerns words which encode the ideational world into language. If the speaker does not use some words, then the speaker will only be talking about a restricted, narrower part of the ideational world.

LIMITED SPEECH

GRAMMAR

VOCABULARY

The fourth and rather general impairment, is the slow rate of language development. The other three impairments of limitations, grammatical structures and vocabulary reflect this overall slow rate; language development generally moves from more limited and simpler language to the more varied and complex. The clinician diagnoses by finding a gap between expressive language and other verbal and non-verbal abilities. Again, since verbal and non-verbal abilities are developmental, a gap with expressive language implies that the expressive language is unexpectedly under-developed. Without information about other verbal and non-verbal abilities, we hear immature language as either part of a general picture of slow development or as a more narrow impairment in expression. To identify which of these accounts is correct, the clinician must know about language abilities from a number of tasks and situations, from direct testing, reports of behaviour across a number of contexts and tasks, or direct observation in a range of naturalistic contexts.

SLOW DEVELOPMENT

4.2.2   Language features

We now detail the three broad kinds of impairment of expressive language disorder. The objective is to characterise Communication Disorders in terms of the features of language that are at stake and the kinds of meanings that result (see Table 4.1). Learning about the meanings speakers with Communication Disorders produce helps us both recognise the disorder and also understand how these speakers have difficulty in social processes. Since there are several different impairments in expressive disorders, we can expect that the effect on the kinds of meaning will also be varied.

Table 4.1	Limitation in use of language	Amount
Expressive language disorder: language features		Vocabulary
		Grammatical structures
	Impairments in grammatical structures	Simplification
		Omission
		Word order problems
		Vocabulary

Limitation in use of language

The first general kind of impairment is limitation; the speaker uses less language and less variety of language. We judge a limitation in the amount of speech in terms of the contexts of the utterances. If a speaker uses widely different amounts of speech depending on the context (is the addressee a friend, peer, superior? Is the context emotionally stressful? What is the purpose of the interaction?), then expressive ability itself is not impaired. Rather, there are unusual contextual constraints on using the ability. That is, a socially based dysfunction is more likely. Selective mutism is such an example. The speakers have full control over the vocabulary and grammar of the language, but in certain circumstances, generally in the presence of strangers or in stressful situations, they speak very little. In less severe cases, a shy or passive individual may say very little despite reasonable control over vocabulary and grammar. Ultimately, however, all language use is language in social context. Therefore, the issue is how much of an effect context has on the amount of language. If across a range of contexts, the individual speaks less than expected given other abilities, then the impairment may be an expressive language disorder. If the limit in expression is restricted to some contexts, then another disorder is, more likely, one tied to specific social dimensions.

Amount

A speaker who talks less than expected is also expressing fewer meanings and consequently limiting the social processes that are accomplished. A limited amount of speech will often not encourage another speaker to develop the interaction. If questions are answered by short answers, if statements are reacted to with shorter than expected responses, the speaker gives the impression of not wanting to contribute to and continue the interaction. On hearing repeated short utterances, another speaker may also participate less, thus curtailing the social process. Overall, we hear short utterances as uncooperativeness, a standoffish attitude, or perhaps guess that there is impaired hearing. We could even suppose a receptive language impairment since the speaker seems to misunderstand what is required in the situation. These short utterances may be similar to the curtailed speech in depression, the lack of communication in pervasive developmental disorders, or the poverty of speech and other negative symptoms in schizophrenia (I am indebted to Dr. Anat Goren for this insight).

Vocabulary

As well as a limited amount of speech, there can be a limited range of vocabulary in Communication Disorders. Vocabulary has the major function of encoding the things and events of the world. Vocabulary therefore gives us the institutional focus of the interaction (see Chapter 2 for more detail about institutional focus and the 'field' that vocabulary sets up). The institutional focus concerns the things and events that are talked about and around which the interaction takes place. Loosely, it can be seen as the topic or subject matter. When vocabulary is limited, then either the speaker will be talking about fewer things or will be giving less detail about the things. The result is that if the vocabulary repeats, the speaker sounds preoccupied. If there is little detail, the speaker sounds shallow. As with limited amount of speech, we must distinguish this limitation of vocabulary and the apparent restriction in topics from the special interests in pervasive developmental disorders, fixed ideas in schizophrenia and perhaps the lack of interest in depression. To distinguish the disorders, the clinician needs information about the language and communicative development of the individual as well as information about the wider range of verbal and non-verbal behaviours that are not simply communication impairments.

INSTITUTIONAL FOCUS

Grammatical structures

Unlike the limitation in vocabulary, the limited variety of grammatical structures does not restrict the subject matter that is at stake. Rather, the limitation in meanings is elsewhere: in the meanings carried specifically by grammatical structures. These meanings are typically of tense and signals of the time of events ('run' instead of 'ran' or 'runs', 'walk' instead of 'walked') and of the number of things mentioned ('table' instead of 'tables'). In some languages, such parts of words give elaborate information. This information can include the gender of the person mentioned, whether the event has been finished or is continuing, whether the talk is about the speaker (first person), the addressee (second person), some other individual (third person), or even some combination of these individuals. Without this information from the grammar, the speaker sounds incorrect or unclear. In addition, the speaker is using a restricted set of meanings such that information of time or number, for example, is narrow or not present. Such language may sound similar to a beginning speaker of second language.

Sentence types

A limit in sentence types introduces yet a third kind of restricted meaning. The limited range of sentence types may be due to cognitive processing difficulties or due to more interactionally based reasons. However, whatever the cause, the effect is to restrict the kinds of interaction. There are usually several ways to word the same meaning. This is especially true for different sentence types conveying a single speech function. The following utterances all give us about the same ideational meaning but do it in different ways:

I don't like broccoli	declarative
No thank you	elliptical, depending on the verbal or non-verbal context
Don't give me broccoli	imperative
Do you really think I eat broccoli?	yes-no question
No broccoli for me	no verb, non-finite clause
No. No. No.	repeated negative term

SUBTLE RANGE OF MEANINGS

A speaker using a limited range of such sentence types does not express certain meanings, again, similar to a second language learner who has not yet learnt some grammatical patterns. However, there are also more subtle effects of limited sentence types. If some sentence types are not used, then other types are used to attain the same effect. For example, if requests are not made with questions ('Could you move the chair?', 'Why don't you see if they are home?'), then imperatives are maybe used rather more frequently ('Move the chair', 'See if they are home'). These imperatives express more direct, less polite, less hedged meanings. That is, the restriction in sentence types is also a restriction in the range of subtle meanings. A speaker who is not using some forms often is over-using other forms and then over-using the meanings associated with these forms. To take another example, a speaker who does not use forms such as rhetorical questions ('Did you really have to do that?') limits the fine-tuning of language for the situation.

In considering sentence types, intonation is also involved. In English, we can ask a question by using a verb such as 'do' ('Do you want to go?') or by rising intonation on what could be a statement ('You want to go?'). Therefore, clinicians must be sensitive to whether there is a restriction just in the grammatical forms of sentences or also meanings carried by other means, such as intonation, rate of speech or hesitations. A general narrowing of meanings suggests the source of the problem is generally avoiding interaction or impaired social or communicative functioning rather than an expressive communication disorder. The speaker may have a limited variety of sentence types but the central issue is that the speaker does not want to interact, to initiate, to challenge another speaker and so on. It is best to consider Communication Disorders as disorders of the ability to create meaning and disorders at lower levels of language such as sounds and stuttering. Here we do not consider how those abilities are used in context. Expressive Communication Disorders are then diagnosed when there is little effect of different situations on the language. Since language can only be fairly assessed in real contexts, information about a range of contexts is needed, either by observation or by reliable reports. To gather information, it is important to give examples of different wordings and different sentence types as well as asking if the speaker sounds repetitive, too plain, or unsubtle. That is, we must consider both the wording and the meaning.

INTONATION

The clinician can notice limitations in amount, vocabulary, grammatical structures and sentence types individually or in combination. The more there are different types of limitations, the more the utterances will sound impoverished and the less the speaker will easily accomplish in social contexts. Consider the following piece of conversation between a teacher (T) and a seven-year old boy (A).

1 T: all right you were just saying you'd like to talk about what goes on in the classroom … can you tell me some of the things that happen in our classroom?

2 A: um you have to read um books and uh lots of stories and we have to write them and … um at recess we we play and then and then we come in and then we're bad

3 T: yeah I noticed your bad … what should you do when you come in? do you know?

4 A: sit down and be quiet

5 T: what story are you reading right now?

6	A:	um Mr. ah … Wish on a Penny
7	T:	is it a good story?
8.	A:	yes
9	T:	what's it about?
10	A:	um … it's some somebody wishes on a penny and she wishes that she could fly up to the in a rocket into up to the moon

The boy's language can be made to sound more like an individual with Communication Disorders by having him say less, use a narrower vocabulary and change the grammatical structures. In this example, there is little opportunity to change the sentence types. The full effect of such changes would require a much longer sample. However there is a noticeable difference even in these few utterances. The passage now sounds as follows:

1	T:	all right you were just saying you'd like to talk about what goes on in the classroom … can you tell me some of the things that happen in our classroom?
2	A:	um you have to read um book write them and … um at recess we we play and then and then we come in and then we're bad
3	T:	yeah I noticed your bad … what should you do when you come in? do you know?
4	A:	sit down sit down
5	T:	what story are you reading right now?
6	A:	um Mr. Penny
7	T:	is it a good story?
8	A:	yes
9	T:	what's it about?
10	A:	um … it's some somebody wish on a uh and could fly up to the in a uh up to the

Impairments in grammatical structures

As well as limitations, a speaker with a Communication Disorder can have impairments in expressing grammatical structures. These impairments compromise how the grammar conveys meaning. As utterances are simplified, truncated or misarranged, less of the necessary structure remains and therefore there is less meaning. We notice the changes in meaning since our on-line grammatical analysis fails and we cannot understand the speaker.

Intact grammatical structures are easy to follow, even if standard speech contains some slips in expected grammatical forms.

Simplification

Simplifying grammatical structures occurs at different levels of grammar and affects different kinds of meanings. At the lowest level of language, the forms of words are simplified by dropping endings or beginnings (happily – happy, discomfort – comfort, comfortable – comfort, untie – tie, changeable – change). Words with simpler structures carry less information in each word even though a speaker can express the same overall meaning combining words ('unhappy' can be expressed as 'not happy' or 'sad'). If, though, speakers also have restricted vocabularies, they may not be able to use a simple word as a substitute and there is overall less complex meaning.

WORDS

At a higher level of language, there can be simplified structure in the groups of words expressing the things, events and circumstances in the world. Nominal groups (groups of words centred around a noun that often can be subjects of sentences, e.g., 'the tall and amazingly sturdy pine *tree*') typically encode the people, objects and concepts of the world. If these groups of words have a simplified structure then less detail is given. The following passage is part of a narrative from a seven-year old girl.

NOMINAL GROUPS

> and this is the next German word I was saying I was I was saying German words and there das … there's un und …und means and and nein is no and ja is yes and there are lots of other German words but there's less German words than there is English words I think … and … so far we've played a few games … and … I've I've I'm ….easier to tell about what I do and everything I have to do spelling my my reading work and my writing every morning (…) instead of gym we have spelling game or math game and we didn't do a spelling game or math game today 'cause we're having gym.

Although there is little structure of groups of words in this passage, as is appropriate for a seven-year old in the context, we can still simplify what structure there is and so reduce the amount of detail. It now sounds as follows:

> and this is the word I was saying I was I was saying words and there das … there's un und …und means and and nein is no and ja is yes and there are lots of words but there's less German … I think … and … so far we've played games … and … I've I've I'm ….easier to tell about what I do and everything I have to do spelling reading work and my writing in the morning (…) instead of gym we have games and we didn't do a game today 'cause we're having gym.

At a yet higher level of grammatical structure, we can simplify parts of the clause by omitting certain elements. A speaker can say 'John is here' or 'John, who I saw yesterday, is here'. To take another example, information can be conveyed in a more complex clause ('She is fast asleep in her bed') or in two simplified clauses ('She is fast asleep.' 'She is in her bed'). With this kind of simplification, we lose the integration of information. These examples show that there is a functional cost to simplified grammatical structures. Either information about the world is not presented or the information that is presented is not integrated. In each case, though, we hear the speaker as presenting less rich information. Simplification of grammatical structure is not just a matter of grammar or the cognitive mechanisms used to produce the grammar. The simplification has an effect on communication and interferes with social activity. This impairment in social activity is what we notice in the disorder.

Omission

Beyond simplification of grammatical structures is the omission of important parts of sentences or the shortening of sentences. To understand the effect of omissions, we have to reconsider the normal elements of sentences and their role in constructing interaction. As outlined in Chapters 2 and 3, there are three main functional elements of the sentence:

(1) the things of the world that are expressed in language as the 'participants' we speak about (but not the speakers, themselves);

(2) the goings-on of the world that are expressed as verbal 'processes';

(3) the surroundings of the events that are the 'circumstances' in the sentence.

A speaker may omit one or more of these three critical kinds of meaning. If they are missing, the utterance sounds incomplete.

However, how incomplete and how disruptive an utterance sounds depends on what is missing. Sentences and clauses are built around the verbs and the events they express. For example, 'die' is used with only one necessary participant. Something alive can 'die' but one cannot say 'A died B'. On the other hand, 'give' implies that there is a giver, a receiver and something that is transferred between them ('A gave B the book'). These different 'processes', worded by verbs, are needed to make claims (technically, 'predications') about the world. Even in telegraphic language, processes are important. In the following example, the processes are in italics: '*Having* good time. *Send* money'. On the other hand, when there are no processes, it is difficult to understand what is happening: 'Mary George. Book George in room'. In this last example, there are participants (Mary, George, book), but no way to interpret what is happening among them. We do not know how they are connected to each other in the goings-on of the world. Usually speakers state processes explicitly or the processes are easy to recover from the context ('Have you seen Bill?' 'Sure'. (I saw him.)). Sometimes, the hearer can infer the relations and infer the goings on. However, if this interpretative process is required more than usual, it can lead to inaccurate understandings of what the speaker wanted to say. These effortful or inaccurate interpretations are what we experience when interacting with a speaker with a Communication Disorder.

Processes, expressed by verbs and talking about the events and goings-on of the world, are thus the most crucial elements of an utterance. When these processes are omitted, there is potentially great misunderstanding. However, participants (the objects, people, places of the world) are closely connected to the goings-on. Each process has certain participants connected to it. A verb of sensing (see, witnessed, etc.) will have: — PARTICIPANTS

(1) a sensor, who is usually an animate being;

(2) something that is sensed (a 'phenomenon').

If the process is present and one or more of the participants are missing, then the hearer may be able to infer the participants. At least, the hearer understands what event is reported. In any case, the omission of participants makes the discourse less explicit about the things of the world even when we can guess at the missing parts.

It is our difficulty in interpreting speech that is the key criterion in assessing the omissions of participants, processes and circumstances. In unfolding interaction and even in more one-way communication such as narratives or descriptions, we can omit many elements of a sentence if they are recoverable from the context. The issue in Communication Disorders, as well as other disorders that are characterised by too little language or omissions of parts of language, is that the hearer fails to interpret what is said. The diagnostic criterion of omitting critical parts of sentences is based on hearers failing to understand. If the information were recoverable, then neither the lay nor clinical communities would notice the absence; the omissions are seamless. The source of the difficulty in expression may be a low-level problem in expression, a cognitive disorder that affects memory, conceptual or syntactic assembly processes or some similar cognitive ability, or a social misunderstanding of what the hearer knows or needs to know.

Speakers express information about the events and processes in the 'circumstances' in the sentence. These circumstances give information about extent in time and place, location in time and place, manner, cause and other information (see Halliday, 1994:149-61, Eggins, 1994: 237-9). Circumstances are less critical to understanding a sentence than the things (participants) or events (processes). Circumstances can frequently be omitted: 'They ran' (into the house) (quickly). However, at a higher level of discourse, we use circumstances to build a setting and for consistency of meaning. Circumstances tell 'where did all this take place?' 'when did all this happen?'. Without this information, the goings-on expressed in processes seem detached from the world. To consider other circumstances, manner and cause are regularly expressed in some contexts. If a speaker is asked why something happened, then information about cause is expected (It fell *because it was placed on the edge and the screws were not long enough for the weight*). We expect messages with a certain level of complexity. When this information is missing, the message is functionally incomplete in context and incomplete in terms of the expectations of other hearers, even when the syntax is intact.

As well as simplified grammatical structures and omission of parts of sentences, expressive Communication Disorders are typified by shortened sentences. What may be shortened in a sentence is similar to what can be omitted. However, there are some additional considerations. There are certain elements that tend to be at the ends of sentences and there are certain functions that are expressed towards the ends of sentences. In English, goals ('John made *the cake*'), phenomena ('Kim looked at *the pictures*'), verbiage ('John said "Hello"') and circumstances ('John ate the cake *in the car as he was driving last night*'). In other languages, other elements may be placed towards the ends of sentences. For example, in languages that typically put the verb at the end of the sentence, such as German, the processes are more likely to be omitted if the sentence remains unfinished. As we have seen, some sentence elements fall at the end of sentences and would be omitted if the sentence were not completed. There are also, though, certain general meanings that fall at the end of sentences. The sentence usually contains information that is assumed to be known to the hearer (given information) and information that comes later in the sentence that is encoded as new to the hearer (see Fries, 2001 for a clear account of this distribution with many good examples). It is thus information that the speaker is coding as 'new' or 'newsworthy' for the hearer that is liable to be omitted. In this way, the truncating of sentences is not just the omission of certain sentence elements but also the omission of a kind of information: new information. When this new information is absent, the discourse seems to have no real point to it. It does not convey any 'news'. Consider the narrative presented above with the ends of sentences, expressing the 'news' deleted and replaced with a pause and 'uh', marked (… uh) in the text.

> and this is (… uh) …I was I was saying (… uh) and there das … there's un und …und means (… uh) and nein is (… uh) and ja is (… uh) and there are (… uh) but there's (… uh) I think … and … so far we've played (… uh) … and … I've I've I'm ….easier to tell about what I do and everything I have to do (… uh) … instead of gym we have (… uh) and we didn't do (… uh) 'cause we're having (… uh)

Of course, this is an extreme example with all the new information removed but it demonstrates how little 'news' is conveyed if these particular final parts of sentences are omitted. Even omitting some of the 'new' information compromises the discourse and makes it sound uninformative.

Word order problems

Unusual word order is also a characteristic of expressive Communication Disorders. The effect of the unusual word order depends on the inherent flexibility of the language. At lower levels of language, the word order tends to be less flexible and so unusual word order sounds worse. For example, changing the word order within a nominal group (a red China bowl => a China red bowl, red a China bowl, bowl China a red, etc.), a verbal group (was going to tell us => going was to tell us, was going tell to us, was tell going to us, etc.), or a preposition phrase (from out of the refrigerator => out from of the refrigerator, from the refrigerator out of, the refrigerator from out of, etc.) is very disruptive and generally hard to interpret. On the other hand, if the unusual word order is at the higher level of the sentence, there is some flexibility and the utterance may sound odd but not completely uninterpretable ('She quickly put the knapsack on the rock next to the gorge.' => 'The knapsack she put quickly on the rock next to the gorge', 'On the rock next to the gorge she put the knapsack quickly', 'The knapsack on the rock she put quickly next to the gorge.'). Because of the looser constraints in word order at higher levels of language, unusual word order sounds less disturbed at these levels than at lower levels. We can use this difference in both functional effect and level of language to listen for the varieties of the disorder and to research the underlying processes.

LOWER LEVELS

HIGHER LEVELS

Vocabulary

ACQUIRING WORDS

Vocabulary is the third set of impairments in expressive Communication Disorders, in addition to limitations and grammatical structures. This limitation in vocabulary may be interpreted as the result of another feature of expressive Communication Disorders: a difficulty in acquiring new words. The acquisition of new content words (nouns, verbs, adjectives, adverbs) takes place over an extended period in childhood and through the adult years. The grammatical, function words (articles, prepositions, auxiliary verbs, conjunctions, etc.) tend to be acquired early. It is the content words that are at stake and diagnostic for Communication Disorders. 'Difficulty in acquiring new words' describes a process. Impairment in the process is measured by range of vocabulary compared to speakers of the same age, intelligence, education and social setting. The limited range of vocabulary may be of the main verbs or nouns. Words (adverbs and adjectives) that typically enrich the meanings of main verbs and nouns may also be limited. In either case, the speaker gives us less specific information about the things and events in the world. A speaker who uses vocabulary that was acquired as a child such as 'tree', 'drink', or 'unhappy' in place of vocabulary that is generally learned later such as spruce, swallow, or gloomy restricts the range and the subtlety of meanings in interaction.

WORD FINDING

The features of word finding or vocabulary errors surface in various ways with different effects on interaction. Using the wrong words ('They found the cat', instead of 'They looked for the cat' or 'They wanted the cat') simply sends an unintended message. Delays before content words, presumably during word finding, produces unevenly paced or even disfluent speech. A word-finding difficulty is indicated by pauses occurring more often before content words than before grammatical, function words (for example, 'to', 'and', 'it', 'more'). Furthermore, the pauses would be expected before uncommon, infrequent words more than before common words. Expressive Communication Disorders can affect both vocabulary and grammatical structures. As a consequence, speakers with the disorder produce both subtle unusual meanings and completely uninterpretable utterances. These differences in effect may be produced by separate underlying processes or more general processes affecting different areas of language. The co-occurrence of the different atypicalities in language requires careful observation and ultimately rigorous study from two perspectives. First, regarding the individual as the unit of analysis, it must be determined if individuals have more than one of the different kinds of impairments. Second, it is important to determined how the impairments distribute relative to each other in a single speaker; for example, do the impairments in word-finding occur in the same utterances as the shortening of sentences or unusual word order?

A possible description or even explanation of expressive Communication Disorders is a slow rate of language development. This difference in rate may apply generally to all areas of language or perhaps separately to one or more areas. If true, the speakers with expressive Communication Disorders will sound younger than their chronological age, assuming that chronological age and mental age are similar in these individuals. However, it is possible that the impairments are different from delayed development. That is, the language may not reflect the normal developmental trajectory. This possibility of atypical language development must be investigated for each area of language.

Mixed expressive-receptive language disorder 4.3

4.3.1 Clinical features

		Table 4.2
Word level	Understanding and expressing beginnings and ends of words	
Clause level	Understanding and expressing connections between clauses	*Mixed expressive-receptive language disorder*

A mixed expressive-receptive language disorder combines features of expressive language disorder (see Table 4.1) with an impairment in reception of language (see Table 4.2). This combination complicates the problems of conceptualising the disorder and describing its linguistic characteristics. The disorder is ultimately defined as impairment in social processes, that is, the usual interference in academic, occupational or social interaction and achievement. The description of the disorder implicates certain causes in order to separate the disorder from other disorders with overlapping behaviours. Thus, for example, there is a discrepancy in language and non-verbal functioning since overall low functioning is indicative of retardation rather than a more specific impairment. Given the need for this discrepancy, special tests may be needed to establish the higher level of non-verbal functioning compared to the level of verbal functioning that is interfering with social processes.

Conceptually then, the disorder can be viewed as:

(1) one or more impairments in receptive verbal functioning;

(2) impairment in social functioning;

(3) a relation of these two possibilities to each other: that is, there are impairments in verbal processing that result in social impairments.

IMPAIRED SOCIAL
FUNCTIONING

This last formulation requires some exploration. Impaired processing may be impaired reception of sounds, words, structures or some combination of them. However, we would not notice these impairments unless there was some impaired social functioning. An impairment on a test of auditory processing could indicate some affected process that is variable in the population at large but not disruptive of behaviour. Furthermore, there may be kinds of processing (perhaps some unexplored areas of verbal memory or word patterning) that we can at present not test. If we cannot now identify the processing source of the impairment in social interaction, then we cannot establish the discrepancy between verbal and non-verbal functioning. A more general disorder, such as mental retardation or pervasive developmental disorder could then be considered. On the other hand, other specific impairments must also be excluded. For example, hearing impairment or a motor impairment affecting speech could appear as a receptive-expressive disorder. That is, there could be an identifiable explanation for the language behaviour that is external to the communication disorder.

Behind the notion of a discrepancy in functioning is the assumption that there are specific abilities that can be selectively impaired. This is a good working assumption that must, however, be examined and re-examined as the clinician learns more about the speaker. An individual who seems to have an impairment in language functioning should be investigated for a specific impairment. However, the failure to find a specific processing impairment that is tied to the impairment in language function is quite ambiguous; there may be a more general impairment or there may be an unidentified, untestable specific impairment. We start the treatment of mixed receptive-expressive language disorder from the phenomenon of failures in social processes (the academic and occupational impairments) rather than from possible causal explanations at the level of difficulties in processing.

4.3.2 Language features

WORD LEVEL

The expressive difficulties of receptive-expressive language disorder affect a number of levels of vocabulary and grammar. At the level of the word, there can be impairments in both understanding and expressing beginnings and ends of words (prefixes and suffixes) that carry meaning. For example, if an individual does not process the sounds represented by the '-ed' of 'walked' or 'talked', then the hearer will not understand important information about the time period mentioned. Similarly, if the 'un-' in 'unexpected' is not processed, there will be serious miscommunication. At the level of whole words, words such as 'fill' and 'file', 'accepted', 'expanded' and 'excepted' must be distinguished although they are close in sound. On a more semantic dimension, words like 'into' 'out of', 'far from' 'close to' must be separated and processed correctly both in reception and production. At a higher level

still, clauses are often combined with other clauses to express a range of
meanings. A speaker or hearer must encode or decode utterances such as
'If you go, then I want to go too' that present grammatical relations and
meaning in complicated ways. Consider that the statement could also be
worded as 'I want to go, if you go'. The hearer must processes the kind of
grammatical relation (conditional 'if-then'), the content of the two parts
of the utterance and the order of the two parts. Such relations apply to
many semantic connections (see Halliday, 1994: 215-73 for much detail
and Fawcett, 2000: 318-30 for a different view). To take another example, a
speaker may say any of:

> Get dressed after you eat.
> After you eat get dressed.
> Eat and then get dressed.
> Eat before you get dressed.
> Before you get dressed, eat.
> First eat, second get dressed.
> Get dressed after you have eaten.

Processing each of these utterances depends on understanding the ordering
of the segments and how connectors (such as 'before', 'after') are used. If the
receptive impairment is mild, then the speaker will come across few trouble-
some structures or semantic problems. That is, in actual social interaction,
few instances will lead to misunderstanding and the resulting behaviour that
indicates the misunderstanding. Sporadic odd behaviour may only indicate
that the receptive impairment concerns an infrequently used part of the
language. In these cases, careful testing may be able to discover the specific
underlying impairment: is the problem with passive sentences, temporal
connectors, negative sentences, etc.?

Individuals who show more severe impairments in behaviour may have more
severe receptive-expressive disorders in at least three ways:

(1) The impairment may be on more frequent structures or sets of words.

(2) The affected areas of language may be more important for communication.

(3) There may simply be more areas of language affected.

An impairment that affects the use or understanding of plural ('stores', 'books'
compared to 'store', 'book') and also of the '-ed' form of verbs ('walk-ed',
'talk-ed') could sound severe since these kinds of meaning are expressed
often. If the affected area is important for communication (such as positive
or negative clauses: 'they did*n't* leave'), then even if there are few occurrences,

the failure in communication will be clearly noticed. Obviously, if there are several impairments, then communication and the success of the social process are more likely to be compromised.

4.3.3 Distinguished from other disorders

There is a problem in discriminating these more severe receptive-expressive disorders from more general disorders such as retardation, hearing impairment and pervasive developmental disorders. As the reception and expression of language is more impaired, so is the failure to attain social goals. This failure then resembles the behaviour of individuals with these various other disorders.

We must also distinguish mixed receptive-expressive Communication Disorders from expressive Communication Disorder. The obvious difference in these two disorders is the additional comprehension impairment in the former. This difference, though, must be inferred indirectly in addition to the more direct evidence for an expressive disorder. The indirect evidence for the comprehension impairment is that individuals seem not to hear, not to pay attention, or to be confused when hearing something. The comprehension impairment is then conceptualised as another problem: not hearing, not attending or being confused. The evidence we have for this impairment in comprehension is the lack of properly contingent verbal behaviour. As described in Chapters 2 and 3, there are various sequences of utterances in interaction; e.g., question – answer, command – response, invitation – acceptance/decline. In these pairs of functions and more generally in the initiation – response pattern, individuals with a mixed receptive-expressive communication disorder do not take the expected verbal role and do not give the expected second slot in the sequence. The contingent behaviour may be either verbal or non-verbal but, in either case, is not appropriate. The response may be too little, too much or the wrong kind. If comprehension is poor, then the speaker fills the second slot in the sequence of conversational functions with irrelevant ideational meaning. This ideational meaning is carried by the content words. For example, if asked, 'What games to you play after school?' an ideationally irrelevant response is, 'We don't like our teacher. He has funny hats and talks too fast.' On the other hand, the interpersonal meanings may be affected, resulting in the wrong kind of response. For example, in response to the question about games, an individual could say 'Well why don't we go and buy some shoes' which is an offer to do something or perhaps an invitation. This utterance is inappropriate to the interpersonal role of giving information that the first utterance requires. It does not give information, relevant or not, in response to a request for information. To confirm that an individual has impaired reception of language, we must test different kinds of input: questions ('Where is your brother today?'), commands ('Bring me the games'), invitations ('Let's go for a walk'), expressions

IMPAIRED
COMPREHENSION

IRRELEVANT IDEATION

INAPPROPRIATE
INTERPERSONALLY

of emotion ('Wow, that's a wonderful idea') and a number of different topics (for children, for example, school, games, hobbies, friends). Furthermore, the structure of the input should be varied to determine if there are some kinds of vocabulary and grammar (e.g., passives, imperatives, complex commands) that the individual has particular difficulty comprehending. Direct assessment of receptive abilities can be done by standardised tests. The underlying assumption is that the difficulties evident in the test situation are the same as those in spontaneous interaction. The clinician can examine this assumption by comparing the clinical assessment, reports from teachers, co-workers and family to the standardised tests.

There are a few specific features of the language of mixed receptive-expressive Communication Disorders. The speaker may be very quiet or very talkative. These two extremes suggest that the mechanism(s) for determining an appropriate response can be affected. In either case, the clinician considers the amount of response in relation to the expected amount of response. A speaker with mixed receptive-expressive disorder may also have difficulty maintaining a topic. The evidence for this difficulty in maintaining a topic is:

(1) drift from one vocabulary set to another;

(2) changes in what is being spoken about by shifts in the pronouns tracking the objects, places and people mentioned.

There may be returns to the topic after minor tangents and distractions, perhaps encouraged by clarification questions from an interlocutor.

Phonological disorder   4.4

Phonological disorder is a communication disorder that affects relatively low levels of language: the sounds (see Table 4.3). The phenomena themselves are inaccurate use of speech sounds by substituting one sound for another, omitting sounds, adding sounds, not combining or blending sounds typically or not pronouncing sounds accurately. The diagnosis is based on excluding explanations from other sources. A phonological disorder is thus the presence of a difference in sounds without an alternate explanation. The alternate explanations include speech-motor difficulties, mental retardation, hearing impairment and environmental deprivation. It is not necessary that the phonological disorders also represent a single aetiology. In excluding other explanations and terming the residue a phonological disorder, we define a disorder that can in principle be reduced even further by new explanations for new subgroups of phenomena.

Table 4.3	**Inappropriate speech sounds from:**	Substituting one sound for another
Phonological disorders: language features		Omitting sounds
		Adding sounds
		Inappropriate combining or blending of sounds
		Inaccurate sounds

There can be extensive disruption in social processes if speech sounds are unintelligible. Speaking with strangers is particularly difficult, since close family and friends may have adapted to the phonological differences of a speaker with a phonological disorder. That is, strangers will hear the impairment more than those who frequently interact with the speaker, much like a foreign accent, that is heard more by strangers than those who know the speaker. Therefore, more formal and structured social processes in which speakers tend to be less familiar with each other are at greater risk for disruption.

In terms of the various levels of language, phonological disorders affect all levels equally. The sequence of turns in an exchange (e.g., question – answer) will be affected as well as the intelligibility of individual words. All of the ideational, interpersonal and textual meanings will be compromised. However, this broad effect on language from the single area of sounds also means that phonological disorders are not likely to be confused with other psychiatric disorders. The clinician will not confuse the general disruption of meaning from a phonological disorder with the more specific effects on meaning and social processes of other disorders. Quite simply, phonological disorders share few features of language with other psychiatric disorders.

4.5   Stuttering

4.5.1   Clinical features

As with other Communication Disorders, stuttering is a well-developed field on its own. The purpose here is to:

(1) show how stuttering interacts with presenting meanings and the patterning of language that can be affected in other disorders;

(2) show the effect of context on stuttering, since it is the effect on the social process that is of concern.

Like phonological communication disorder, stuttering is also at the level of sounds. However, stuttering interacts with situation and interacts with other language areas (see Table 4.4). In this way, stuttering is both more concrete in its expression than phonological disorders and more socially sensitive than phonological disorders. Stuttering covers a wide range of fluency and timing patterns in speech. It may even be more accurate to speak of classes of stuttering rather than one entity. The range of phenomena includes excesses such as repetition, circumlocution, interjections, prolonged sounds and extra stress and restrictions such as pauses. These phenomena, further, may occur at a number of levels, such as pauses within words or pauses between words, prolonged sounds or prolonged syllables, repetitions of sounds or repetitions of words.

		Table 4.4
Textual meanings	Given and new information signaled by intonation	*Stuttering: language features*
Interpersonal meanings	Repetition Interjection	
Ideational meanings	Circumlocution	

4.5.2 Textual meanings

Stuttering interacts largely with textual and interpersonal meanings rather than with ideational meanings. Stuttering particularly affects signalling information as given or new. When we signal information as given or new we are fitting the utterance into its context. We do this in part by taking into consideration what the other speaker may know. New information is usually signalled by sentence stress towards the end of the clause. This stress is physically a combination of pitch change, volume and pace. Stuttering, though, can change these physical characteristics by prolonging sounds thus making a syllable sound stressed and by using excessive physical tension in producing a syllable. The syllables or words receiving stress as a result of the stuttering are then heard as 'new' or even as surprising (contrastive stress). If the stuttering occurs towards the end of sentences, then it is likely to interfere with stress that signals new information. The message of new or contrast will be even stronger if the stressed element is early in the clause. For example, the ideational message of 'THEY arrived yesterday' is that the hearer knows that someone arrived and that the people identified by 'they' are known. However, the stress on 'they' means that, contrary to expectation, it was these people who arrived. If the stutter on 'they' contributes unusual stress, then this subtle interpersonal message will be sent when it is not appropriate for the context. Similarly, if stuttering produces a stress is on 'n't' in 'They didN'T receive the package yesterday', then the message will be heard as 'I think that it is surprising to you that the package did NOT arrive'. Again, this may not be the appropriate message in context and the hearer will wonder why the speaker sent such a message.

4.5.3   Interpersonal meanings

As well as textual meanings, stuttering affects interpersonal meanings. One of these meanings is the speaker's estimate of how clear the message is for the hearer. In repeating words or even syllables, the speaker is telling the hearer that the speaker thinks these speech elements were not heard clearly. It is as if the speaker repeatedly announces, 'I think you have not heard what I said so here it is again'. Similarly, pauses may be interpreted by the hearer as extra time to interpret the speaker ('You probably need more time to take in what I said'). Interjections add yet a different kind of interpersonal meaning, 'I want to tell you about my attitude to the ideational meaning presented'. For example, in the utterance 'I saw the *well* greatest television programme last night', the interjection 'well' helps intensify and emphasise what follows. If such interjections are added to utterances, they add extra meanings that again may neither be intended nor appropriate to the context.

4.5.4   Ideational meanings

CIRCUMLOCUTIONS

In addition to textual and interpersonal meaning, ideational meaning may be affected by the use of circumlocutions in stuttering. Circumlocutions may be produced to avoid words that are long or complicated or words with sounds that are difficult for the speaker. These circumlocutions may facilitate the smooth production of words, however, at the cost of avoiding the most usual and expected expression. The reaction of the hearer may then be 'This is an unusual way to word the utterance. What special meaning is the speaker intending by using this wording?'. As with other departures from typical patterns of using language, the hearer searches for some reason for the wording and the meaning it carries. When there seems to be no special purpose for the wordings and meanings, then understanding of the interpersonal and even ideational, meanings is compromised.

4.5.5   Effect of context

As outlined, stuttering interacts with the textual, interpersonal and ideational metafunctions and may affect those meanings. Stuttering also is sensitive to the context of the speaker and the utterance. To explore this effect of context requires considering how language is related to context by field (the topic of the language), mode (the channel of communication) and tenor (the roles of speakers). See Chapter 2 for details of these concepts. Stress and anxiety may exacerbate stuttering. The stress and anxiety may derive from different aspects of the situation. The field may be one cause of anxiety. If the topic is about school grades, for children, or occupational performance or rewards for adults, then there is likely to be more anxiety. The channel of communication may also induce anxiety. A telephone conversation may induce less anxiety than speaking to a group face-to-face. That is, the mode used to communicate may create anxiety and the consequent stuttering. Lastly, the roles of the speakers can influence stress and anxiety. When speaking to a superior in the social context, then there is naturally more anxiety. For example, teacher – student, boss – worker, clinician – patient and police officer – motorist roles are all asymmetrical and may cause stress in the junior partner. Even on a micro level, taking the role of answerer or receiver of an order to do something can induce stress. On the other hand, pretend interaction with inanimate objects or verbal interaction with animals is unlikely to induce stress and anxiety since there is little feedback and little evaluation of the speaker's interaction.

Stuttering, in summary, can interact with other patterning of language to affect textual, interpersonal and ideational meaning. This range of meanings, when affected together, can seriously impair the social processes of the individual with stuttering. Furthermore, the effect of a number of elements of context may exacerbate the stuttering just when it is socially most necessary to be easily interpretable. For each individual, the effects on the metafunctions need careful study to assess and then mitigate the consequences of the stuttering. Similarly, close study of the context, including the field, mode and tenor factors can identify causes of stress and anxiety that induce stuttering in some individuals.

Chapter 5 contents

Pervasive developmental disorders

Overview of pervasive development disorders   5.1

Pervasive developmental disorders are defined by three kinds of severe and pervasive impairments: impairment in reciprocal social interaction skills, impairment in communication skills and stereotyped behaviour interests and activities (Table 5.1). These impairments are closely tied to the failure to achieve social goals. Language is usually used to make things happen in the social world, to attain our social goals. When these social goals are not accomplished, language is usually responsible. The speaker has just not used language in a way that effectively gets things done in the world. Of course, the underlying deficit is not in the use of language but it is in language that we see the deficits. There is a set of skills and behaviours that are impaired that lead to the overall poor social functioning. We do not attribute the impairment in the skills in terms of the phenomenology to an intrapsychic state, such as poor Theory of Mind, or to some other concept such as mood, contact with reality, associative or memory processes. Although more abstract concepts may be explanatory in pervasive developmental disorders, they should not be part of the description of its diagnostic features. Rather a thorough understanding of the communication and language behaviour of those affected is needed to construct hypotheses about the underlying impairments and lead to insight into the biological substrata.

Table 5.1	**Impaired social interaction**	Impaired peer relationships
Pervasive developmental disorders: clinical features		Impaired spontaneous sharing
		Lack of social or emotional reciprocity
		Impaired non-verbal skills
	Impaired communication skills	
	Stereotyped behaviour, interests and activities	

5.2　　Clinical features

SOCIAL INTERACTION

The three impairments in social interaction skills, communication skills and stereotyped behaviour and interests are 'middle-level' categories, middle-level between the level of the disorder and the level of diagnostic criteria. Each of these impairments compromises achieving social processes. The first impairment, 'impairment in social interaction skills', attributes the failure in social processes to the individual's not knowing what to do in a social situation. We can understand this 'not knowing what to do' by considering an individual who is parachuted into a foreign culture and cannot determine what must be done. It could even be that the individual does know what must be done (e.g., getting food) but does not know how to do it; for example, is food obtained by exchanging beads, pieces of tree bark, greetings, promises, etc. A less extreme parallel is entering into an unfamiliar religious ritual, even within one's own language and social group. An individual may not know whether one is to bless, receive blessings, enter into a religious act by speaking, or by remaining silent, etc. An individual with a pervasive developmental disorder may act like such a religious novice in the most ordinary of social situations. We attribute the unusual behaviour to the impairment in social interaction skills.

COMMUNICATION

As well as an impairment in social skills as just discussed, pervasive developmental disorders are characterised by impairment in communication skills. This diagnostic criterion attributes the failure in social processes directly to the communication of the individual. In a word: the communication does not advance social processes.

STEREOTYPICAL BEHAVIOUR

The third major impairment is stereotyped behaviour, interests and activities. This impairment is the replacement of typical behaviour, with unusual behaviour. Typical behaviour is reduced or eclipsed by the stereotyped, idiosyncratic behaviour. The individual displays less of the typical and more of the unexpected verbal and non-verbal behaviour. Conceptually, then, we take the criterion of 'stereotyped interests' as an explanation of some verbal and non-verbal behaviour: the individual says certain things and behaves a certain way because there are underlying stereotyped interests. Our objective later in this chapter is to identify the language that leads to conclusions of stereotyped interests.

The three middle-level categories are not on the same level of abstraction. A hierarchical relation among the categories is proposed later in this chapter. The three impairments of impaired social interaction, impaired communication skills and stereotyped and idiosyncratic behaviour are manifested by a variety of more specific diagnostic criteria. Since autistic disorder includes all three of these impairments, the discussion starts with this disorder.

Autistic disorder   5.3

5.3.1   Social interaction: clinical features

The first characteristic of autism is impaired social interaction. We notice impaired social interaction since some individuals do not seem to accomplish the social processes usually found in the community. The social processes may be as simple as meeting a new neighbour, saying hello to a passer-by, or buying a newspaper or as complex as buying a house or voting in an election. Those individuals with autism characterised by impaired social interaction do not use verbal and non-verbal signals to accomplish the social processes within the community. There can be an underlying disturbance in social ability that produces the lack of social reciprocity and social accomplishment. Yet more basic precursors may be difficulties in understanding the demands of certain situations, difficulties in cognition or perhaps other IMPAIRED COGNITION underlying factors. These individuals may have a developmental delay in comprehension or expression and perhaps in reading the interaction signals of other speakers. We need not see social and cognitive impairments as separate entities, one causing the other. It is certainly easy to conceive of a cognitive impairment in memory, perception, association or production as a cause for an impairment in social functioning. However, the reverse is possible: a social impairment blocks cognitive development by blocking IMPAIRED SOCIAL involvement in those environments that lead one to learn from functional ABILITY communication and social experience. The position taken here is neutral to a single causal direction. Rather, both kinds of causation can be accepted and their operation can be simultaneous or even interacting.

Clinically, the impairment in social interaction is composed of four sub-categories, in fact, the diagnostic criteria:

(1) impairments in peer relationships;

(2) impairments in spontaneous sharing;

(3) impairments in reciprocity;

(4) impairments in non-verbal behaviours (Table 5.1).

These subcategories are at different levels of analysis. The failure to develop appropriate peer relationships (Feature 1) may be brought about by and identified by lack of spontaneous sharing (Feature 2) and lack of reciprocity (Feature 3). Furthermore, the individual's use of language leads us to identify all of: impairment in peer relationships, spontaneous sharing and social and emotional reciprocity (see Table 5.2). Similarly, the impairment in non-verbal behaviours is how the clinician identifies the other impairments. That is, the impairments in non-verbal behaviour are parallel to the impairment in language: an impairment in a signalling system used to construct social interaction. The four diagnostic criteria for impairment in social interaction are discussed in turn.

Table 5.2	Clinical feature	Language features
Pervasive developmental disorders: impaired social interaction – language features	Failure to develop peer relationships	what is spoken about: field language fit with channel of communication: mode relationship among speakers: tenor linguistic reactions of interlocutor initiations and responses with others
	Lack of spontaneous seeking to share	lack of initiating speech roles lack of 'giving' and 'information' meanings combined (especially in a range of contexts)
	Lack of social or emotional reciprocity	lack of expressions of emotion (attitudinal epithets, expressive stressed intonation) lack of second turn of adjacency pair in sets of turns lack of follow up moves lack of continuity with ideational meaning of other speakers inappropriate coding of information as 'given' and 'new' infrequent repetition of other speaker's words

5.3.2   Social interaction: language features

Failure to develop peer relationships

The first specific diagnostic criterion of impaired social interaction is a failure to develop peer relationships appropriate to the individual's developmental level. As indicated above, this social impairment arises from impaired spontaneous sharing, reciprocity and non-verbal behaviour. To explore the evidence for impaired peer relationships (see Table 5.2) we return to the model of language as a set of choices or potentials, some of which are used at specific times and in specific contexts. There are culturally typical interactions that individuals have with their peers. In particular, there are kinds of activities that an individual 'can do' and kinds of meanings that can be expressed ('can mean' possibilities). In practice, a list can be drawn up of activities appropriate to a particular culture and age group. If a child's activities are not typical of the peer group, then peer relationships will not be developed. When a speaker says about an activity that it 'is most of my time out of the house', the activity should be assessed in terms of how typical it is for others in the same situation. More subtly, a speaker may 'mean' differently from the peer group. For example, if a speaker sounds too formal or pedantic because of the choice of formal vocabulary ('I desire to' instead of 'I want to'), then the speaker will not sound like his or her peers. Notice that the language can contribute to the lack of peer relationships and also be a marker of that lack.

To determine the failure to develop peer relationships, the clinician must consider the relative frequency of certain language behaviours. Some language characteristics in autism occur more frequently than usual (for example, slow or pedantic speech) while other language characteristics occur less frequently than usual (for example, age and culture appropriate slang). In a clinical setting with no interaction among peers, it is difficult to determine such atypicalities in frequencies. Similarly, just asking about specific interactions may not be enough to assess an individual's peer relationships. By asking the child directly about social activities, asking parents and caregivers about social activities and even by asking about specific activities at specific times ('How did you spend the weekend?'), the clinician can get a fuller picture of peer interactions. Some of this picture is then built from direct observation and some from the speaker's reports of activities.

FREQUENCY OF BEHAVIOURS

There are several specific aspects of a speaker's language that indicate poor peer relationships. Largely, the issue is how the speaker's language fits into the situation. At stake are the following aspects of language: field, mode and tenor. The 'field' is the kind of material that is spoken about and that is

SPEAKING IN CONTEXT

centred on social activities. For example, children at each age have activities that form the basis of peer interactions. If a child has an atypical interest (for example, the colour of subway cars or the texture of surfaces), then the language will focus on that interest and exclude activities more usual for the peer group. 'Mode' has to do with the channel of communication. Face-to-face conversations, group interactions and telephone interactions, for example, each reflect different kinds of peer relationships and require different language. 'Tenor' concerns the relationship between speakers. Language encodes whether an interaction is formal or informal, aggressive or relaxed and the roles taken by the speakers. A child who adopts an atypical role, such as being the boss of peers or perhaps of consistently being the junior member of relationships, uses language to enter into these roles. In fact, to close the circle, language largely creates such social relationships. These three aspects of language (field, mode and tenor) can each reflect a speaker's poor peer relationships.

To assess possible departures from field (the kind of material for an interaction), tenor (the interpersonal features of language) and mode (the channel of communication), the clinician ultimately considers the wider notions of culture and genre. Any given use of language, no matter how repetitive, pedantic or stereotyped, may be reasonable in the proper context. The underlying issue of unusual or absent peer relationships arises when language does not map onto the specific situations and social processes.

SPEAKING ABOUT PEERS

As well as looking directly at the language in social interactions with peers, the clinician can examine how an individual speaks about peers. Does the speaker spontaneously speak about activities with peers? Can such talk be elicited? It is important to note that an individual who speaks about restricted kinds of interaction or is repetitive may have another characteristic of pervasive developmental disorders: repetitive and stereotyped behaviour (see below). Such restricted speech may, on the one hand, focus on peer relationships or, on the other hand, limit talk about peer relationships. Even when an individual does speak of peer relationships, the variety of interactions and the kinds of social activities can indicate that peer relationships are atypical. For example, an individual may speak about only one aspect of relationships, such as clothing, or may speak only of certain kinds of interactions, such as what happens in one classroom or on one school trip.

REACTIONS OF PEERS

In addition to the social interactions with peers and what an individual explicitly reports about peer relationships, there is a third source of information for poor peer relationships: the reactions of peers to the individual. An atypical prevalence (either more or less than expected) of arguments, loss of friendships, long telephone conversations or interactions in a particular locale could indicate that peers regard the individual as being not part of the group, of being an 'odd' kid.

To conclude the discussion of peer relationships, we must note that in pervasive developmental disorders the overall pattern of peer relationships is atypical. This atypicality may be found in different ways. There may be a series of language and interactional features that together indicate the impairment. In other cases, one linguistic feature may impinge on features in both language and in interaction more generally. For example, infrequent initiation of interactions limits the number of social processes that the individual is involved in, further limiting the development of peer relationships. Even though the pattern of peer relationships is atypical in pervasive developmental disorders, it must be stressed that there may be wide variability of language and social behaviour in the community itself. Within this variability, children with pervasive developmental disorder themselves are quite a heterogeneous group in terms of the social interactions and peer relationships.

Lack of spontaneous seeking to share

'Lack of spontaneous seeking to share enjoyment, interests or achievements with other people' (American Psychiatric Association, 1994), as a characteristic of pervasive developmental disorders, is social behaviour that upsets the usual pattern of interactions. Initiating in a conversation without being explicitly prompted is one part of interacting. Who initiates and under what circumstances may vary with social roles and across different cultures. In some cases, teachers initiate but students do not, while in other cases it is the reverse. However, an individual who does not initiate has a restricted inventory of social behaviours that results in rather imbalanced social roles and social interactions. The lack of social initiation may reflect restricted verbal and non-verbal behaviour. The non-verbal behaviour may include not approaching others and not establishing the eye contact that is a precursor to verbal interaction. The linguistic aspects of lack of spontaneous seeking to share are outlined below (see Table 5.2).

INITIATING
INTERACTION

In terms of language, we find the lack of spontaneous seeking to share in the interpersonal meanings (see Chapter 2): the meanings concerned with the roles speakers take in interaction. Most clearly, individuals who do not seek to share information are failing to combine the social role of 'giving' (as opposed to 'demanding') with what is being given: the information at stake. Since the impairment is in 'spontaneous' sharing, the speaker may give

INTERPERSONAL
MEANINGS

information after another's questions. Specifically, however, the speaker does not give information when not asked for it, in other words, in contexts in which some other speaker has not previously taken the role of 'demanding' information. Since the sharing may involve non-verbal material as well (for example, showing a new gift or pointing out objects in the environment), the impairment may be generally not giving either information (through language) or goods and services (mainly non-verbal) spontaneously.

CONTENT-BASED
INITIATION

To take the analysis of language to a lower and more specific level, the speaker who is not spontaneously sharing may be attending (that is, creating the conditions for interaction) and so responding to greetings and to calls from others and may even initiate greetings and calls. However, when it comes to more content-based interactions, the speaker just responds to the initiations of others and rarely initiates on a matter of substance. Naturally, the amount and kind of initiation expected depends specifically on the context and social processes. Only in some social activities is it typical for a child to spontaneously share interests or ideas. For example, an adolescent would not be expected to spontaneously share information of poor grades or poor athletic performance with peers, especially of the opposite sex. That is, the field (subject matter of the social interaction) and the interpersonal relations normally influence variability in spontaneously sharing and so must be taken into account. For the listener, one clue of impairment is finding little initiation in a wide range of contexts. In these cases, the impairment is characteristic of the speaker instead of merely a variable characteristic of language in situations. However, the more the situation calls for sharing information, the more the absence of the sharing is noticed. In summary, then, there is a 'hole' in the distribution of speech functions since certain content-based initiations are largely absent. The speaker is using only a restricted range of the socially possible and typically expected speech functions.

STARTING EXCHANGES

SHARING

To detail yet further the lack of spontaneous seeking to share and to help identify it, consider the kind of information that is not being shared. Depending on the age of the speaker and the situation, the material that is not being shared may be verbal information (what can be directly shared through language, e.g., a story about what happened at school) or non-verbal goods and services (objects or actions, e.g., an offer to start playing a game or an offer to share a meal). In addition, the problem may be either in the spontaneity or in the sharing. These two aspects are expressed somewhat differently in language. If the issue is spontaneity, then, the gap in the speech functions will be in starting certain kinds of exchanges. On the other hand, if the issue is sharing, then we would expect that the elements missing in language include getting the attention of others ('Mary, George, come over here'), certain social activities that necessarily involve sharing (e.g., games that involve a number of players), language that indicates that the speakers share social space (e.g., slang, expressions that signal knowing a game or activity) and signals of the speaker's attitude (e.g., absolutely, you bet, certainly, usually). Of course, the aspects of sharing and spontaneity should come together in speech and their absence at the same time helps to indicate that the speaker is not involved in an important part of social interaction.

Lack of social or emotional reciprocity

If the previous category of 'lack of spontaneously seeking to share' speaks mainly of initiation in interaction, the current category involves the reaction of the speaker and how the individual builds interaction with others. In social processes, we typically find careful coordination of verbal and non-verbal behaviour such that even short delays or overlaps are noticed and can be exploited for humour or sarcasm. Such coordination is context sensitive. There may be rapid coordination in waiter-customer interactions (Customer: I'll have my egg with toast; Waiter: White or brown toast; Customer: White, please) but a slower and more deliberate interaction in a bank when withdrawing a large amount of money (Cashier: How do you want it? Customer: I'll take it half in 100s and half in 1,000s; Cashier: That will be 40 100s and four 1,000s, right? Customer: Right.). The speaker must identify the cultural and situational norms and perform the required on-line processing to produce coordinated interaction with others.

The notion of reciprocity involves the mutual construction of social processes: action by action, utterance by utterance. The speakers must each contribute different moves to the interaction and through the moves (e.g., offer services, provide services etc. in the above examples) build up exchanges that accomplish the social processes (the food is ordered, eaten, paid for, etc.). Also inherent in reciprocity is echoing the role of the other speaker. If an individual only takes one role (initiating or responding) in interaction but not the complementary role, then the interlocutor will feel that the interaction is one-sided. For example, if one speaker provides all the specific information, asks all the questions, or provides all the emotional content, then the other speaker may feel that the first participant is not reciprocating. At a lower level of analysis, if one speaker regularly repeats or clarifies the actions and language of the other, but there is no repetition or clarification by the second speaker, then there will be a lack of reciprocity: one speaker will be doing all the interactional work of a certain kind, repairing misunderstandings.

MUTUAL ACTIVITY

In autism, there is a lack of reciprocity in social and emotional interactions. The social reciprocity is engaging in activities sanctioned by the cultural. This coordination among individuals is crucial to many activities and its absence leads to the devastating social impairment in autism. Both the exchange of information and the exchange of goods and services are affected and thus a wide range of social activities is not accomplished. Specifically, the lack of reciprocal emotional interactions involves a subset of information that is rarely exchanged. That is, speakers rarely speak of emotional topics. These topics, as with field (the institutional focus or topic of talk) in general, are identified by sets of content words; here, emotional ones. In addition, these speakers may infrequently use expressive intonation that usually carries emotional state (e.g., 'We REALLY liked that movie'). Aside from the direct use of language to convey emotions, language can accompany non-verbal expressions of emotions. For example, when comforting a friend by touching, there may be words of comfort ('There, there things will be better', 'It's not so bad', 'I know you must be feeling awful about it'). Thus verbal and non-verbal signals, alone or together, may indicate the absence of emotional reciprocity.

CONTENT WORDS

INTONATION

There are specific linguistic features that mark the lack of social or emotional reciprocity in autism. These features are found in a number of areas of language. This is the case since the difficulty is in how the speaker coordinates different aspects of language in context. The lack of coordination is most noticeable in those parts of the interpersonal functions of language whose normal role is to build interaction. Therefore, as we have seen above, the interpersonal structures of speech functions, moves and exchanges are particularly at risk. To identify this diagnostic feature, the listener's attention should be centred on these interpersonal aspects of language (see Table 5.2b, a part of Table 5.2).

Table 5.2b *Linguistic features of 'lack of social or emotional reciprocity'*	**Lack of social or emotional reciprocity**	Lack of expressions of emotion (attitudinal epithets, expressive stressed intonation) Lack of second turn of adjacency pair in sets of turns Lack of follow up moves Lack of continuity with ideational meaning of other speakers Inappropriate coding of information as 'given' and 'new' Infrequent repetition of other speaker's words

However, the listener hears the lack of reciprocity in other aspects of language as well. The ideational function largely encodes the institutional focus of the interaction including what is being talked about. If a speaker does not follow up on the subject matter of the other speaker, particularly if that subject matter is emotional, then the interaction will lack a reciprocity that may slow or stop the interaction. Similarly, language constructs messages in terms of what the other speaker is assumed to know or not know (coding given and new information in the textual function). If a speaker does not make the correct assumptions, then there is no reciprocity in terms of which information is regarded as shared.

Aside from the three metafunctions of interpersonal, ideational and textual, language can signal lack of reciprocity at the low level of how meanings and functions are worded. Typically, a speaker repeats the words of another speaker as well as repeating grammatical structures. It is a sign of coordination ('Do you want *supper* now?' '*Supper*, for sure!') and wordings ('He really *thinks he's great!*' '*Thinks he's great*, does he?'). If such repetition is infrequent, then the speaker is signalling common ground less than anticipated. At worst, we hear the lack of repetition as one speaker repudiating the wording or meaning of the other. In response to 'Do you wanna play cards now?' 'No. I don't like cards' (with a repetition of 'cards') sounds more reciprocal than 'No, I'll get bicycles'. A speaker who repeats words is showing that he or she has interpreted the other speaker appropriately. If a speaker hears his or her words being repeated, then the speaker feels that the two speakers understand each other and their roles in interaction. However, with little repetition, one starts to doubt that the speakers are building the same social process.

WORDINGS

5.3.3 Communication

As indicated, autism is characterised by the three middle-level categories of difficulties in social interaction, communication and stereotyped behaviour. There are four basic kinds of impairments in communication. These impairments in communication overlap with and to an extent, signal the impairments in social interaction of autism.

Delay of spoken language

The first specific impairment in communication is a delay or lack of development of spoken language with no effort to compensate by developing an alternative communication system (Table 5.3). The underlying and fundamental issue is that there is no evidence of a desire to communicate. The assumption is that there are two deficits: (a) the means of communication (mainly, language) which is separable from (b) social interaction. However, the major evidence for impaired social interaction is, in fact, the impaired communication. Communication, verbal or non-verbal, is a prerequisite for social interaction. The normal social development of the profoundly deaf, or those with severe physical impairments of the speech apparatus show that the social interaction is the necessary characteristic of individuals without autism and that the communication can be largely non-verbal. However, we do not have to establish either social interaction or communication as primary; the mutual dependence just must be appreciated. In pervasive developmental disorders, the delay in spoken language is evidence for the impaired means of communication rather than evidence for the result of the impaired communication, the impairments in social interaction. Nevertheless, the clinician must also determine that there is no alternate means of communication (an elaborate non-verbal signalling system) that would indicate a desire to communicate. The evidence must then be no spontaneous communication by whatever means, no social approaches that are the basis for needing a communication system.

Table 5.3	Clinical feature	Language features
Pervasive developmental disorders: impaired communication – language features	Delay of spoken language	No evidence for wanting to communicate No non-verbal approaches to communicate No non-verbal signalling system
	Impairment in initiating conversation	Infrequent demanding of information, goods & services Infrequent initiating of exchanges Infrequent wh-questions, yes-no questions, imperatives
	Impairment in sustaining conversation	Lack of second turn of adjacency pair in sets of turns Lack of response speech functions Inappropriate coding of information as 'given' and 'new' Infrequent use of pronouns to continue participants Infrequent conjunctions to develop messages Infrequent repetition of vocabulary of self and others
	Stereotyped language	Fixed language expressions (nominals, verbs, adverbs, etc.) Imitated expressions from others
	Repetitive language	Repetition of content words, repetition of longer phrases
	Idiosyncratic language	Fixed and unusual openings and closings to interactions Fixed and unusual vocabulary
	Lack of make-believe and social imitative play	Infrequent use of nominals, verbs, adjectives to encode unreal things, events and qualities of the world Infrequent copying of speech roles and vocabulary of others

Impairment in initiating or sustaining conversation

A second impairment in communication, in addition to delayed or lack of development of communication, is an impairment in initiating or sustaining conversation. Although the impairment is stated as an 'inability' to initiate or sustain conversation, we draw a conclusion about ability from our observations of language. The question is which specific language behaviours provide us with the evidence for this impairment. Initiating conversation and sustaining conversation involve different features of language and will be outlined individually. As indicated for impairments in social interaction, initiating in conversation derives mainly from the interpersonal function of language and involves constructing the appropriate speech functions, moves for each utterance and exchanges of utterances from one speaker to the next (see Table 5.3a). The grammar of utterances is also at stake since one would expect as initiating moves, wh- questions ('Where will they find them?'), yes-no questions ('Did they find them?') and imperatives ('Leave!'). That is, these grammatical structures form the related speech functions of requesting information and ordering. If there is a general impairment in initiating in conversation, then this impairment will be found in a variety of these grammatical patterns. At another level, the level of context, we would expect to find the failure to initiate rather generally across situations rather than just in specific situations.

Impairment in initiating conversation	Infrequent demanding of information, goods and services	Table 5.3a
	Infrequent initiating of exchanges	
	Infrequent wh-questions, yes-no questions, imperatives	

Table 5.3a

Pervasive developmental disorders: impairment in initiating – language features

A social consequence of relatively fewer initiations in conversation is that other speakers decide on the social processes and also then the institutional focus, including the subject matter of the conversation. At a basic level, other speakers determine the flow of information and 'goods and services'. Initiation is also mapped onto social roles. If a speaker initiates infrequently, then the speaker will take fewer social roles. For example, a speaker who infrequently initiates will only infrequently be the organiser of a new game or the leader of a new social activity. Overall, the lack of initiation in conversation may also contribute to the impression of personality characteristics (shy, passive, etc.).

LIMITED SOCIAL ROLES

As well as initiating, in autism there can be an impairment in sustaining interaction. We notice an impairment in sustaining conversation by noticing that less language is semantically connected and operative in social context. Conversation is sustained by building conversation on what the other speaker has said or on what the current speaker has said earlier. In each case, the speaker must be able to understand how the social process is unfolding and contribute appropriately. It follows, therefore, that if the speaker does not typically sustain the conversation, then the social process

IMPAIRED SUSTAINING INTERACTION

itself will not be accomplished. In particular, the speaker must contribute to conversation in a way that recognises the stages (generic components) of the social process. If, for example, there is a conversation about events at school, there are typical components that may be added: how a similar event happened to the speaker, the background to the event just described by another speaker, what someone else said about the event at the time. If a speaker contributes unexpected or apparently unconnected information, then the social process of describing, evaluating or developing the event will not be completed. Furthermore, there may be negative social consequences for the individual who appears to end the development of the conversation. If adding inappropriate information is not the difficulty, but rather the speaker does not contribute at all, then the speaker may be left out of the social process as others develop the interaction. As well as seeing the impairment as one of communication, some individuals may not have learned the social processes or how they are implemented by language. That is, the failure to sustain conversation may be the linguistic consequence of other impairments. In this latter case, we must consider a general impairment in social interaction.

SUSTAINING IDEATION

SUSTAINING TEXT

The specific linguistic evidence for not sustaining conversation is found in the three functions of ideational (the subject of the interaction), interpersonal (how the language establishes the relationship between speaker and hearer) and textual (the relation between the language and the context)(see Table 5.3b). That is, different kinds of meanings indicate that conversation is not being sustained. In terms of ideation, a speaker must continue to talk about the institutional focus that is present in the conversation. If the conversation is about school grades, teachers, weather or clothing, then the speaker should likely stay within the same realm. Interpersonally, if an exchange is being developed ('Do you know George?' 'Which George? Sam's friend?' 'Yeah, I saw him yesterday'), then the speaker should advance the typical exchange structure rather than abruptly end it. The textual function is concerned with how one stretch of language relates to another and to the non-verbal context. For example, conversation is sustained by using pronouns ('they', 'our', 'it') that signal that the speaker is talking about things the hearer knows about. The textual function also encodes information as given and new by using word order and intonation. A speaker uses given and new information to build a conversation utterance by utterance, signalling what the hearer is expected to know and signalling to the hearer which information is expected to be new. In summary, the inability to initiate or sustain conversation is primarily a statement about the linguistic elements used for interaction. As outlined, by not using some of these linguistic elements speakers with autism speak with gaps in the meanings. As well as gaps, there can be an overabundance of other meanings. These meanings and how they are worded are the evidence for the diagnostic criterion.

		Table 5.3b
Impairment in sustaining conversation	Lack of second turn of adjacency pair in sets of turns	*Pervasive developmental*
	Lack of response speech functions	*disorders: impairment*
	Inappropriate coding of information as 'given' and 'new'	*in sustaining – language*
	Infrequent use of pronouns to continue participants	*features*
	Infrequent conjunctions to develop messages	
	Infrequent repetition of vocabulary of self and others	

Stereotyped, repetitive and idiosyncratic language

A third characteristic of the impairment in communication (after the developmental impairment and the difficulty in initiating and sustaining conversation) is stereotyped and repetitive use of language or idiosyncratic language (see Table 5.3). There are three characteristics here: stereotyped, repetitive and idiosyncratic that separately and together create poor communication and help produce the impairments in social interaction. These three characteristics can apply to almost any functional component of language. That is, if repeated or used in unusual ways, almost any functional element will sound noticeably odd.

A speaker who favours certain sets of recurrent meanings creates the impression of stereotyped language. These sets of meaning may be those that recur for the individual speaker such as set phrases ('you really oughta have been there', 'you really oughta have seen it') or set kinds of meaning (e.g., much hedging: 'I *thought of doing* it', 'I *may* have done it', '*Probably* did it'). Stereotyped speech may also involve imitating sets of meanings from the culture, such as a famous politician, television personality, or sports figure. A speaker may adopt set phrases ('You don't say', 'Well I bet') or, more extensively, set patterns of meaning (e.g., commands: 'We oughta do that', 'Let's start now', 'Let's get going', 'You do X and I'll do Y'). In more limited cases, speakers may imitate language from another context making the current speaker sound pedantic, scholarly, or out of a science fiction description of another civilisation.

Sometimes a speaker may use set phrases over and over giving the impression of repetition rather than of stereotyped language. That is, if specific words and grammatical structures are used, the hearer will immediately be struck with the similarity of the expressions. The speaker will be saying the same things, whether or not the meaning is the same. For example, 'I know' has various meanings such as a hesitation marker (parallel to 'Um', 'Let me think for a second'), a statement of cognition (parallel to 'I am convinced that') and a term of agreement (parallel to 'I agree that you are correct'). However, even if a speaker intends 'I know' with different meanings, merely using the same phrase will sound repetitive. In addition, repeating the same vocabulary root morpheme, even in different forms (e.g., rent, renters, renting, rented, rent out), will give an impression of repetition. In terms of the processing involved, repetition may indicate that the speaker is tied to the sounds of words rather than the meanings they convey.

Idiosyncratic use of language is noticeable and may disturb the flow of conversation. However, such language is nevertheless interpretable in context. Language may be idiosyncratic:

(1) in the meanings chosen;

(2) in the way those meanings are worded (e.g., President Kennedy's phrase 'I would like to say this about that', instead of many other possible wordings such as, 'I would like to comment on what you say').

For example, a speaker may always try to initiate a conversation by asking a personal question, or by asking a question that is too personal or inappropriate (e.g., 'Why did you come over here to visit us?' 'Where did you abandon your children yesterday?' 'Did you get to play with Kim yesterday afternoon?'). An individual may typically use such openings rather than the full variety of patterns in the speech community. As mentioned, idiosyncratic language is not too different from the typical language in the speech community and as such is interpretable. The reaction of the hearer will not be 'I do not understand' but 'This is the way this speaker often sounds' and/or 'This is somewhat of an odd way to say things'.

Lack of make-believe and social imitative play

The fourth kind of impairment in communication is a lack of varied, spontaneous make-believe play or social imitative play. As with the previous impairment of stereotyped, repetitive and idiosyncratic use of language, this criterion is a specific type of social behaviour that is characteristic of the disorder. Communication is involved since both verbal and non-verbal communication are typically part of make-believe and imitative play. The social activities themselves are defined as 'varied' and 'spontaneous' and so the hearer expects to find these characteristics in an individual's interactions. In terms of the use of language, the two kinds of social behaviour (make-believe play, social imitative play) are rather distinct. In make-believe play the speaker uses language to construct a reality that is not physically real (being the captain of a space ship, a dragon or a movie star) and to engage others in the world being created. Social imitative play, on the other hand, requires copying patterns of language from one established context into another context. In both cases, we do not find the use of symbols during play. In the usual case, though, these symbols gather meaning by being referred to by language ('This is the magic tree. When you touch it you can't be taken prisoner'). Individuals use language in all these cases to construct a reality that is usually not assumed. The participants use language, as well as non-verbal signalling to some degree, to build a temporary shared reality.

The four impairments in communication:

(1) delayed or lack of development of communication;

(2) impairment in initiating or sustaining conversation;

(3) stereotyped and repetitive use of language;

(4) lack of make-believe or social imitative play;

all contribute to a middle-level category of impairments in social interaction. As well as impairments in social interaction and impairments in communication, a third middle-level category characterises autism: markedly restricted repetitive and stereotyped behaviour, activity and interests. This overall category is in large part realised through language. That is, language is a clear, observable phenomenon that accompanies or creates the activities and interests that are repetitive or stereotyped. When the repetition of language seems to be the main factor, then the problem is interpreted as a problem in 'communication'. However, even if the repetition is non-linguistic, there may still be aspects of language that are repetitive. The repetitive stretches of language may be used to direct the hearer's attention to the non-verbal repetitive activity. For example, an individual who speaks about playing cards may also repetitively shuffle or count cards. Since repetition, both verbally and non-verbally, is so noticeable, it has an immediate effect on the successful construction of social processes.

5.3.4   Summary

The clinician finds three middle-level categories of impairments in communication, social interaction and repetitive behaviour to be distinct although they are closely interrelated in terms of language. There may be common components of cognitive processing underlying these categories. For example, being insensitive to macro or micro contexts of social interaction, or having a restricted inventory of verbal behaviours could be the underlying cognitive impairments that are observed as problems in social interaction, or more specific problems in communication. Since autism need not include a general intellectual delay, there may be a subset of cognitive functions underlying the specific social and linguistic impairments, rather than an overall cognitive deficit.

From the perspective of language, we must try to understand autism in terms of how it sounds, regardless of the known or unknown substrates and the specific diagnostic categories. In the speech community, the issue is: what part of a speaker's interaction and language creates a specific impression? There may be a hierarchy of features. If the language seems interpretable, then we see the problem as one of social interaction rather than 'communication'. Similarly, if the behaviour and specifically the language behaviour, is repetitive, stereotyped or idiosyncratic, then we think of the 'repetitive, stereotyped or idiosyncratic' category rather than, more generally, the categories of impairment in communication or impairment of social interaction. Furthermore, a number of atypical verbal and non-verbal characteristics may be aligned to create the impression of impairment in communication or repetitive-stereotyped behaviour. It is this alignment of a number of characteristics that creates the impression of the middle-level categories. At the extreme, the alignment of numerous impairments in communication results in no spoken language at all. If there is less alignment of various difficulties, then there may be language but perhaps specific impairments in initiating and/or sustaining conversation. In terms of the overall impression of a speaker's language and interaction, some characteristics are very noticeable; for example, unclear reference in schizophrenia, or first and second person pronoun reversals in some speakers with autism. Other characteristics may contribute to the overall impression but not be immediately identifiable (for example, atypical stress patterns in some speakers with pervasive developmental disorders). The clinician must be aware both of the separate language features that are at risk and how the features line up with each other to create more or less severe symptomatology and social impairment.

5.4 Asperger's disorder

5.4.1 Clinical features

Asperger's disorder is defined as the characteristics of autism without the specific impairments in communication. Nevertheless, we find language that leads to the middle-level categories of impairments in social interaction and repetitive stereotyped behaviour as well as some specific problems in language different from those in autism. These include a clinically significant delay in language development. In any case, the impairments in communication in autism are not so noticeable in Asperger's disorder and do not characterise the disorder. The social interaction is nevertheless at a low level but with, perhaps, sufficient language resources to accomplish some social processes.

We must then reconsider the interrelation of the three middle-level categories of social impairment, communication impairment and repetitive activities for Asperger's disorder. A central question is: what is an impairment in social interaction without an impairment in communication/language? Although social interaction is created by language, in Asperger's disorder, the potential for communication is present in terms of the vocabulary and grammar. However, speakers do not use these resources to build social interaction. Some of the time, the use of language is repetitive, stereotyped or idiosyncratic and for those reasons does not build the expected social interactions. In Asperger's disorder, compared to autism, there is less alignment of the atypical uses of language. For both Asperger's disorder and autism the non-verbal signals are not used typically and thus contribute to the impairment in social interaction and repetitive behaviours. However, the greater verbal abilities of vocabulary and grammar in Asperger's are not exploited normally. That is, language that typically is used to create social interaction is used but seems to fail in its primary function. Rather, language seems to parallel the non-verbal signalling system in that both fail to create social interaction and both may be repetitive, stereotyped and idiosyncratic. With no clear and strong vocabulary or grammar impairment in Asperger's disorder, attention will be focused on the stereotyped and repetitive behaviour of the disorder as it unfolds in the construction of interaction (see Table 5.4). This stereotyped and repetitive use of language replaces more typical and functional language, compromising the speaker's contributions to social processes.

Clinical feature	Language features
Stereotyped language	Fixed language expressions (nominals, verbs, adverbs, etc.)
	Imitated expressions form others
	Fixed intonation patterns
Repetitive language	Repetition of content words, repetition of longer phrases
	Repetition of grammatical structures, intonation patterns

Table 5.4

Pervasive developmental disorders: restricted repetitive, stereotyped behaviour, activities, interests – language features

5.4.2   Language features

STEREOTYPED
LANGUAGE

Stereotyped language is the language specific to a particular speaker. It is repeated unusually often. For example, some speakers may talk about aeroplanes or weather patterns (certain subjects of interest), may be stereotypic in asking questions or making comments about the world around them (aspects of the interpersonal function), or may consistently sound as if they are speaking from a written text (aspects of the channel of communication). At yet a lower level of analysis, we hear these stereotypes as repeated vocabulary items, repeated grammatical structures or intonation and repeated patterns of stress and vocabulary that sound formal or 'written'. The denser the atypical features of language, the more disruptive the stereotyped language seems.

REPETITIVE
LANGUAGE

Repetitive language, as opposed to the stereotyped use of language, involves a wider range of activities. In stereotyped language, it may be easy to identify the speaker: 'That is John, since he always talks about trains', 'That is Mary since she always asks the same kinds of questions'. However, for repetitive language, the speaker may repeat any issue or repeat various meanings, wordings or intonation. Since language accompanies many non-verbal activities, an individual who repeats activities or actions may nevertheless use repetitive language at the same time. For example, if a child has specific routines such as dressing in a certain way or eating in a certain way, then there may be accompanying repetitive language. Similarly, the preoccupation with parts of an object may be associated with repetitive language concerning those parts. We can distinguish speakers with Asperger's disorder who have such repetitive speech from other speakers with pervasive developmental disorders who may have more general problems in communication.

In Asperger's disorder, language itself reveals the impairment in social interaction and/or the restricted, repetitive and stereotyped behaviour. The language is not a serious impairment of its own. There is a problem of interpretation here. We may find that the perception of intact language in Asperger's disorder is in comparison to the obvious and striking problems that other speakers with pervasive developmental orders have in social interaction and repetitive behaviour. If these two impairments are less severe, then the observer notices that language does function to some extent but that language also expresses the two other impairments: social interaction and repetition. If the impairments in social interaction and repetition are very severe, then we see that language is also involved, since the speakers can hardly accomplish any social goals. We relate the impairment in communication to the other impairments. It is quite possible that the language atypicalities in Asperger's disorder are different from those in other forms of pervasive developmental disorders such as high functioning autism in which there is also some use of language. Research is needed to explore what aspects of language are associated with the subcategories of restricted, repetitive and stereotyped patterns of behaviour and what aspects of language are central to the general impairment in communication found in autism. In particular, then, a difference may emerge between the impairment in autism of initiating and sustaining conversation and the lack of make-believe or social imitative play.

Chapter 6 contents

Attention Deficit Hyperactivity Disorder

Overview of Attention Deficit Hyperactivity Disorder 6.1

Attention Deficit Hyperactivity Disorder (ADHD) is widely diagnosed and is one of the few disorders of childhood that is also widely treated by medication. The clinician uses both language and non-verbal behaviours to recognise the disorder. In fact, both verbal and non-verbal behaviours are part of the definition of the disorder as we will see below. Although there is no specific evidence, the verbal and non-verbal characteristics may be correlated. ADHD is made up of various cross-cutting diagnostic categories. Furthermore, the disorder has substantial co-morbidity with a number of other disorders including anxiety disorder, conduct disorder, mood disorders and language impairments. At the moment, the clinical community sees ADHD as a conceptual entity with much co-morbidity. However, even if this conception is modified, the following account in terms of language remains relevant since the analysis dwells on the diagnostic criteria, specific features and the middle-level categories of inattention, hyperactivity and impulsivity. The phenomenology is always present despite the various ways the features may be combined.

This chapter outlines the characteristics of ADHD in terms of the language that is indicative of the disorder, the three middle-level categories of inattention, hyperactivity and impulsivity and the specific diagnostic criteria within each of these middle-level categories.

As our examination of the diagnostic criteria for ADHD shows, language is used in establishing the diagnostic criteria (e.g., butts into conversations) but we do not take language to be causal in any manner. The language is not the cause of the disorder, whether in terms of hyperactivity, inattention or impulsivity. However, language is critical for monitoring the activity of individuals with ADHD and particularly important in indicating the effect of medication or other treatment.

In terms of language, the clinician and others have the impression that children with ADHD talk more than normal. This main observation is associated with the overall impression of children who seem to be moving more than usual, active more than usual and still or quiet less than usual. Teachers and parents seek assistance because of these impressions. The individual seems to have unaccomplished or disturbed social processes. Obviously, in a non-social context, children who are more active than usual are not disruptive. To narrow the task, we must understand how the language and other behaviours are noticeable and disruptive. It further follows that the language of children with ADHD seems excessive against a background of the usual role of language in context. This argument leads to considering the typical use of language as a control measure. As with other disorders, this normal control is the implicit intuition that the speech community and the clinician bring to observing children. For ADHD, the clinician's task of observation is especially difficult because of the range of co-morbidities. In particular, the co-morbidities also present us with atypicalities in language. For example, conduct disorders and language impairments implicate language implicitly and explicitly, respectively. We use two approaches below to explore the relationship of ADHD to language that both derive from the clinical view of the disorder:

(1) exploration from the concepts that are used to explain the verbal and non-verbal behaviour; namely, inattention, hyperactivity and impulsivity;

(2) exploration of phenomena as laid out in the diagnostic criteria.

The clinician will find the familiar categories explored one by one.

Clinical features   6.2

The categories of inattention, hyperactivity and impulsivity are middle-level between the level of the disorder and the level of individual diagnostic criteria. These categories group the diagnostic criteria, since each criterion appears under only one of the middle-level categories. The middle-level categories are used to explain the specific criteria and behaviours in the following way. Inattention, for example, includes nine symptoms or specific diagnostic criteria. These nine symptoms are the operational definition of inattention. Implicitly, there is a common cause for these nine symptoms: lack of attention, a cognitive concept. To extend the model, we can see the middle-level categories as hypotheses of neuropsychological functioning. The hypothesis is that there is a process or entity corresponding to a middle-level category that is perhaps affected by treatments. We explore in detail below the diagnostic criteria in each middle-level category. We are interested in the functional characteristics of language for each diagnostic criterion. This exploration of language helps us to understand the middle-level categories as hypotheses of neuropsychological functioning as we build bottom up from the language to the diagnostic criteria and further upwards to the middle-level categories.

MIDDLE-LEVEL CATEGORIES

Language features   6.3

6.3.1 Inattention

Inattention, the first middle-level category, covers a number of observations about behaviour. A central concept is engagement with aspects of environment. When the engagement is limited or shifting, then inattention is said to be the cause. Language is particularly important in assessing this engagement since we create social activities mainly through language. We can view the impairment in social activities, that is the criterion for a psychiatric disorder, as either a gap in the social activities themselves or in terms of the cognitive process of inattention. The purpose here is to understand the behaviours that are taken as evidence for inattention and then to examine how specific parts of language create these behaviours. The concept of inattention itself is not directly at stake. A broader or narrower notion may eventually be needed to explain the phenomena in ADHD. That endeavour will depend on much

ENGAGEMENT WITH CONTEXT

neuropsychological data across various contexts and include both language and non-verbal behaviour. Here, we explore the phenomena relating to engagement with the context that tend to co-occur in the behaviour of a set of individuals, largely children, who have ADHD.

Sustaining attention

There are several individual criteria grouped as inattention. The observation that the individual 'often has difficulty sustaining attention in tasks or play activities' is quite wide and implicates a number of language factors (see Table 6.1). The key concept is the 'sustaining' of attention. We can temporally put aside the neuropsychological aspect of attention as an explanation. What remains at the level of behaviour is 'sustaining' conceptualised as consistency of activity. We must see this consistency within the social situation, since the language should reflect consistency in terms of the social process.

Table 6.1	Clinical feature	Language features
Attention deficit hyperactivity disorder: inattention – language features	**Sustaining attention**	Jumps in social processes Jumps in stages of social processes Changes in topic of interaction (ideation) Unannounced changes in things, people, events, location, time
	Focus on interaction	Topic of interaction (ideation) • changes in things, people, events, location, time Interpersonal focus • inappropriate second pair in adjacency pair • inappropriate responses to initiations • inappropriate level of certainty Compatibility with context – textual focus • incompatibility of 'new', 'given' by intonation, word order • incompatibility of starting point (theme) by word order • changes in things and people by inappropriate pronouns • changes in things, people, events by not repeating vocabulary • infrequent use of earlier information by ellipsis/substitution
	Follow through on activities and other non-verbal indicators	Direct expression of incompletion of activity Inappropriate response speech functions to exchanging goods and services

Social process

The social process itself is one overall entity. For example, playing a game, finishing an academic task in the classroom, or returning a borrowed article may be activities that reflect consistency of purpose, material objects and perhaps time and location. Lack of consistency will result in the incompletion of the social process. The clinician or lay observer may attribute the incompletion to the individual's inattention, a cognitive approach, or lack of sustained engagement with the environment, a behavioural approach.

INCOMPLETION OF SOCIAL PROCESSES

To take the approach from verbal behaviour, social processes are composed of stages or subcomponents that are usually produced in order (see Ventola, 1987). To continue the examples above, a game may have stages such as selecting teams, determining the rules and establishing the starting time or event. An academic task may have stages such as determining the goal, assembling the materials needed, checking if the goal has been met and receiving assessment. Returning a borrowed article may involve determining the owner, locating the owner, determining if the owner wants the article returned (perhaps it is to regarded as a gift) and delivering the article. Each stage of a social process can have its own consistency. Therefore, lack of consistency is at risk even for rather short stages of social activity. In terms of language, each stage of an activity has its own consistency of language. For example, when enquiring who owns a borrowed item, the language will be in past and present time rather than in future time. A child may say 'Did you give it to me?' 'Was it the blue one or the brown one?' 'Did you give it to me in a bag?' 'Is it yours or your sister's?'. The enquiring will also tend to be in major clauses with a process (e.g., from the above examples 'give', 'was', 'give', 'is') rather than, for example, elliptical 'yes', 'no' or 'well'.

STAGES OF SOCIAL PROCESSES

The criterion for 'sustaining' is the socially accepted amount of consistency given the age and social position of the speaker and given the demands of the social process. If there is not enough sustained activity, verbal or non-verbal, then the social goal will not be attained. It is a common complaint that children with ADHD do not complete school assignments or do not finish errands. They start the activity but shift to some other activity before all the stages of the first activity are finished. A child starts an activity in one book but then starts watching some friends, becomes involved in a discussion about another activity or just picks up a different book.

Children regularly engage in staged activities at home and in school. These situations are conventionalised in that there are frequent staged activities such as work and play patterns in school and household tasks that involve other members of the household. Staged social activities by their nature flow from one component (greetings, statement of process, trying to accomplish process, etc.) to another. The individual must constantly update a personal map of dos and don'ts as the social activity unfolds. For language, the stage of the activity influences how an utterance will be interpreted. If at the stage of greetings, an individual says, 'We are going to play this new game', the speaker can be interpreted as inattentive in not continuing the greetings. Rather, the speaker is jumping to another stage. At a later stage in interaction, the same utterance will not seem to be inattentive, unengaged or inconsistent. The more flexible the activities are, then the less the child with inattention will stand out. That is, we will notice less the shifting and the incompletion of activities. Ultimately, though, the child is evaluated by the achievement of social processes. This criterion of sustaining attention is further specified as 'often has difficulty sustaining attention in task or play activities'. Here again there is an implied normal range of consistency for social processes. Two particular social processes are specified: task or play activities. These processes largely derive from the home and school situations mentioned. From the point of view of language we are interested in what aspects of language create consistency in the social processes and what aspects of language indicate that the consistency is less than we expected. The linguistic evidence may be at a number of levels. At the most abstract level, lack of consistency involves language that jumps from one social process to another. That is, there are components of social processes that must be ordered and completed to achieve the social goal. For example, in a team game, there are the components of dividing the players into teams, assigning the players to specific roles or locations, establishing the rules, agreeing on the starting point of the game, etc. An individual must be present and correctly order the components. If these components are not accomplished or misordered, and they are usually accomplished largely through language, then the social process will not take place. There will be no game. From the cognitive perspective, such a breakdown could be attributed to failure 'to sustain attention'.

Topic of interaction

At a somewhat less abstract level than the entire social process, when a speaker changes the institutional focus, evident as a change in the topic of conversation, the clinician may conclude that individual is failing to sustain attention (see Table 6.1). Even within a single social process, such as buying a dessert, if the speaker moves unusually quickly or suddenly from one kind of item to another or from one aspect of the item to another aspect (from flavour to cost, for example) then the speaker does not seem to sustain attention. For example, 'Well, I want a chocolate one, no a chocolate one with sauce, with vanilla maybe with two kinds of sauce no, does it cost more with another flavour? Does it cost more here or across the street?' Jumping

JUMPS IN TOPIC

from speaking about flavours to speaking about cost and then again to costs in another store creates the impression of attention. One or two jumps in attention do not identify a speaker as failing to sustain attention. A consistent pattern of such behaviour does, though, disrupt social processes and makes the clinician suspect impairment in attention. It must be pointed out again that the frequency and amount of change is measured against the expected changes for peers in the same situation.

The specific language features that indicate the changes in social processes are vocabulary shifts that signal a change in topic (in the earlier example, the change from 'chocolate', 'vanilla', 'sauce' to 'cost', 'cost'). Different combinations of conversational moves also signal that a speaker is shifting unusually to a different social process or a different part of a social process (for example, discussing the roles for players in a game before the teams have been chosen). Even focusing on a new part of the physical environment ('What's that over there?') can disrupt an ongoing social process. In all these cases of shifts within or across social processes, the language is a rich and subtle source that indicates if an individual is on-task.

VOCABULARY SHIFTS

The linguistic evidence for sustained attention is inherently based on unusual frequencies of features of language rather than on language that is qualitatively different from what we expect. That is, the 'sustaining' characteristic is a description of a consistency in language and non-verbal activity. There is a change in frequency of language features, rather than the presence of extraordinary language features such as vocal tics. The threshold for the change in frequencies is the degree that it is 'maladaptive and inconsistent with developmental level'. Consider the following interaction of a teacher (T) with two seven year-olds (P and N).

T: do you agree? What does that have to do with math?

P: oh I forgot math [I'd rather play ball now]

T: you were thinking of writing.. OK think about shopping

P: uhh uhh [are they coming to play now?]

T: when do you need math when you're shopping?

P: oh when you need some pencils and a rubber and something else [balls and shoes are what I need to play with now]

T: how do you use math when you're shopping?

N: oh it's easy you bring a math book with

P: [let's go play now]

The utterances by P have had material added to them (in brackets [ ]) to show how language can pull the conversation in a new direction and indicate lack of attention. The last utterance explicitly attempts to cut off the social process (discussing the practical use of mathematics) that the teacher is developing.

Focus on interaction

As well as difficulty sustaining attention on tasks and play, the clinician notices inattention when an individual 'often does not seem to listen when spoken to directly'. The individual is inattentive since he or she seems to be processing other stimuli or perhaps no stimuli. There may be non-verbal indications of such inattention, such as looking away from the speaker, flat affect, or body movements unrelated to what the interlocutor is saying. However, there is a rich set of verbal clues that lead to a conclusion of inattention to what another is saying. The linguistic evidence for not listening or hearing when spoken to directly involves the three functions of ideational, interpersonal and textual linking of language to the context. In general, a speaker must mesh the three kinds of functions to contribute appropriately to ongoing activity. Each of these functions is outlined in turn. Aside from direct evaluation of an individual's language, in a naturalistic context, the clinician can gather important evidence by listening to the other speakers in the interaction. If other participants repeatedly ask questions, or give orders to the affected speaker, then one infers that others in the social situation think that the individual is not participating appropriately.

Topic of interaction – the field

OFF-TOPIC NOUNS,
VERBS, ADJECTIVES

A clear indication that a speaker is not listening is that the individual speaks off-topic. It is the content words in language, the nouns, verbs and adjectives, that encode information about things and events in the world, establishing ideational continuity from one speaker to the next. If an individual is not listening, then it sounds is as if the two speakers are drawing their meanings from separate, only slightly overlapping, sets of meanings. The affected speaker may continue with his or her meaning without acknowledging the different ideational focus of the other participant(s). Again, it will be mainly the nouns, verbs and adjectives that do not overlap. We particularly notice off-topic speech when the structure of the interaction tightly constrains what a person should say. For example, after an invitation ('Can you come over later?'), an acceptance ('Sure, when?') or decline ('Not today.') of the invitation is expected. After a greeting ('Hi'), a response to the greeting ('Hi') is expected. If something else is said, the listener appears not to be listening or, perhaps, intentionally ignoring the speaker.

Interpersonal focus

As the last example shows, ideational signals interact with the interpersonal, interactional patterning to create the impression of inattentiveness. At the level of conversational interaction, one speaker must generally say things that are contingent on another speaker's talk. For example, if a question is asked, then we take the next utterance by the other speaker as being relevant to the question even if it is not a direct answer. Similarly, a statement by one speaker is usually followed by a statement by another speaker that supports or challenges that first statement. A statement that is unrelated may indicate that the speaker was not listening. The point is that utterances are grouped into sets of exchanges such that there is a dependency of one kind or another from one speaker's contribution to the next. If this conversational dependency is lacking, then the speaker will not appear to be listening. We feel the lack of connection since any individual will, at a minimum, contribute the right kind of contingent utterance whether or not this second speaker is accepting the content of the first speaker's utterance.

CONVERSATIONAL DEPENDENCY

More subtly, but still interpersonally, a speaker must contribute to an interaction by relating to the level of certainty expressed by other speakers. A speaker who asserts that it is raining outside is usually responded to differently than one who 'suggests', 'thinks' or 'guesses' that it is raining or says something like 'It is *probably* raining'. In the following stretch of conversation, two students 'P' and 'N' ('T' is the teacher) use verbs such as 'should', 'have to' and 'won't' and the expression 'you know' to indicate how strongly the statements are to be taken. If the conversation then continues without such interpersonal signals of uncertainty, as indicated by the last utterance (Q), then there is a change in interpersonal tone from 'do you hear my suggestions and ideas' to 'this is what I have to say'. We hear the speaker as inattentive to the interpersonal meaning of the other speakers and perhaps not listening.

P: when you go shopping you *should* never wish for clothes because you always *have to* wish for food

T: tell Norman

P: I was first you *should* always get food before 'cause when you run out of food then you *won't* got and that's more important than toys

T: so what do you think?

P: and money isn't everything *you know* Norman

[Q: money goes a long way… it gets you what you want … it is much better than anything else]

In all of these cases of interactive or interpersonal signals, the clinician must carefully consider the language of both speakers. It is only in relation to what the other participant has said that the affected speaker's contribution indicates lack of listening. If there are pairs of utterances that usually form an exchange, such as question – answer, greeting – response to greeting, or invitation – acceptance/decline, then the clinician must notice if the first utterance in the set must be repeated or explained. Furthermore, there may be back channel utterances that clarify ('Is that what you meant?' 'What?') and confirm ('Sure', 'Ah ha', 'You're kidding') what was said. These clarifications and confirmations give clues to how well the speaker was listening. At yet a more obvious level, attention-getting devices such as calling the speaker's name or raising one's voice to the speaker indicate the lack of attention. The clinician must thus carefully consider the interactional roles and contributions of both speakers in order to conclude that there is inattention to what is being said.

Compatibility with context – textual focus

The third kind of meaning we must notice in considering inattention, in addition to the ideational and interpersonal meanings, is the compatibility of the language to the verbal and non-verbal context: textual meanings. This area of meaning includes what the speaker decides to encode as given information (usually at the beginning of a clause) and what to encode as

NEW INFORMATION

new information (usually at the end of a clause or with intonational stress). If a speaker presents some information as 'new' when that information was just mentioned, then it will seem that the affected speaker was not listening. For example, if one speaker says 'John is doing his arithmetic homework in the bedroom' then we will usually assume that that information is available to those that heard the statement. If such a hearer then says 'JOHN is doing his homework' (with added emphasis on 'John') then this statement is interpreted as meaning that 'John' is new information and that the other hearers are assumed not to know this. In other words, it seems that the speaker has not heard or taken into consideration what the first speaker said. The emphasis on 'John' can, though, be interpreted as surprise that it is John (rather than George) who is doing homework. In this case, it is the unexpected identity of John that is 'new', not merely the information that it is John who is working. We hear such subtle misunderstandings and incompatible signals as signs that the speaker is not attending or is awkward in communicating. As such messages from the speaker are repeated, others in the context will feel that the speaker is not attending to the issues of the social processes (the 'given' information) and is not then extending that strand of information. We can add emphasis (in CAPITALS) to certain words of an earlier example, to change what is expressed as 'new' information in order to make the speaker sound as if he is not attending to the other.

> P: when you go shopping you should never wish for clothes because you always have to wish for food
>
> T: tell Norman
>
> P: I was first YOU should always get food before 'cause when YOU run out of food then you won't got and THAT's more important than toys

With emphasis on 'you' and 'that', the speaker is signalling these pieces of information as new or contrastive when they do not otherwise seem to be. If repeated, the speaker sounds out of touch with the conversation. This disconnection could be attributed to inattentiveness.

Similarly, a speaker who does not use pronouns to continue what another   PRONOUNS
participant has said will seem to be not attending to the language of others. For example, after the statement 'John is doing his arithmetic homework in the bedroom', a speaker may say either 'I haven't seen *him* work so hard in months' or 'I haven't seen *John* work so hard in months'. In the first utterance, when 'him' is used, the speaker is displaying that he or she has heard the utterance of the first speaker and is implicitly drawing on it to identity 'him'. In the second utterance, the use of 'John' stands independent of what the other speaker has said. It is as if the speaker has not heard the other participant's earlier utterance. In the following interaction between a teacher (T) and a seven-year old (S), there are a variety of devices that link back to the teacher's contribution, indicating that the seven-year old attended to what was said. In the second version of this passage these signals of attending (in *italics*) have been removed to create an example of being out of touch with the teacher.

> T: you were talking about different countries maybe you could tell me about some of the other things that happened last night (International Night at the school)
>
> S: like um ... a person ... that *they* took a hat and *they* stuck it out um *they* only took ah money to have a party for for *the teachers* because they made up *International Night* and like they took up a hat for *the teachers* who made up *the International Night*
>
> [S: like um ... a person ... a hat was used ... it was stuck out ... took money to have a party for some teachers because they made up a play and money was collected for teachers who made up the party]

Another linguistic device that signals appropriate attending to other speakers is ellipsis (see Chapter 2). Ellipsis can only be used successfully when the individual is attending to other speakers. In response to the question 'They use these things today?' a student replied 'Um no'. The use of 'no' is interpreted as ellipsis of the full clause: 'No they don't use these things today'. When attending is compromised, such ellipsis will not make sense or convey the wrong message ('That was very nice Doug, don't you think so?' 'No' (I don't have any pencils here).).

As with pronouns, the signalling of 'given' and 'new' information and the use of ellipsis, if a speaker fails to repeat some of the words of other speakers, gives the impression that these other speakers have not been heard. In the following example, there is repetition (in *italics*) of vocabulary across speakers that signals attending. Repeating vocabulary words signals that the speaker has heard what was said and is even acknowledging and accepting the wording of the interlocutor. When the repetition is reduced (as in the altered version in brackets [ ]), the language is again distanced from the interlocutor with the possible explanation that the speaker is not attending.

> T: what do you like to read Lois? What is your very favourite book?
>
> L: um well about those *read*ing *books* [um well about those home activities]
>
> K: well I mostly like adventure *books* [well I mostly like adventure games]
>
> L: cat *books* [cat activities]
>
> T: why do you think Kim likes adventure books Lois?
>
> L: mm because she really likes to *read* them [mm because she really likes to look at them].

These several cases of linguistic markers from the textual metafunction (using given and new, pronouns, ellipsis, repetition) signal not hearing another person. The affected speaker does not continue the language of another speaker. We may hear this discontinuity in a number of different areas in language. It could be that some speakers show the discontinuity in one way and other speakers show the discontinuity in another way.

Follow through on activities and other non-verbal indicators

Still within the inattention characteristic of ADHD, an individual may often 'not follow through on instructions and fails to finish schoolwork, chores, or duties in the workplace'. The interactional evidence for this diagnostic criterion is largely non-verbal. However, there may be some evidence in language. The signals will be language that is incomplete in achieving the social process. As well as the direct expressions of incompleteness ('I do not want to finish this', 'This is too hard to finish now', 'I'm going to do something else'), individuals use language to accompany tasks. This accompanying language will track the completion of the task. Negotiations over the purchase of an item or the enquiries about whether tickets are available for a specific film are largely done by language. The completion of the expected language patterns indicates the completion of the social process. Even when language is only used with some essential components of the social process, such as when playing a game of ball or doing household chores, then language may still signal the incomplete social process ('You can't leave now', 'That is not what I said to do', 'There is more to be done after that', 'Let's finish this job first', 'Remember what you should do next').

The other diagnostic criteria that form the inattentive category include: difficulty organising tasks, dislike for tasks with sustained mental effort, losing necessary objects, easily distractible and forgetful. Again, these criteria may be evident in language by the overt expression of the difficulty ('Not history again', 'Oh where is the ruler', 'I can never find my red socks'). The language of distractibility may be more indirect by referring to extraneous, outside stimuli. For example, after an interruption from a telephone call, the individual may not return to the topic at hand, or may say 'Where was I?' In any case, the social process is interrupted. The interruption may be noticeable (a telephone ringing, noise from outside the immediate context) with the speaker then not returning to the interrupted social process. Other, focused, speakers may complete the interactional exchange, the utterance or even the phrase they had started before the interruption. In the following example, speaker A returns to the topic and speaker B follows the return as well. If speaker B had started discussing the content of the announcements (as in the altered version in brackets [ ]), then the outside stimulus would have led to a distraction.

A: What do they do that's different or what do they have that's different from our country?

B: well um they usually do war um they do war all the time and

(school public address system gives announcement)

A: all right we just had a little interruption do you want to continue with what you were saying B?

B: well I think I've forgotten when I was listening to the announcements
[well I think that we should stop school early and all go to the game or go home]

A: I think you were talking about different countries …

Inattention, in general, is characterised as how the affected speaker says something after the contributions of others. The most extreme case is of not responding at all when a contribution is expected. The less extreme cases, the speaker says something that does not adequately fit with what has gone before, leading to the conclusion that the speaker was not attending to the social process as it was unfolding.

6.3.2 Hyperactivity

RATE OF SPEECH

We now move from the first general category, inattention, to the second general category of ADHD: hyperactivity (see Table 6.2). The rate of speaking, quite simply the number of words per minute and shorter or less frequent pauses indicate hyperactivity. In particular, the pausing may be shortened either from utterance to utterance within the speaker's turn of speaking or may be shortened at the transitions from one speaker to another. We can feel the effect by reading the above examples rather quickly and especially by not pausing at the intuitively usual places at the end of clauses and at the end of utterances. Another aspect of the hyperactivity is the amount of talk. Speakers continue with what they are saying and seem to add more information than expected. They may add information by stringing conjunctions one after another ('and', 'but', 'or', 'then', etc. as indicated in *italics* below). For example, if the above conversation is extended as follows, especially if said rather quickly, it sounds as spoken by a child with hyperactivity.

AMOUNT OF SPEECH

> T: you were talking about different countries maybe you could tell me about some of the other things that happened last night (International Night at the school)
>
> S: like um … a person … that they took a hat *and* they stuck it out um they only took ah money to have a party for for the teachers *because* they made up International Night *and* like they took up a hat for the teachers who made up the International Night to thank uh to make a party for them *and* mis mister um *well* Mrs. S she got a bouquet of flowers *and* mister miss I don't know his name *but* he got a pack of chocolates *and* that's for the um the thanking for making International Night *and* um different countries people do different stuff than us *like* the Holland people they wear wooden shoes *and* Scotland people they wear funny dresses *and* these horns that they play …

A speaker who repeats vocabulary items gives the hearer the impression of going on rather longer than usual on the same topic. In the following brief segment, the speaker repeats 'you', 'your', 'ask', 'mother'.

I know what … *you ask your mother* un to um why don't *you ask your mother* if *you* could stay go … until June why don't *you ask your mother* and all that until May the 25th if *you* could stay in *your* proper house …

Even repeated grammatical structures (one statement, question or exclamation after another) indicate the excessive talk in hyperactivity. If the above passage is spoken with a questioning, rising tone on each statement, the repetition of the intonation and of the questioning meaning makes the passage sound even more hyperactive.

Clinical feature	Language features	
Difficulty playing quietly	rate of speaking loudness of speech amount of speech	
'On the go'	rate of speaking • few and short pauses domination of ideational meaning • things, people, events, details of events	

Table 6.2

Attention deficit hyperactivity disorder: hyperactivity – language features

Difficulty playing quietly

One specific diagnostic criterion for hyperactivity implicates a generally noisier child: 'often has difficulty playing or engaging in leisure activities quietly'. In these cases, language accompanying the activities is at stake. That is, the speaker is saying too much even when language does not necessarily accomplish the activities. This verbal excess is parallel to the excessive motor activity of these children. Although the clinician may not be able to directly observe the excessive verbal activity directly in a clinical context, informants should be able to accurately compare the affected child's verbal activity to that of peers.

'On the go'

A second specific diagnostic criterion describes the child with hyperactivity as 'on the go' or acts as if 'driven by a motor' or 'often talks excessively'. In these cases, the clinician primarily notices the interpersonal function of language. That is, another speaker finds it hard to contribute to the interaction since the affected speaker continues on without pausing or even signalling for another person to speak. There can also be an ideational component to this 'on the go' description of hyperactivity. If the affected speaker dominates the interaction in terms of the topic, then other speakers will hear the speech as excessive. A speaker dominates the topic of interaction by using restricted, narrowly focused vocabulary items. Furthermore, such items may be densely packed into utterances. The more these features of language coincide, the more the hearer will experience the talk as excessive. The following piece of a conversation between an eight-year old and a nine-year old girl shows how speaker L, the older girl, dominates the conversation and controls the topic of conversation by introducing and repeating vocabulary items ('play', 'ball', 'kid', 'come over', 'swing', 'fixed') related to one topic. Under some circumstances, this density of vocabulary items from one speaker may indicate the ideational dominance of a speaker who 'talks excessively' or who has language that seems to be 'driven'.

L: we we went on this we went out and we played on the swings and everything and we really had a ball um … oh ya like there's this rough kid next door you know … and he came over … and we sa we um … my sister she broke the swing she was sitting in it and then pow the swing fell you know and … then my sis and then my ah and then my friend fixed it but it wasn't that fixed you known and we called um … the little boy next door over and he really was so rough … and he came over and he and um … he … we said Col um … we said Colin that's the boy's name you know we said Colin try the swing oh it's beautiful … you know and so … cause but it was …

M: did he try it?

L: yes he tried it and he fell right on the floor … and then my friend fixed it again so that … he would fall again and she goes Colin come and um try the swing … it's really good now … I fixed it

M: how old was the boy?

L: grade one … and … so she we he went on it and he was he got pushed a little bit on the swing you know and then … pow … down he falls and then we called his brother over … he was the really really rough and … he was really light too and um he went on the swing and … and my girlfriend you know she put it in again and we said come on um I don't know I … forget the boy's name … but we … told him to come over and sit on the swing you know … and so he came over he came over and he sat on the swing and so uh

As with other descriptions of the language of psychiatrically affected populations, the clinician must establish the elements of the context that influence the atypical use of language. For hyperactivity in general and excessive talk in particular, the clinician must, in particular, consider the expected social roles of the speakers. In some contexts, speaking quickly or at length will not be unusual and will not be noticed. Similarly, some contexts typically have one speaker dominating the interaction. To consider another dimension, age or other markers of status may greatly influence how much a speaker contributes to an interaction. In some circumstances, the channel of communication (face-to-face, by telephone, one-to-one, or one-to-many, etc.) will influence how a clinician assesses excessive talk. Despite all these considerations, if the speaker's language still sounds excessive, then it is likely that the speaker himself or herself is more generally hyperactive. The more one finds different contexts with the excessive speech, the more general will be the impression of hyperactivity.

6.3.3 Impulsivity

After inattention and hyperactivity, the third basic characteristic of ADHD is impulsivity. Impulsivity is largely described in terms of the interpersonal function of language. Speakers who show impulsivity use atypical meanings in organising the turns of talk with other speakers. We hear impulsivity since the speaker is presenting meanings that interrupt and generally disturb the expected verbal flow. The most general diagnostic criterion is 'often interrupts or intrudes on others (e.g., butts into conversations or games)'. There are three linguistic characteristics of this criterion: overlapping, change in topic and initiating an exchange out of place (seeTable 6.3 and Appendix B). The impulsivity is especially noticeable when these three characteristics co-occur.

Clinical feature	Language features
Overlapping speech	interactants speak at same time
Changing topics	infrequent repetition of vocabulary infrequent pronouns signalling same things, people, place
Initiating interaction	frequent first pair partners in adjacency turns often expressed as question or imperative

Table 6.3

Attention deficit hyperactivity disorder: impulsivity – language features

Overlapping speech

Overlapping is the speech of one speaker simultaneous with the speech of another speaker. In the flow of interaction, overlapping is created when one speaker starts before another speaker has finished. In social interactions, there are predictable moments when another speaker may enter the interaction. A speaker can explicitly signal these moments ('Joan, what do you think about that idea?'). Other moments are signalled more subtly by a slowing of the rate of speech at the end of an utterance or by a pause. In any case, these possible points of transition from one speaker to another rarely come in the middle of a linguistic unit such as a phrase or clause. That is, the exchange structure of the interaction, intonation and grammatical structure all signal the likely moments of transition from one speaker to the next. When a speaker frequently overlaps at other points, then the speaker is not aware of, or is not using, such information and will be heard as interrupting or intruding.

POINTS OF
TRANSITION

The usual points for entering a verbal interaction are illustrated in the following section of conversation repeated from above:

1   L: we said Colin that's the boy's name you know we said Colin try the swing oh it's beautiful … you know and so … cause but it was …

2   M: did he try it?

3   L: yes he tried it and he fell right on the floor … and then my friend fixed it again so that … he would fall again and she goes Colin come and um try the swing … it's really good now … I fixed it

4   M: how old was the boy?

5   L: grade one … and … so she we he went on it and he was he got pushed a little bit on the swing you know

In this interaction, speakers start after the previous speaker has completed a clause. The exception is the transition between turn 1 and turn 2. Turn 1 ends with an incomplete clause ('cause but it was …'). However, speaker L pauses and speaker M enters the conversation without overlapping speaker L. In essence, speaker M enters during a pause. Since speaker L uses a number of incomplete linguistic units (e.g., 'you know and so…'), speaker M can assume that there will not be a competed structure this time as well. Speaker M's turn then sounds less intrusive than it could have sounded if speaker L was speaking fluently without pauses and incompletions. Turns 3 and 5 start appropriately in terms of the conversational structure since speaker M has asked questions that turn the floor over to speaker L. These questions also have a clear ending in terms of their clause structure. Nothing further is expected (in contrast to an incomplete question structure such as 'What do you think happened to…'). To create a sense of impulsivity, the example above can be read or acted with one speaker starting before the end of the previous speaker's turn creating overlap.

Changing topics

As well as overlapping, a speaker sounds impulsivity by changing topics during interaction. Topics naturally change when we speak. However, when a speaker unexpectedly and without notice changes topics, then the change sounds impulsive. Taking the above example and adding some off-topic utterances (turns 2a and 5a below) creates the sound of impulsivity. We recognise off-topic utterances since they will likely not repeat vocabulary items or use pronouns signalling that the same things are spoken about. In turn 2, 'he' refers to 'Colin' in turn 1 and 'it' refers to 'the swing' from the same turn. However, turns 2a and 5a do not have such references to elsewhere in the interaction.

1	L:	we said Colin that's the boy's name you know we said Colin try the swing oh it's beautiful … you know and so … cause but it was …
2a	M:	teacher, Kim took my hat
2	M:	did he try it?
3	L:	yes he tried it and he fell right on the floor … and then my friend fixed it again so that … he would fall again and she goes Colin come and um try the swing … it's really good now … I fixed it
4	M:	how old was the boy?
5	L:	grade one … and … so she we he went on it and he was he got pushed a little bit on the swing you know
5a	L:	put back my book … you thief

Initiating interaction

A third linguistic characteristic of impulsivity is using initiating turns, in contrast to responding turns. As outlined in Chapter 2, initiating turns (such as invitations, questions, offers) start an exchange structure that continues for a few utterances, requiring speakers to take turns and provide conventional meaning step-by-step. Specifically, initiating turns define the kind of response required from the other speaker: acceptance of invitation, answer to question, etc. A speaker is heard as impulsive who:

(1) often initiates turns;

(2) overlaps turns with other speakers;

(3) changes the topic.

The speaker cannot wait for an appropriate moment to take control of a topic in conversation. Turns 2a and 5a above are not only off-topic but also are initiation turns, 2a is a statement that implicitly demands an action from the teacher and 5a is a command that explicitly demands action from the hearer, another student. If turn 2a also overlaps with the previous turn, then the three linguistic characteristics of overlapping, change of topic and initiating co-occur and the speaker sounds especially impulsive. As usual, the frequency of such linguistic features is important for creating the impression of impulsivity.

WAITING FOR A TURN

Aside from interrupting and intruding on others, there are two more specific diagnostic criteria for impulsiveness: blurting out 'answers before questions have been completed' and 'difficulty waiting a turn'. The former is a more specific case of the latter. Therefore, we start with the general case, waiting a turn. As just outlined, verbal turns are often organised into short exchanges of two or three turns. Typically, the first turn in the exchange initiates the type of exchange by asking for information ('What time is it?'), giving information ('It's cold outside'), making an exclamation ('That's great!') etc. The next turn in the exchange is a reaction to the first turn and is usually closely coordinated with the first turn in terms of information given or the emotional reaction. There is sometimes a third turn in the exchange that confirms or challenges the second turn. Of course, conversations may be made up of many exchanges and even exchanges embedded within exchanges (see Chapter 2). We hear impulsivity when a speaker of a second or third turn does not wait for the prior turn to be finished or when a speaker of a first turn (question, command, statement) does not wait for the prior exchange to be finished. For example, if one speaker says 'I want some milk with cookies and pretzels' and another speaker says 'Me too and I want it now', there will be a sense of interruption and impulsiveness if the second speaker starts too soon. Some overlap of turns is not uncommon in spontaneous speech, but if the overlap of speech starts too early or if the overlapping is frequent, then we clearly hear the interruption.

Questions and answers are a specific set of turns that are particularly closely related. Specifically, after a question, there is a restricted amount and kind of information that is expected. Furthermore, the ends of questions are relatively easy to predict since the intonation patterns (rising in some cases: 'Did you see him?' and falling in other cases, 'Where do they go Friday mornings?') and the grammatical structures give clear clues to the end of the turn. If, with such clear signals, the affected speaker starts an answer too soon, then the interruption will be disruptive since such early answers are generally infrequent. Impulsivity, then, can be heard as a disruption to the interpersonal function of language with its sets of exchanges and turns. When a speaker enters into another's turn or disrupts the taking of turns in usually well-managed series of exchanges, then others may attribute impulsivity to the speaker.

Summary 6.4

This chapter has described ADHD through its diagnostic criteria as these criteria are divided into the three middle-level categories of inattention, hyperactivity and impulsivity. Each of these middle-level categories can occur alone or in combination with the other categories. More concretely, the individual diagnostic criteria can occur in various combinations and in different degrees of severity.

The amount of co-occurrence both of middle-level categories and of diagnostic criteria is an important marker of the severity of the disorder. At the level of language, the more the linguistic markers recur and are combined with the linguistic markers from separate diagnostic criteria, the more affected the speaker will sound. The view of ADHD from the perspective of language places the emphasis on the interactional characteristics of the disorder, on how individuals act and sound. Nevertheless, the language reflects the formulation of the concepts of inattention, hyperactivity and impulsivity. There is, however, overlap of linguistic characteristics across these three concepts and certainly with concepts and behaviour from outside the disorder. Closer examination of the language in many speakers could well establish that these middle-level concepts of inattention, hyperactivity and impulsivity should be replaced with other wider or narrower categories. These categories also reflect a cognitive description of speakers as having difficulties in cognitive mechanisms associated with attention, activity level and impulse control. The examination of language use in context offers a way to explore these cognitive processes in detail and to build the concepts carefully out of specific language behaviours.

Chapter 7 contents

Psychotic disorders

Overview of psychotic disorders 7.1

In this chapter we explore how schizophrenia can be expressed through spoken language. The surface phenomena, mainly in language, may give rise to the diagnosis of schizophrenia and may be the reason why society bothers with the phenomena. Our goal is to understand schizophrenia from the social interface that language constructs. This verbal social interface is largely what draws schizophrenia to the attention of others. More broadly, we interpret psychosis as discontinuity with the context in several ways. The discontinuity is evident largely in how some speakers use language.

Psychotic disorders are the psychiatric disorders most studied from the point of view of language (see Section 7.2). Furthermore, by far the greatest amount of research and thought about psychosis has been done on schizophrenia. For these reasons, this chapter is structured differently than the other chapters. Our focus here is on schizophrenia, although there are examples from other forms of psychosis. The clinician can apply much of what we say here about the psychosis in schizophrenia, with some adjustments, to other kinds of psychosis. There is a range of conceptualisations of schizophrenia both from a linguistic approach and from more standard psychiatric approaches. A synopsis of some of these linguistic and non-linguistic approaches is first given (Section 7.3.1). Then the concept of psychosis itself is discussed in terms of functional linguistics (Section 7.3.2). Finally, the detailed characteristics of schizophrenia are expanded and interpreted in functional linguistic terms (Section 7.4).

The linguistic approach to schizophrenia uses the linguistic concepts and terms introduced earlier to characterise how speakers with schizophrenia construct meaning in social contexts. As indicated in these earlier chapters, the linguistic terms sometimes overlap with the terms used in clinical description. However, the value in the linguistic descriptions is that they are designed to cover the full range of meanings and wordings that could be used, rather than to give an account of the particular unusual uses of language important for clinical description. They can, at a certain level of detail, show why hearers notice the features included in clinical descriptions. The linguistic approach also specifies both the kinds of meanings that are atypical in context (and thus are part of the clinical descriptions) and also the words, structures and sounds that convey those noticeably atypical meanings. For clinical purposes, we need to notice these wordings as the direct signs of schizophrenia.

The approach to schizophrenia through the verbal social interface does not exclude a cognitive or psychopathological approach (see the various discussions of the role of language in schizophrenia in the context of other impairments in Chaika, 1974; Chaika and Lambe, 1985; Chaika, 1990; Lanin-Kettering and Harrow, 1985). However, we see these problems in the community through language and other behaviours. Although there are no convincing overall accounts of the neurophysiology, aetiology and transmission of schizophrenia that relate to the behaviours, we must first closely describe the behaviours in order to map possible causes onto the behaviours that are so evident and non-functional. The linguistic approach details the phenomenology in order to create a picture of the dysfunction in the community and to simultaneously outline the phenomena that must be explained cognitively, biologically or otherwise. There may be several mechanisms and several aetiologies underlying schizophrenia. Therefore, it is even more important to have detailed understandings of the verbal phenomena so that some phenomena can be associated with one mechanism and perhaps other phenomena can be associated with another mechanism.

In the following account, we do not assume any unity in either the phenomena being described or in their underlying sources. The language phenomena may be distributed in various ways across individuals, just as the diagnostic criteria are variously distributed across individuals. In fact, the distribution of the detailed language phenomena may itself suggest underlying mechanisms. That is, the co-occurrence or disassociation of linguistic phenomena in schizophrenia may well lead the clinical community to understand which individuals are similar with possible common mechanisms for the disorder. This problem of grouping affected individuals frustrates the search for causes since unlike cases are incorrectly regarded as similar. It is then not surprising that common elements are not found (see the discussion of the parallel problem in the study of aphasia: Caramazza, 1986; Caramazza and McCloskey, 1988; Zurif, Gardner, Brownell, 1989).

Clinical features

Schizophrenia is the focus of this chapter since it includes the major characteristics of the other psychotic disorders and is the most studied disorder. The structure of the current clinical description of schizophrenia (American Psychiatric Association, 1994) is of a number of positive symptoms (delusions, hallucinations, disorganised speech, disorganised or catatonic behaviour) and negative symptoms (flat affect, restricted fluency and productivity of thought and language, restricted initiation of goal-directed behaviour). The disorder is diagnosed on the basis of the patterning of these symptoms rather than the presence of one or the other of them. Characteristics such as disorganised speech or restricted content of speech obviously implicate language directly. Other characteristics (e.g., delusions, avolition) usually involve language but only indirectly in the reporting of sensations or feelings.

Synopsis of schizophrenia and language

7.3.1 Approaches to schizophrenia and language

Reviews of approaches to the language of schizophrenia are found in Rochester and Martin (1979); Chaika (1990); Fine (1994) and more generally in Beitchman, Cohen, Konstantareas, Tannock (1996); especially Caplan (1996). The Rochester and Martin approach was first outlined in Rochester and Martin (1977) and then more fully in Rochester and Martin (1979). Like Rochester and Martin, this chapter focuses on language as it is used in context and on those characteristics of language that compromise the connection of language to its context.

Rochester and Martin (1979) developed a functional linguistic approach to the description of the language of speakers with schizophrenia. The approach starts with the principle that people talk to create social reality. A speaker typically contributes to an interaction by relying on the context that has been built up and agreed on: what has happened up to this point in the interaction. Hearers attempt to make sense of what is said in terms of this context. However, the language of speakers with schizophrenia fails to build social reality. The source of this failure is that the language is not, from the hearer's perspective, connected to the assumed shared context. The language is uninterpretable because it does not fit with the hearer's sense of context.

Rochester and Martin found specific linguistic differences in interactions of speakers with thought-disordered and non-thought-disordered schizophrenia and normal controls. In general, the speakers with schizophrenia used less cohesion, that is, less connection to earlier speech (he, she, it, and, afterwards) than normal controls. In particular, the language of speakers with thought-disorder had more unclear referring (using 'she' or other pronouns when the hearer could not identify the person being spoken about) and more repetition of content words ('bird', 'pill') that created a false sense that the topic of conversation was continuing.

On the other hand, there was more signalling about information in the physical non-verbal environment (exophoric reference) such as 'I', 'you', 'that chair'. These signals connect language to information that the hearer can interpret since it is in the physical environment. It is not, however, information that was specifically mentioned. Speakers with schizophrenia used fewer signals that indirectly imply that the hearer and speaker share the same world ('the dam ('you know which one I mean, the one on the river I mentioned, although I haven't explicitly mentioned the dam')' (implicit reference, bridging)). This combination of patterns in the language of speakers with thought-disordered schizophrenia creates language that does not fit into its context as we would expect and therefore does not create a shared world. Viewed as a process, the step-by-step contributions to interaction do not build on the language and the meanings that the hearer experiences. These findings of Rochester and Martin have been extended and reviewed in a range of studies (see summary in Fine, 1994; criticised, Alverson and Rosenberg, 1990; reply in Fine, 1995; related to other discourse elements, Caplan, 1996).

Chaika has also developed a major approach to the language of schizophrenia. In early papers (Chaika, 1974; Chaika and Lambe, 1985) she noted the atypicalities of the language of speakers with schizophrenia at the discourse, semantic, syntactic and phonological levels. Chaika (1990) presents an extended treatment of psychotic speech. Psychotic speech, she points out, is intermittent and affects the phonetic rules of language (the sounds that are used), word formation (the presence of neologisms), discourse (the associational chaining, clang associations), syntax (the production of word salad) and processes of perseveration (repetition) and intrusion (jumping from topic to topic). These various levels of disturbance, according to Chaika, arise from the lack of control over the linguistic processing levels (a failure in linguistic competence) and from the intrusion of irrelevant material. The result is a speaker who cannot order and organise material. Chaika sees the interpretive problem as a difficulty in being able to create a mental representation from what a speaker says. In contrast to Rochester and Martin, Chaika postulates mental representations that must be created by the hearer. The speaker whose language is disordered fails to send the signals to create appropriate representations.

Caplan (1996) also sees the disturbances in the language of speakers with schizophrenia as occurring at different levels. Caplan divides the impairments into problems with the overall communicative plan (macrostructures), problems with words and sentences (microstructures) and problems of socially appropriate speech (pragmatics) that include turn-taking, level of formality and amount of speech. Three principal components emerge from this work on childhood schizophrenia:

(1) discourse measures that link within language;

(2) loose associations and verbal comprehension;

(3) illogical thinking and reference to physical context (exophora).

Caplan found that most discourse measures are not associated with formal thought disorder. However, the use of reference to the physical context is related to the clinical category of illogical thinking and both may indicate a basic impairment in information processing. In terms of communication, Caplan (1996: 173) sees a macrostructure deficit involving 'poor organisation of topic maintenance and inadequate reasoning' and a microstructure deficit involving 'impaired use of linguistic devices that link the contents of contiguous and neighbouring sentences'. Together these deficits seriously compromise communication.

7.3.2   Schizophrenia in functional linguistic terms

The linguistic approach in the current chapter is different from these other approaches in several ways:

(1) First, we wish to capture the whole range of the diagnostic categories that define schizophrenia, rather than focusing on one or two.

(2) Second, our primary goal is to account for the impairment in social functioning rather than to explore the cognitive underpinnings of the disorder. It is quite likely, though, that exploring the impairment of social functioning will lead us to an understanding of the cognitive underpinnings.

(3) Third, we consider a wide range of language phenomena to describe how a speaker with schizophrenia sounds.

(4) Fourth, the linguistic approach is functionally based. It is therefore directly tied to language use in context and what language can accomplish in interaction.

This chapter describes the language of schizophrenia in order to detail why the language sounds atypical and why the speakers are not able to accomplish normal social goals. This description, can, though, be taken as the data that a cognitive approach needs to account for. The linguistic approach, as opposed to a clinical descriptive approach, uses concepts, categories and descriptive terms that have been developed for understanding how language usually works in social contexts. The categories and descriptions are not developed ad hoc for the atypicalities found in schizophrenia. Rather the language characteristics of the disorder are seen against the backdrop of how language usually functions. The approach then has specific and direct clinical implications: the clinician learns how the language of the speaker with schizophrenia is different from more typical uses of language.

Clinically, schizophrenia is defined by the positive and negative symptoms and especially by prominent hallucinations and delusions (American Psychiatric Association, 1994). These symptoms lead to the impairment in normal functioning that is so severe. In the description of schizophrenia, there is a combination of cognitive description and social impairment. Neither of these is to be taken as cause or effect. Sometimes, for research or clinical purposes, however, it is useful to think primarily from one perspective or another. The following sections describe the phenomenology of schizophrenia from the social perspective since it is the dysfunction in the community that is available for observation, diagnosis, treatment and the phenomenon that demands a causal explanation.

Although the focus is on the social dysfunction, the clinician cannot ignore the perspective of the individual. The disorder may or may not be discomforting. The individual may have no insight into the positive symptoms and not be aware of the negative symptoms (for example, not be aware of poverty of content of speech). On the other hand, the hallucinations may be acutely disturbing (voices that do not stop) and even endanger life. The individual may also feel discomfort if he or she notices that others avoid interaction, take the interactions trivially or seem not to understand. This sense of isolation further suggests that the speakers do not share a social reality. The individual's subjective feeling of the disorders thus interacts with the social impairments that characterise the disorder from the community's perspective.

To return to the social basis of schizophrenia, clinicians reliably observe and identify the positive and negative symptoms. They can also be taught from one generation of clinicians to another. That is, the characteristics have a stable social reality. Essentially, individuals are identified as behaving atypically, in a range of verbal and non-verbal ways (the signs). There may be:

(1) atypical meanings (for hallucinations, 'that voice I hear', delusions 'I am the King of Siam', poverty of content of speech, etc.);

(2) atypical ways of wording the meanings (blocking, unclear speech, derailment) or

(3) both of the above.

Hearers judge the atypicality of a comment in terms of its context. We most clearly hear atypicality in meanings (the ideational metafunction) in hallucinations and delusions. The speaker is heard as contradicting the ideational reality of the speech community. Sometimes, the disconnection with context is more directly with the wording of language in the context. In this case, the textual metafunction is compromised resulting in disorganised speech, blocking, poverty of speech and poverty of content of speech. In other cases, the disconnection with the context is in terms of interpersonal factors (the interpersonal metafunction) with resulting flattening of the affect normally expected (see Table 7.1 for some examples of the kinds of discontinuity). Taken together, these disconnections with context result in language that codes loss of ego boundaries and problems in reality testing. The degree of the atypicality can be slight or infrequent. To take a non-schizophrenic psychosis as an example, in a Korsakoff psychosis there may be only a few examples of fabrications that set up a reality that is not shared (see a linguistic description in Fine, 1994, Chapter 4). If the atypicality is severe, then interaction is scarcely possible, as in severe thought-disordered schizophrenia. If the language that is produced is quite unexpected, then the hearer may consider that the speaker did not comprehend: 'if the other person really understood what I said, then such an interaction is not likely'. That is, the hearer cannot interpret the response in the context and then attributes the problem to the speaker's comprehension rather than to the speaker's complete failure to fit language to the context.

DISCONNECTION FROM CONTEXT

Kind of disconnection	Linguistic functions	Examples of corresponding clinical categories	Examples of language
Disconnection of meanings	Ideational metafunction	Hallucinations, delusions	I am the King of Siam.
Disconnection of wordings	Textual metafunction	Disorganised speech, blocking, poverty of speech, derailment	I saw the cow, brown cow, cow over the moon. That was the cowboy.
Disconnection of speakers	Interpersonal metafunction	Flattening of affect	I guess that's OK. (in a monotone)

Table 7.1
Kinds of disconnection from context

There is no absolute level of typicality expected in language nor an absolute level of how easy it should be to interpret a speaker. Rather, the ease of interpretation varies according to the situation and the social process. For example, we expect bank transactions to be accomplished quickly and with a very high degree of accuracy. Each speech community and each social process may have different amounts of tolerance for variation. For example, in schools, some teachers or schools expect behaviour that is very close to a specified standard while others may permit, expect, or encourage a wider range of behaviour. Hearers instinctively weigh any difficulty in interpreting a speaker against the standard in the situation and the amount of variation expected.

Language is normally connected to contexts. However, there are different aspects of a situation that a speaker must continue in order to avoid sounding detached and psychotic. Firstly, the subject matter or institutional focus of the talk (the field) must be continued or, if there is a change, it must be signalled. Jumping from topic to topic will sound as if there are intrusions or derailment. Secondly, we expect that the actual things mentioned by one speaker should be continued by the next speaker with a given frequency. A speaker who just continues to talk about hobbies in a general way without talking about the very same games or objects as another speaker will sound rather fuzzy and disconnected. Thirdly, the language must fit into the series of turns that different speakers take. The language must be contingent on the immediately preceding turns in terms of appropriately responding or initiating and in terms of the selection of words. An individual who lacks connection in any of these ways fails to build social reality by not continuing meanings. Schizophrenia appears as the failure of the speaker to connect appropriately to the context. Much of the display of the connection is by way of language and so language is largely the evidence for schizophrenia. This evidence is in terms of both positive symptoms (delusions and hal- lucinations) and negative symptoms (blocking, poverty of content of speech, derailment, etc.).

The above interpretation of schizophrenia is quite general in its call on disconnection from context as the crucial factor. The task now is to link the specific features of schizophrenia to this disconnection. The remainder of this chapter outlines each of the diagnostic criteria and features of schizophrenia in terms of the functional linguistic approach to show how language conveys different kinds of disconnection. Through such detailed presentations, the study of language can add precision both to clinical concepts of disorder and to the description of clinical phenomenology.

Detailed characteristics of schizophrenia in functional linguistic terms   7.4

This section describes the characteristics of schizophrenia in three categories:

(1) the cardinal positive symptoms of delusions and hallucinations (Section 7.4.1);

(2) disorganised speech (Section 7.4.2);

(3) the negative symptoms of blocking, poverty of speech, poverty of content of speech and flattening of affect (Section 7.4.5).

The term 'speech' here is borrowed from the clinical descriptions. No fundamental distinction between the terms 'speech' and 'language' is implied. The diagnostic criteria for schizophrenia are related to the major functions of language which are at stake (the metafunctions) as listed in Table 7.2.

Diagnostic criteria	Metafunctions of language at stake
Delusions and hallucinations	Ideational
Disorganised speech	Ideational, textual
Negative symptoms	Ideational, interpersonal

Table 7.2

Relation between diagnostic criteria for schizophrenia and the metafunctions of language at stake

7.4.1 Delusions and hallucinations

Delusions and hallucinations are similar clinically since, if severe, they clearly indicate schizophrenia even without the presence of other symptoms. They have a similar jarring effect. Linguistically, delusions and hallucinations are similar in signalling atypicality in the ideational metafunction of language. That is, these symptoms are expressed in language that does not encode the experiential reality in typical ways. This encoding of experiential reality is the most obvious part of our understanding of schizophrenia: the disconnection of meaning from context.

Delusions

Delusions are defined clinically as 'false belief based on incorrect inference about external reality that is firmly sustained despite what almost everyone else believes' (America Psychiatric Association, 1994: 765). Furthermore, the belief is not accepted by the culture or subculture. The clinical definition then is in terms of beliefs. The concept of 'beliefs' is extrapoled from the verbal and non-verbal behaviour of the individual. Clinically and from the point of view of language analysis, we must identify the aspects of language that lead hearers to identify such false beliefs. The ideational metafunction of language encodes into language three main types of reality: the people, places and things of the world (things), the events of the world (events) and the information surrounding events (circumstances). We hear a delusion when one or more kinds of information do not match with external reality as the rest of the community understands it (see summary and examples in Table 7.3).

Table 7.3

Schizophrenia: delusions – language features

Clinical feature	Meaning in world at stake	Language features	Examples
Delusion	people, places, things	nominals modification of nominals	You are the *king of England*. The *six kilometre* spaceship *made of butter*.
	events	verbs	I *jumped up* to the moon.
	details of events	circumstances worded as:	
		• adverbs	They built it *carefully*.
		• prepositional phrases	They ate *at noon*.
		• clauses	They considered it *because it was important*.
	firmly sustained belief in delusion	added stress attitudinal adjuncts	He *WAS* born on the moon. He was *certainly* born on Mars.

THINGS

The 'things' encoded in language may not match reality in a number of ways. When the speaker gives the speaker or hearer identities that are not generally accepted (the Queen of England, Napoleon), then the hearer has clear evidence that the speaker is introducing 'things' directly into the conversation that are rejected by others. In detail, the speaker is giving identities to first person pronouns (I, we, mine, etc.) and second person pronouns (you, yours, etc.) that are deemed to be impossible. Somewhat more remote from the interaction, identities of things not part of the interaction will be atypical. Calling an automobile 'a space ship', or a bedroom 'a dungeon' and acting accordingly expresses delusions beyond the interlocutors and so sounds less disturbing than strange identities for the speaker and hearer themselves. A speaker can also present 'things' that mis-match reality by being completely fictional. An individual who talks about visits from extra-terrestrial beings or unicorns with a certainty of their reality expresses delusions that are more troubling than merely conveying the belief that one real object is in fact another real object. At a more subtle level, the problem with expressing things can be in terms of the thing itself ('I', 'spaceship', etc.) or in terms of how the thing is described in language ('The *six kilometre long* spaceship *made of butter*').

As well as the 'things' of the external world, delusions can centre on the events of the world that are usually encoded into verbs. In the statement 'I flew to the moon', we can accept the identity of the things 'I' and 'moon' but we normally do not accept as reality the event of flying involving 'I' and 'the moon'. As with things, the events may be wholly fictional ('I was born weighing 50 kilograms'), or possible but not real ('You were born a genius on the level of Einstein'). The third category of ideational information is information of time, place, cause, etc. (circumstances) that fills in the details of events. This circumstantial information can convey complete contradiction to external reality. The following statements sound delusional because the circumstances (in *italics*) contradict reality, not because the things or events are false:

EVENTS

CIRCUMSTANCES

> I was born *on the moon.*
> Those people were my friends *in 1650.*
> *While I was a baby,* I bought three houses and built up my business.

As these examples show, the combination of things, events and circumstances conveys a delusion even if each one of them is real. That is, the language expresses a delusion by encoding and combining parts of reality that the community does not accept as a possible combination; infants do not make business decisions, people do not have friends from hundreds of years earlier. Reality is socially constituted and hearers broadly agree about the departures from their reality. A question that needs careful research and clinical attention is whether the reality constructed by the speaker with schizophrenia is itself internally consistent; that is, are the statements implicating delusions in themselves consistent?

As well as a mismatch between the reality created by language and the reality of most other members of the community, speakers with delusions firmly believe in the delusional ideation. This belief is encoded by statements such as, 'Yes, I WAS born on the moon' (with added stress on 'was') that confirm an earlier statement and reject contradictions of the speaker's unusual reality. The clinician can expect to find such pairs of utterances with the affected speaker rejecting challenges to delusional statements. Certain adverbs (attitudinal adjuncts), such as 'really', 'certainly', 'definitely', also convey the strength of the beliefs ('I *certainly* was born on Mars'). Depending on the severity of the delusions, the clinician may hear several linguistic markers of ideational disconnection and also the markers of conviction of the unusual reality.

Some of these examples of delusions may sound like metaphors. Usually, we recognise metaphors as making points indirectly, by saying something that we recognise as not having a literal interpretation. In the language of some speakers with schizophrenia, the metaphoric sounding language is not intended to have a metaphorical interpretation. The speaker does indeed intend the literal interpretation and will affirm the literal interpretation if questioned and reject attempts to assume a metaphoric interpretation. Metaphor usually works exactly because hearers can reject the literal interpretation as being unreasonable ('That murderous tyrant is running this company to the ground') and therefore construct some interpretation that does make sense in the context ('That self-important, uncaring, unsympathetic boss is managing this company in a way that will lead to bankruptcy'). Speakers with schizophrenia do not carefully match and mismatch their impossible meanings with the context to create metaphor. When there is mismatching with context ('I am Napoleon'), the intent is not to draw attention to the unreality of the literal meaning and force a metaphorical interpretation. The intent is, in fact, to send the literal meaning.

Hallucinations

Hallucinations, as well as delusions, are mainly expressed through the ideational metafunction of language. In contrast to delusions, we hear hallucinations directly in a speaker's talk of reality. There is no need for a concept of 'beliefs' intermediate between the language and the reality the speaker experiences. A hallucination is 'a sensory perception that has the compelling sense of reality of a true perception but that occurs without external stimulation of the relevant sensory organ' (American Psychiatric Association, 1994: 767).

Individuals may or may not know that they are having hallucinations. As with delusions, the language expresses things, events and circumstances that the rest of the speech community rejects (see Table 7.4 for a summary and examples). Rather than characterising the problem as a false belief (as in delusions), clinically the problem is formulated as a false perception that is then expressed in language. The clinician hears a statement about perception which is then rejected as an unrealistic perception. That is, the impairment is not an atypicality in language but in perception. Language merely enables the hearer/observer to know what the perception is. An impairment in expression could be interpreted as an expression of a hallucination; for example, by confusing words, a speaker may say 'I saw a blizzard in the summer sky' instead of 'I saw a buzzard in the summer sky'. In general, though, the unreality of false perceptions repeats systematically, ruling out sporadic impairments in expression. Careful clinical listening and a few probing questions can distinguish impairments in expression from hallucinations.

Clinical feature	Meaning in world at stake	Language features	Examples	Table 7.4
				Schizophrenia: hallucinations – language features
Hallucination (auditory, visual, gustatory, olfactory, somatic, tactile) often with restricted focus	Sensations of things, events, details of events	Mental verbs of sensing, perceiving	I *see* the creatures. I *hear* them coming.	
		Relational verb + object	There *are* some *unicorns*!	
	Lack of insight	Reference to external reality	*The* voices in the room. *This* light is bothering me.	
		Given-new information expressed by sentence stress	You *SAW* them come in.	

We hear the language of hallucinations in a restricted ideational focus (a field of discourse). This ideational focus reflects the kind of hallucination: auditory, visual, gustatory, olfactory, somatic or tactile. In turn, these ideational foci are worded into language by verbs that present the events of sensing (hearing, seeing, tasting, etc.). As explained earlier, it is the combination

IDEATIONAL FOCUS

of ideational meanings that expresses the delusion or hallucination. For hallucinations, it is the verbs of sensing (technically, mental verbs, Halliday, 1994) combined with what is sensed (voices, the smell of rotten eggs), at what time (when no one else senses them), that present unreal experience. In language, then, there is a clustering of ideational meanings that are not related to context in the usual way.

Expressions of hallucinations are unlike other kinds of talk in that only specific ideational foci are involved. An auditory hallucination can be expressed without other disconnections from reality and without the speaker expressing other atypical ideational. For example, an individual with schizophrenia may speak about voices that are heard and be able to describe the quality and content of the voices, but still be able to engage in conversation with a clinician and perform many daily activities. Even if the individual 'speaks' to the voices, much other talk and activity may be typical. In many cases, the restricted domain of the hallucination (auditory, olfactory, tactile, etc.) and the distinctive content of the hallucination (threatening voices, the smell of sewage), as well as their unreality, set the language of hallucinations apart from other uses of language. As a result, the speaker sounds reasonable much of the time. At the level of wording, pronouns and nouns represent the person, places and objects (the things of the world) that the speaker claims to experience and verbs represent the events of the world as the speaker with schizophrenia perceives them. In the statement 'I feel these snails crawling up my leg', the pronoun 'I' encodes the speaker, the nouns 'snail' and 'leg' encode objects and the verbs 'feel' and 'crawl' encode two events, one of sensing and one of a material action. A close examination then reveals whether things or events are central to the hallucinations.

INSIGHT

A speaker may or may not have insight into hallucinations. This insight is also expressed through language. Essentially, an individual with insight into the hallucinations can distinguish shared reality from the reality that the individual understands is inaccessible to others. In language, then, the speaker distinguishes between 'voices' or 'smells' that are regarded as personal and those that are shared. The speaker with insight into the hallucinations can then, in fact, describe the sensual perceptions to try to convey the experience to others. If there is no insight into the hallucinations, the speaker expects others to have the same perceptual experiences and so uses language that does not describe but rather assumes common information. For example, instead of describing the 'voices in my head' or the 'voices that I hear' an individual may talk directly to the voices or talk about 'the voice' or 'what we just heard', assuming the interlocutor had the same perceptual experience. Often, the definite article 'the' (when used for demonstrative reference) or the words 'that' and 'this' signal information that the hearer is assumed to know: 'What's *that* cat doing there?' '*This* light is bothering me'. Intonation and sentence stress also encode either assumed or new information for the hearer. The exact patterns are outlined in Chapter 2. Assumed information is usually at the beginning of clauses and new information is towards the end, with new information receiving sentence stress by loudness and pitch. In general, the meanings of the intonation patterns are easy to distinguish: the hearer notices that the information seems assumed when he or she does not know what the speaker is talking about. To summarise, the insight into hallucinations is an insight into the two different perceptual worlds of the speaker and hearer. The speaker can then separate these two realities when talking about perceptual experiences.

7.4.2 Disorganised speech

When the speech of an individual with schizophrenia is difficult to follow in context it is called disorganised speech. The clinical understanding of disorganised speech is as either derailment which is taken to be an across clause phenomenon or incoherence which is taken to be a disturbance within a clause (American Psychiatric Association, 1994). These two categories thus differ in terms of the segment of language at risk, either a group of clauses or just one clause in itself. In terms of the disassociation from context, derailment is disassociation from a neighbouring clause and incoherence is disassociation within a clause. This section outlines both the characteristics of language that create derailment and incoherence and the impairments in meaning and social activities that result (see summary in Tables 7.2 and 7.5).

Derailment

Derailment, also known as loosening of associations, is defined as 'ideas slip off one track onto another that is completely unrelated or only obliquely related'. 'In moving from one sentence or clause to another the person shifts the topic idiosyncratically from one frame of reference to another and things may be said in juxtaposition that lack a meaningful relationship' (American Psychiatric Association, 1994: 766).

We hear derailment as inconsistency and unusual transitions in how the external world is encoded in language (mainly, the ideational metafunction). We now explore derailment from the language itself on upwards to the social processes. This orientation upwards from the details of language to the social processes is presented first to show how we recognise derailment in language. In a following section, the orientation down from the social processes to language is outlined to show how the social processes themselves are not accomplished.

Table 7.5

Schizophrenia: disorganised speech – language features

Clinical feature	Meaning in world at stake	Language features	Examples
Derailment (between clauses)	Continuity of people, places, things	Inconsistent nominals, verbs, adjectives, adverbs	See section 7.4.2
		Lack of reference to people, places, things already mentioned	
		Incorrect reference to people, places, things already mentioned	My father and brother like basketball. *He* is tall. The *other* (?) river.
	Continuity of time and place frames	Adverbs Nominals Prepositional phrases	Yesterday Three years ago After the sun set, in the hole
Incoherence (within clauses)	Random meanings of people, places, things, events	Incongruent nominals, verbs Impaired word order	The night in the kitchen doesn't go around. Wet not to wear boots.
	Details of people places, things	Incongruent modifiers of nominals	Loud idea Thoughtful banana Banana in the concept

As outlined in Chapters 2 and 3, the external world is mainly encoded into language by nouns and pronouns for the people, places and objects of the world, verbs for the events of the world and prepositions and their objects ('into the house', 'around noon') and adverbs ('quickly', 'suddenly') for the details of the events. It is the consistency of these things, events and circumstances across clauses that is at stake. In the following story, a normal control subject first introduces the person 'lady' into the story and then sustains the character through the story by references to: '*her* husband', '*she* wanted', '*she* was afraid', '*she* thought', '*she* would play', '*she* decided'. Similarly, 'a tiger's whisker' is introduced and then referred to again by '*the* tiger's whisker'. When such chains of people and things are not used across clauses, the talk seems to shift topics.

> Well there was once a lady and *her* husband was sick and to make him better *she* wanted a tiger's whisker to make medicine… now *she* was afraid of tigers so *she* thought *she* would play a trick and get *the* tiger's whisker. So *she* decided to take some food…

In contrast, when a speaker introduces several people, places and things that are not continued through the text, it sounds like ideas slipping off the track. The following stretch of language spoken by an individual with schizophrenia (repeated from Chapter 3) introduces several such things ('they', 'the pill', 'organism', 'diabetes', 'the kids', 'things', 'a school building', 'the girls', 'the boys', 'this half', 'you', 'a school', 'problems') most of which are not referred to again.

> It was back in fifteen hundred when they took the pill actually and it created some kind or organism and diabetes and things like this you know… the kids they're all actually fine you just gotta know how to talk to the kids and how to associate things with the kids right? Like you separate a school building and keep the girls on this half you keep the boys on this half and if you ever criss-cross a school then you run into all kinds of problems

The consistency of things must usually be extended from one speaker to another in order to create interaction dynamically with each speaker contributing to the context. In the following conversation, speaker W uses 'them' to refer to the rocks that speaker K has mentioned and speaker W uses 'that trip' to refer to the trip implied by speaker K when saying 'the museum'. Speakers are linking the 'things' of the world across speakers thus establishing continuity. There is no derailment here.

CONSISTENCY OF THINGS

> K: her father is a scientist so she has a whole bunch of rocks and so we were looking at those and I saw one that was almost the same as one that was in the museum.
>
> W: did you see *them* all? Do you remember *that* trip?

Sometimes a speaker develops the interaction on similarities of sound instead of continuing to talk about the same things in the world. In this case, the derailment is based on 'clang associations'. If a speaker says: 'I went down in my plane' and the next speaker says 'but there was *plain*ly nothing to do', the repetition of sounds from 'plane' to 'plainly' shifts the interaction from one ideational object ('plane') to another ideationally irrelevant topic.

CLANG ASSOCIATIONS

As well as consistency of things, there must also be a certain consistency of time and place of events we speak about. Hearers cannot clearly interpret talk

CONSISTENCY OF TIME, PLACE

if the frames of time and space change without warning. If a hearer cannot readily understand if an event happened three days ago or three years ago, then the language sounds detached from the world and uninterpretable since the time frame is not clear. There is much detailed research to be done in this area. The clinician must listen for and the researcher must study the consistency of time frames and how they are expressed. The information about time is expressed by time words that are adverbs (yesterday), nouns (three years ago) and in prepositional phrases (at that time, during the space race, after the sun set).

CONTEXT OF SPEECH

We now move from how consistency is expressed to consider the context of the speech. The extent that a speaker is 'on track' or 'off track' depends on the context of the interaction and the social processes involved. If there is a casual question of 'How are you?' then the consistency of the interaction needs to be sustained only briefly. On the other hand, if the interaction concerns tasks at work, hearers expect the ideational consistency and the continuity of the things in particular, to last much longer. There is no absolute, independently definable length of 'being on track'. Rather, slipping 'off track' is assessed in terms of the social processes involved (in language, the genre that is unfolding) and the relation to the context (technically, the register, see Chapters 2 and 3).

Of course, interactions and even monologues do naturally move from topic to topic. However, there are typical signals that are used to warn hearers of the changes. A speaker who does not use these signals sounds psychotic. A stretch of language can be probed for derailment by inserting some explicit signals, 'boundary markers' (discussed below), to see if the derailment improves. The following interaction between Interviewer (I) and Patient (P) demonstrates how a sudden shift in topic from one clause to another is improved when the speaker explicitly signals the transition by saying 'to look at the causes' or 'to think about the money'.

I: hmmm what are the changes like? (at the university)

P   (with thought-disorder): OK I'll restrict myself to the campus scene because well in sixty eight there was a lot of anti war demonstrations ant Che Guevara demonstrations there was student multi student power

I: ya

P: there wasn't much (xxx) in sixty eight that came later but (*'to look at the causes', 'to think about the money'*) now it's because any economy was quite good ... see minimum wage was a dollar an hour ... and the difference is now is the higher employment students who are occupational oriented because they fear they won't get jobs if ...

As this example shows, there is a continuum of relatedness from clause to clause. Not all transitions can be clearly labelled as derailment or not. As interactions unfold, even minor derailments will be noticed if they closely follow each other in a series. The clinician suspecting derailment must listen both for the severity of the derailment and the frequency of minor shifting from one track to another.

So far we have presented the details of language and how they affect social processes, a bottom-up approach to derailment from language. Now the approach is reversed to consider how the social processes define 'slipping off the track' and to consider the social consequences of such derailment, a top-down approach. As outlined in Chapters 1, 2 and 3, language accomplishes various social goals in context. If the language, and non-verbal behaviour as well, is not connected typically to the context, then the speaker sounds psychotic. This disconnection from context impairs achieving social goals. We then find the social/occupational dysfunction that is the underlying criterion for psychiatric disorder.

SOCIAL PROCESSES

Social processes are staged activities that accomplish social goals. The patterns of language that actualise these activities are the genres. We can see the disconnection from context in schizophrenia as atypically combining parts of different social processes or a disturbance in the order of the elements within a social process. When different social processes are combined, none of the social goals may be achieved. An individual who first tries to order a meal in a restaurant but interrupts it to express political opinions may neither eat nor convince the hearer about politics. If the elements within a social process are disordered, then again the social goals will not be attained. Saying 'Good-bye' or 'I really have to leave' when meeting an acquaintance will quickly break off a potential interaction and social process. In a less extreme case, telling a travel agent how much money is available for a trip before stating the purpose, destination or dates of the trip may compromise the social processes since the ordering of the elements departs from the typical.

We now continue down from the social process to language. Although the components of the social processes may be disconnected from each other and from the context, we must also notice whether the social processes and their staged components are expressed typically or atypically in language. That is, the individual can have difficulty in constructing the language (the genre) to accomplish the social goal. To distinguish these two possibilities, we can look to non-verbal evidence for atypical understanding of the context and contributions to interaction. Giving money to strangers in a public place or directing traffic on a busy street usually indicate atypical social processes but the evidence is non-verbal. If the evidence is completely non-verbal, then the clinical impression is of grossly disorganised or even catatonic behaviour. On the other hand, if the components of the social processes seem in place, but the language seems to slip from topic to topic, the conclusion is likely to be of derailment with the locus of the impairment in the expression of the social process through language (the genre). For example, if an individual approaches a restaurant counter, orders an ice-cream cone, pays for it, but at the same time talks about several unconnected topics (medications, solar eclipses, the ice floes in Antarctica), the individual will accomplish the social process of obtaining an ice-cream cone but the language used will be largely inappropriate. When the language of the social process itself is more clearly impaired (for the above example, ordering an ice-cream cone of ten kilograms), then the clinician must attend to the atypical meanings and how they are worded.

We can think of the meanings in social processes as an alignment or configuration of the topic or institutional focus (the 'field' related to the ideational functions of language), the social roles of the speakers (the 'tenor') and the role of language or the channel of communication, spoken, written, etc. (the 'mode') (see Chapter 2 and Martin, 1992: 497-502). A speaker who 'slips off the track' combines the unannounced changes in topic with more or less intact meanings conveying social roles and the channel of communication. The unexpected changes in topic are out of context with what has been spoken before and/or the physical context of the interaction. Since the other two basic kinds of meaning (interpersonal and the channel of communication) are more intact, the clinician notices the disturbances in topic. The specific parts of language that change the topic in derailment may involve:

(1) the sounds of language, as in clang associations;

(2) the vocabulary and sentence grammar of language;

(3) large units of language equivalent to paragraphs or whole sections of talk that seem out of place.

The signals in language that mark the derailment can be related to the psychiatric categories. Caplan's work (summarised in Caplan, 1996) suggests that reference to the physical world (exophora) is associated with illogical thinking but that loose associations are not associated with either reference to the physical world or the continuity of people and objects in the discourse by referential cohesion (the table, they, it, etc.). The macrostructural elements in these studies (formal thought disorder and information processing) were not found to be directly related to how they are expressed in language.

Continuing the discussion of 'slipping off the track' from a top-down perspective, we can ask the question: how could impaired processing of the context result in the language of slipping off the track? This processing of context is both a way to conceptualise the impairment and a way to identify the impairment even if the processing deficit hypothesis is rejected. The issue in terms of context is: which level of context is at stake? Slipping off the track can be in terms of the genre (there is movement from one genre to another, from telling a story to buying a newspaper), an element of a genre (saying 'Thank you' before deciding on the flavour of ice cream), or even a very atypical channel of communication (the mode) (such as writing a message when it should be spoken, or using a very formal tone when it is out of place). See Malcolm (1985) for a technique called phasal analysis that captures many of these changes.

Topic shifting

We have now explored one part of disorganised speech: slipping from one track to another that is unrelated or only tenuously related. A second kind of disorganised speech is clinically described as shifting topic idiosyncratically from one frame of reference to another across clauses and juxtaposing things that lack a meaningful relationship (American Psychiatric Association, 1994: 766). With shifting topics idiosyncratically, the pattern of ideational changes is not typical since the events, people, places and things change without due warning. As outlined for slipping off the track, the changes in shifting topics may involve the social processes, parts of the social processes or how the language fits the external physical context. The juxtaposition of unrelated things also involves the ideational metafunction. Some have conceptualised this unrelatedness as lack of a higher-level macrostructure that enables the hearer to understand the connection between two ideas (see Caplan, 1996; Fine, 1994: 111-2; Hoffman, Stopek and Andreasen, 1986). Of course, this lack of a higher-level organisation is another way of saying that the language is disconnected from the context. From the hearer's perspective, there does not seem to be a reasonable context that would create a meaningful relationship between the two ideas. There is a lack of perceivable or inferable continuity of meaning.

This clinical description of shifting topics as a between clause disturbance may just be a more concrete description of 'ideas slipping off the track'. If the source of the slippage is easily identified, then it is more clinically apparent and accessible. For example, hearing a speaker say contradictory things ('I was born in 1967 and my mother was born in 1969'), hearing a speaker talk about 'that chair' when no chair has been mentioned or is apparent, or hearing two remotely connected ideas linked by 'because' leads the hearer to identify the precise point of disturbance between clauses. A disturbance in referring (*that* (unidentifiable) chair) and a disturbance in how language is linked from clause to clause could implicate different underlying processes. In summary, the across clause disturbances make language uninterpretable because the topics and parts of topics do not fit with a conceivable context and social process.

Incoherence

The first kind of disorganised speech, described as slipping off the track, is a between clause disturbance. A second kind of disorganised speech is a within clause disturbance, clinically labelled incoherence. Incoherence, like the between clause disturbance of slipping off the track/derailment, characterises talk that is uninterpretable in context. The speech is incomprehensible because there are no meaningful or logical connections between words or phrases. Much of the discussion of incoherence, then, dwells on the ideational metafunction, the meanings of the experiential world encoded in language. We perceive the disturbance as incomprehensibility of the talk; therefore, the focus must be on the impairment in conveying meaning. Of course, language conveys meaning by the vocabulary and grammar and there will therefore be atypicality of vocabulary and grammar. The approach here is then to describe the impairments in functions or meanings and at the same time describe how those meanings are worded in the vocabulary and grammar.

Before detailing incoherence in linguistic terms, we turn briefly to the relationship between language and thought. Our concern in this chapter is with the disturbance in the use of language. However, these disturbances of incoherence are sometimes attributed to disturbances in thought. Such a connection is not essential, though, for accounting for the phenomena of schizophrenia. On the other hand, the linguistic account of incoherence provides the details needed to explore the specifics of disturbances in thought. As alluded to at the beginning of this chapter, there is discussion of the distinction between language and thought in schizophrenia and whether there is one disturbance (then, which one is it?) or two disturbances (see Chaika, 1974; Chaika and Lambe, 1985; Chaika, 1990; Lanin-Kettering and Harrow, 1985; Rochester and Martin, 1979). In most cases, language is the evidence for disordered thinking. If there is independent evidence for intact thinking accompanied by disordered speech, it is found in non-verbal behaviour such as appropriate facial expressions, non-verbal comprehension, non-verbal neuropsychological testing and even verbal comprehension as indicated by appropriate short responses in interaction.

To return to characterising incoherence, the basic question is: what makes the within clause relationships 'essentially incomprehensible'? As the clinical description indicates, the problem is logical or meaningful connections. That is, the hearer in the speech community and the clinician do not detect the usual logical and meaningful connections. The issue is not the grammar as grammar but how language fails to signal these connections. To be comprehensible, language within a clause must have reasonable connections to other parts of the clause, as that clause operates in its situational and cultural context. At a more detailed level, then, it is the combinations of meanings (more technically, the language functions) that are at stake. We can refine the basic question as: what combinations of meanings are incomprehensible? In Chomsky's famous example, 'Colourless green ideas sleep furiously', meanings are put together atypically: ideas usually do not have colour, the colour 'green' is usually not colourless, ideas do not usually sleep and the event of sleeping is usually not describable as happening 'furiously'. We can hear such unusual combinations of meanings as poetic, since in some situations or cultural contexts, some or all of these combinations are interpretable, perhaps with a certain amount of effort. The central problem in interpretability here is that the world encoded in language seems impossible ('colourless green', 'green ideas', etc.). For a poetic interpretation, the hearer constructs a new world or interprets the meanings metaphorically ('green' when describing 'ideas' means 'fertile', 'original', 'new', 'fresh', etc.). This point of the poetic/metaphoric impression of some utterances leads us to the more general issue of how the utterance fits into a particular social process. The social processes implied by a telegraph, poem or political chants at a demonstration, for example, impose different constraints on both how an utterance is worded and how it should be interpreted. The clinician must assess the social process and the language that is used within it. If the hearer needs effort to interpret the language, including poetic sounding utterances, then the fit with the social process is at least strained.

At the extreme, word salad can be understood as meanings and the words that encode them, chosen almost randomly from different sets of meanings (different fields or foci of ideational activity). Caplan, (1996: 166) gives the following example of incoherence: WORD SALAD

> Interviewer: What happened next in your story?
>
> Child: The day witches no day goes.

The words 'day', 'witches', 'goes' seem random. 'Goes' is a very general word expressing an event. It can then be construed as fitting with either 'day' or 'witches' among many other entities. The difficulty is that even if the utterance can be interpreted, it seems to fit no context. The utterance can be made worse by increasing the different sets of meanings it draws on: 'The day witches no day goes the bedroom the clothes in the mineshaft'. As there are more different kinds of meaning, it becomes harder for us to construct a context in which the utterance is interpretable.

WORD ORDER

As well as selecting an unusual combination of meanings, incoherence is created by serious impairments in word order. If word order is disturbed, then some meanings will not be presented clearly. If someone says 'Wet not to wear boots', it may be interpreted as 'It is wet outside but I won't wear boots'. However, if the word order is disturbed, the intended message could be 'Not to wear wet boots'. Specifically, if 'wet' is not before 'boots', then the meaning of 'wet' modifying 'boots' will be lost and the utterance will be misleading and perhaps incomprehensible. In general, then, disturbances in word order require the hearer to attempt in different ways to interpret the utterance in the context. Some of these attempts will fail completely and some attempts may lead to unintended interpretations. The clinician must listen for possible infelicities in word order to determine both what could have been intended and how the message has been deformed.

IDEATIONAL MEANING

Incoherence as a within clause phenomenon presents a range of atypicalities in ideational meaning that creates the sound of schizophrenia – the disconnection from context. In fact, to explore within clause ideational phenomena, requires considering the clause in its context. That is, clauses are ideationally atypical and incomprehensible only in relation to their contexts. The major meanings in the clause are the 'things' mentioned (the participants, see Chapter 2), the events (worded as processes) and the circumstances surrounding the events. Less centrally, the modification of the 'things' and the events is at stake. As outlined in Chapters 2 and 3, contextualising utterances starts with considering the possible and typical processes in the culture. Only from this top-down perspective is it clear whether an utterance is incomprehensible. For example, we must think of the social process to assess reports of going to the moon and back or even strange combinations of meanings within a clause. In recounting mythology, going to Hades and back is possible and interpretable. The incomprehensibility arises when the social process (such as recounting a myth) is not signalled or is inappropriate in context. Much then depends on signalling the shifts and boundaries of social processes. The language of schizophrenia sounds disconnected from its context partly because this signalling of shifts and boundaries is not present. Again, the extreme case is a word salad with disturbed word order that seems to fit no context.

7.4.3 Disconnection from social reality in ideation, interpersonally and channel of communication

The disconnections of the individual and his or her language with social reality are the common elements of delusions, hallucinations and disorganised speech. The culture opens up various social processes that are largely accomplished through language. When an individual does not clearly accomplish these social processes (for certainly there is a continuum from successful to unsuccessful instances of social processes), then the clinician considers schizophrenia as a diagnosis, especially if the lack of success stems from a perceived discontinuity with the context. We must understand this discontinuity in terms of the normal kinds of continuity with the context (what is expected) and how changes in continuity are usually signalled. Then we can understand what is not signalled in schizophrenia.

Disconnection in ideation

The language of social processes must be ideationally consistent, must be interpersonally relevant to the context and the explicit verbal ties to the context must be appropriate (the textual metafunction). Social processes unfold in stages and these stages also are largely signalled by language. Greetings ('Hi', 'Hello') are followed by other greetings and usually only afterwards do speakers discuss more central issues. When a speaker presents these stages in the wrong order, then we hear disconnection from the context. Furthermore, if the kinds of meanings that usually go together are separated, the social process may be jeopardised. If a financial transaction (a kind of ideational meaning) is discussed in very informal terms, including slang and cursing (elements of interpersonal meaning), then the social process may be affected. Of course, the appropriateness of such combinations of meaning depends on contextual factors such as the relationship between the speakers. When the combination of meanings is atypical, then the speaker is presenting a reality that does not match the wider community's version of reality. To sound psychotic, though, the unusual combinations must be quite atypical. Otherwise, a speaker will just be heard as 'odd' or 'off', too often sounding as a preacher, sounding too formal, off in another world, etc.

Each kind of meaning (ideational, interpersonal and textual) leads to sounding disconnected from the context in different ways. Delusions and hallucinations are expressed through unusual ideational meanings. Recurring talk about religion, somatic complaints and experiences indicates disconnection from the context as most of the community experiences it. However, even with these ideational atypicalities, there may be considerable appropriateness interpersonally and even in the formal connection of language to the context (cohesion and other elements of the textual metafunction).

Disconnection interpersonally

In other cases, there may be interpersonal atypicalities as well as atypicalities in the ideational use of language. These interpersonal atypicalities, in fact disconnections in their own right, may involve addressing people who are not present, speaking in the third person ('He would not like that' meaning 'I would not like that'), using a royal 'We', addressing others as religious followers, servants or in some other inappropriate role. The hearer finds the linguistic signals of these connections in the terms of address ('Sir', 'Lady', 'comrade', 'butler') or even formal or stilted expressions, intonation or grammar ('It has been drawn to my attention…'). As well as atypical roles, a speaker may also be disconnected from the context in terms of an interpersonal dimension such as intimacy. Speaking about subjects that are too intimate or never speaking about intimate subjects sets up a discontinuity with the context. Furthermore, the discontinuity may be in the combination of the ideational meanings and the interpersonal meanings. For example, speaking about intimate subjects in very formal terms (with formal, stilted intonation, long, technical and low frequency words) sets the speaker apart from the context. The reverse is also possible: discussing a formal topic, such as a tragedy in the daily news, in jovial, dismissive or intimate terms. Again, it is the combination of ideational and interpersonal meanings that conveys the discontinuity with the context.

The extreme examples of interpersonal discontinuity with the context are hallucinations and delusions. The language of hallucinations and delusions often signals a bizarre identity or role relationship with other speakers. As outlined, a speaker with schizophrenia may adopt a role that others do not consider at all real. As well as the role itself, speakers may adopt atypical interactional goals (functional tenor) even if the role they are taking on is not completely imaginary. For example, a speaker may seem overly authoritative or meek. These characteristics will be conveyed, for example, by using an atypical number of imperatives ('Bring me the newspaper'), rhetorical questions ('Why on earth did you do that?') or unqualified statements ('They are all losers') for the context. More subtly, such atypicalities in interactional goals will be evident as longer social processes unfold and we notice the length of the speaker's contributions and the method of development. For example, a speaker who frequently talks about causes for every action will seem to have a particular goal that is forced in terms of the context, if not totally disconnected.

Disconnection in channel of communication

As well as ideational and interpersonal discontinuity with the context, atypicalities in the channel of communication (technically, the mode of discourse as outlined in Chapters 2 and 3) contribute to our apprehension of schizophrenia. The channel of communication constrains who can interact and what messages they can send through the channel. A speaker with schizophrenia may speak loudly to drown out other individuals or may be addressing or answering voices that others do not hear. Furthermore, if an individual assumes that certain people can overhear interactions, the language and behaviour in general will be affected. A speaker will speak in a monologue instead of a dialogue if the speaker assumes that the hearer is a constant unanswering presence. On the other hand, monologic language, telling a story, describing an event or feelings, can atypically become dialogic if the speaker hears voices that demand answers. Even paralinguistic signals connected with the supposed channel of communication, such as shouting or whispering, may send atypical messages. As with ideational and inter-personal meaning, it is the combination of meanings that makes the speaker sound particularly disconnected from the context. For example, shouting requests in certain contexts ('Stop the bus. I want to get off') will be much more disruptive of the social process than merely saying them in a regular tone of voice that assumes the usual channel of communication.

7.4.4 Avoiding discontinuity: the marking of boundaries and how it can fail

This chapter has presented the discontinuity of language with context as indicative of the verbal behaviour of speakers with schizophrenia. Furthermore, the discontinuity is presented clinically as within clause phenomena (incoherence) and across clause phenomena (derailment). Of course, though, speakers do regularly change the social process they are developing, jump from topic to topic and even change in midcourse how a clause will be presented. Aspects of the psychotic sounding discontinuities are not present in these other cases. One aspect is simply the rate of the apparent discontinuities. All speakers create occasional errors and seem to make uninterpretable verbal jumps. The cooperative hearer tries to accommodate these slips and reconstruct the missing links. If the rate of the missing links becomes too great, then the hearer starts to notice how much repair work is needed. As well as the rate of discontinuities, another aspect of changing direction in interaction is how the speaker signals these changes. This process is called boundary marking. As long as a speaker signals a change in direction, the language and activity seem continuous with the context. The boundary markers say to the hearer 'I know that you think I am changing topics, but I am aware of the impending change and I know that I should signal that this change is about to take place'. Just as the

RATE OF
DISCONTINUITIES

SIGNALS OF
DISCONTINUITY

discontinuity of language with context may involve different levels of analysis from the social process down to the clause, so the boundary markers also create connection at different levels. Absence of these boundary markers is a phenomenon that needs both clinical attention and specific research.

The key notion for boundary marking is signalling a change of meaning. We need to signal changes of meaning at the level of social process, the level of ideational, interpersonal and textual meanings (register) and at the level of the wordings in language. Atypicalities in signalling changes at these different levels reflect different characteristics of schizophrenia. In general, people speak in real contexts and they speak to convey meaning. The issue is then, do hearers recognise the connection between the context and the meanings of the speakers? The hearer can judge a speaker to have schizophrenia when the hearer does not recognise the social process and other connections in context. Somehow, the language fails to make these connections clear enough. We now turn to each level of meaning to describe the importance of signalling changes in meaning and the consequences when a speaker fails to do so.

Boundaries of social processes

At the most abstract level, human activity derives from cultural patterns that achieve certain purposes: the social processes that can take place. These staged social processes are then reflected in patterns of language called genres. When the boundaries of these social processes are not clear, the individual appears to be jumping from one social process to another, from ordering a pizza to discussing politics, from welcoming guests into one's home to teaching a child. Typically, such transitions are signalled so that the hearers can fit the language and non-verbal behaviour into the social context; e.g., 'Excuse me while I ...'. There are many formulae that are immediately recognised as signalling these changes in social processes: 'Wait a minute I forgot to ...', 'Just wait while I ...', 'To change the subject ...', 'That reminds me ...', 'Let's move on to ...', 'But we have to ...', 'Now listen to me ...', 'Next, let's ...'. If an individual hears 'I am terrible happy/upset with what happened', but cannot determine if it applies to the welcoming of guests or the teaching of a child, then the speaker appears disconnected from the context. At this level of analysis, a speaker who omits a boundary marker makes it difficult for the hearer to determine what the social process is. The consequence for the hearer is confusion over his or her social role in the interaction. That is, if it is not clear what the speaker is doing, then it is difficult for the hearer to know what role to take. In such a case, it is difficult indeed to construct a joint social process. This failure leads directly to the impairment in social and occupational function that defines mental disorder.

Boundaries of different meanings

As well as the social processes themselves, there are ideational, interpersonal and textual meanings that must be consistent or marked as changing. These configurations of meaning (register) are then mapped onto various contexts. As with the social processes, if important changes in meaning are not overtly signalled, the hearer perceives disconnection from the context. The clearest cases of lack of boundary markers are the jumps in ideation from topic to topic. Here again is a passage from a speaker with florid schizophrenia.

IDEATIONAL
BOUNDARIES

> It was back in fifteen hundred when they took the pill actually and it created some kind or organism and diabetes and things like this you know… the kids they're all actually fine you just gotta know how to talk to the kids and how to associate things with the kids right? Like you separate a school building and keep the girls on this half you keep the boys on this half and if you ever criss-cross a school then you run into all kinds of problems

There is a jumping from an ideational focus (the field) on the 'pill' to a focus on 'the kids' to a focus on 'a school building'. If some boundary markers are added, as below, there is less disconnection between the language and the context, resulting in less disruptive talk:

> It was back in fifteen hundred when they took the pill actually and it created some kind or organism and diabetes and things like this you know… *To consider now what happened to* the kids they're all actually fine you just gotta know how to talk to the kids and how to associate things with the kids right? *Moving on from talking about the kids to where they go to school,* like you separate a school building and keep the girls on this half you keep the boys on this half and if you ever criss-cross a school then you run into all kinds of problems

When there are inadequate signals of the changes in interpersonal meanings, we also hear the discontinuity in schizophrenia. Again, some of this discontinuity results from not using markers to warn the hearer of changes. The changes of interpersonal meaning are changes in the roles in interaction. By not marking the changes in roles, an individual can sound disconnected from the immediately preceding role. In the following excerpt from an interview with a clinician (I), a speaker with schizophrenia (L) first describes himself as a woman lawyer (turns 3, 7), then challenges (turns 5, 22, 24) the questioning of his identity (turns 4, 21, 23) and later challenges the role of the clinician (turn 26).

INTERPERSONAL
BOUNDARIES

1   L: I was in the Sounds of Music back then. I was ah the maid that come
         from the ah Mormon Temple from Chicago to Nebraska

2   I   um mmm to Nebraska

3   L: I have ah wrote books … I've sung songs ah ya I come I come from
         Nebraska State University …in other words I've graduated from
         lawyer's school

4   I: you're a lawyer?

5   L: ya I'm a lawyer

6   I: are you?

7   L: I'm a woman lawyer and ah all I like to keep my books and my phone
         calls separate and everything …

(several turns are omitted here)

21 I: I was interested L, why did you say you're a woman lawyer? The reason
         I'm interested in it is that you don't look like a woman to me

22 L: I don't look like a woman?

23 I: no

24 L: are you certain I don't look like a woman?

25 I: no I'm certain you don't look like a woman to me.

26 L: we can talk about your doctor degree too

This speaker takes on a number of identities 'maid' in the Sound of Music,
writer of books, lawyer all without explicitly signalling the changes. Turn 3
would sound more in touch with the context if the changes in interpersonal
role were signalled as in:

3a L   I have ah wrote books … *but* I've sung songs ah ya I come I come
         from Nebraska State University …in other words *in fact* I've graduated
         from lawyer's school

Later on, the speaker changes his role in the conversation, rather than his
identity, by challenging the interviewer instead of just answering questions:

26 L: we can talk about your doctor degree too

Again, an unsignalled change of interpersonal role in the conversation
(from answerer of the clinician's questions to challenger of the clinician's
identity) creates discontinuity. Although the disruption is not great in this
case, repeated changes of role loosen the connection of the language with
the context as it is built up step by step.

Though, unlikely, unsignalled changes in channel of communication (associated with mode of discourse) may occur, contributing to the discontinuity
in schizophrenia. These are cases in which the speaker seems to switch
from talking directly to the hearer, to talking on a telephone, through a
megaphone, in a whisper or perhaps to voices. Although such changes are
possible in reality, when they are not explicitly signalled, the interaction will
seem disconnected from its context.

We have separately outlined the effect of not using boundary markers when
configurations of meanings change for the ideational and interpersonal
metafunctions. The general effect of these unexpected changes is now outlined in terms of context. When there is a change in the apparent connection
of the ideational and interpersonal meanings of language to the context, the
hearer wonders about the reason and effect of such a change. If the meanings
are inconsistent, we first suppose that there is some purpose, in terms of
social process or subtlety of the message, for the change. If there is no such
apparent purpose, then we listen for an explicit signal or boundary marker
that the meanings are changing. That is, the boundary markers justify apparent discontinuity with the context and thus make the language sound less
psychotic. With no boundary markers, the hearer considers: 'why is there a
change in the ideational and interpersonal meanings, since the context itself
does not seem to have changed from my perspective? The speaker should
be signalling why there is such a change'. Unsignalled changes in each of
the ideational and interpersonal areas (and to some extent in relation to the
channel of communication) create different kinds of discontinuity, topic or
subject matter and social roles, respectively. The boundary markers for ideational and interpersonal meanings thus co-ordinate relatively long stretches
of language (usually longer than a clause) with the context. Omitting such
signals makes language and speakers sound detached from context.

Boundaries of wordings

So far, this chapter has outlined boundary marking at the levels of the social
process and at the level of ideational and interpersonal meanings (parts of
the register). There is also boundary marking at the level of the wordings
of language itself. The patterns of vocabulary, grammar and sounds must
themselves show a certain amount of consistency as a discourse is built
up. When one part of the discourse is inconsistent with another, there will
be an apparent change in direction or emphasis even if the social process
is largely consistent. For example, a speaker who regularly uses signals of
uncertainty (verbs such as would, should, might, may; adverbs such as possibly, probably, perhaps) but shifts without warning to very definite statements
can seem inconsistent with respect to the context. The hearer finds that

nothing in the context correlates with the change in level of certainty. Using a boundary marker such as 'I'm more certain of this ...' builds connection even when there is a change in emphasis or certainty.

On the level of language, we have seen that there are wordings in the grammar and vocabulary for boundary markers. However, there are also important signals in intonation and pseudo-words such as 'um', 'uhum'. These other boundary markers at the level of language include slowing at the end of various units, diminishing loudness, hesitation markers that show that the speaker is thinking of the next thing to say (that may then be a change of direction), throat-clearing or just silence. In some cases, pausing will indicate that another speaker is free to enter the interaction, marking an interactional boundary. The usual subtle hesitations, such as speeding up and slowing down or falling intonation at the end of clauses, all indicate that the language has different kinds of units, topics and contexts. What we find disturbing in the speech of schizophrenics is the free flow of speech from topic to topic or through other changes without any of these boundary markers. The lack of boundary markers signals that the speech is all one unit, although the hearer experiences difficulty in connecting the units together.

Failing to signal boundaries at the level of language, of course, also contributes to the failure to signal boundaries at the level of social process and at the ideational and interpersonal levels. The levels of meaning interact with each other and support each other. Hesitation markers and other boundary markers indicate both a local change of direction and perhaps also a new social process that will emerge.

In characterising disorganised speech, we have stressed the importance of boundary markers since it is precisely boundaries between actions and between sections of language that create some of the discontinuity in schizophrenia. The boundary markers signal a speaker's change in direction. If these signals are appropriate, then the language sounds connected to context. If the signals are not present then the language sounds more disconnected. Of course, schizophrenia is not the lack of boundary markers. Rather, speaking without boundary markers in the specific linguistic sense presented here contributes to the construction of disorganised speech. Looked at the other way round, lack of boundary markers helps define what disorganised speech is. The clinician who listens specifically for boundary markers of different kinds will notice how the speaker is disconnected from the context and why the speaker does not accomplish the social processes of everyday life.

7.4.5   Negative symptoms through language

The negative symptoms of blocking, poverty of speech and poverty of content of speech are all conveyed directly by language. In fact, they are descriptions of language behaviour. This section describes these symptoms in detailed functional linguistic terms to both explain the impression of the symptoms and to give guidelines for recognising them (see Table 7.6).

Clinical feature	Meaning in world at stake	Language features	Examples	
Blocking	Incomplete ideation	Incompleted language structures:		Table 7.6 *Schizophrenia: negative symptoms – language features*
		• words	Dis . . . (interested)	
		• phrases	In a family with . . .	
		• clauses	There are events that . . .	
			They tried to help her and . . .	
Poverty of speech	Less said than expected	All language areas potentially reduced, (see Appendix B) simplified grammatical structures		
Poverty of content of speech	Less information than expected	Fewer subordinate clauses	(see Section 7.4.5)	
		Less modification in nominals	A (large, yellow) boat, the house.	
		Fewer details about events	They left.	
		Ambiguous vocabulary	They're finished.	
Flattening of affect (see Table 7.7)				

Blocking

Blocking is understood clinically as blocking of thoughts, describable as pauses in the flow of speech (see Andreasen, 1979a; 1979b). More generally, other phenomena such as distractible speech, dysfluency and even pressure of speech can result in incomplete segments of speech (see Baltaxe and Simmons, 1995). Speakers with blocking pause unduly within a variety of grammatical formations (see Table 7.6). There may be pauses at the beginning of a clause ('there are events that …'), after a conjunction ('as if they tried to help her and …'), between verbs ('I am not … (going)'), or after a preposition ('my mother lived in a family with …') (examples from Goren et al., 1995). It is important to note that such blocking depends not only on the affected speaker but also the interlocutor. If a speaker is not given the opportunity to display a long pause, then the blocking is covered up. In active conversation, pauses of five to seven seconds are soon filled by another speaker who feels that the first speaker has stopped. In clinical settings, it is important to avoid entering the conversation and filling a pause. By waiting for the speaker to continue, the clinician can observe the frequency of the pausing and the severity of the disruption in interaction. The disruption of pausing in 'pressure of speech' can result from false starts, perseverations and overeagerness to speak (Baltaxe and Simmons, 1995). The smaller the grammatical unit that contains the pause, the more disruptive is the effect. For example, pausing or interrupting speech completely within the middle of a word ('dis … (interested)') is generally more disruptive than a pause or incompletion within a phrase ('with … (my sister)') or within a clause ('They decided… (to leave)').

Poverty of speech

A second negative symptom described by language is poverty of speech. In interaction, speakers with poverty of speech simply say less than is expected. There are typical amounts of information that are given after a speaker initiates in interaction (e.g., by a question or a statement) or responds to another speaker's contribution. When there is less talk than expected, we hear a terseness, perhaps sounding as if the speaker does not want to interact or cannot interact. There may be simple one-word answers or simplified syntax (see review of studies in Baltaxe and Simmons, 1995).

Poverty of content of speech

The third negative symptom we consider here is poverty of content of speech. Speakers with poverty of content of speech fail to build up semantic information as the utterance, or interaction, continues. Caplan et al. (2000) note that even for children the failure to elaborate on a topic after two or more utterances constitutes an unusual poverty of content of speech. In cases where there is elaboration, using expressions that are vague creates poverty of content of speech. For example, responding to questions with 'it depends' or 'could be the case' or using ambiguous vocabulary ('They're finished', meaning either 'completed' or 'destroyed') creates poverty of content of speech (Goren et al., 1995). Simplified grammatical structures, such as few subordinate clauses convey less meaning also resulting in poverty of content of speech. For example, in the following interaction, the speech can be enriched by adding information with subordinate clauses, in parentheses.

> I: I see what kind of job would you be doing?
>
> S: assembling the steel parts together [which are already cooled] or working with boxes on the assembly line … [as the boxes come down] I would put a clamp on it or something or put stamping on it and well do with a whole bunch of parcels and boxes [that need finishing]

The negative symptoms of blocking, poverty of speech and poverty of content of speech, as we have seen, reflect a reduction in the usual flow of language either by interruption or by sparseness of the usual grammar and semantics of speech. The language of these negative symptoms creates discontinuity with the context giving the hearer the impression of schizophrenia. Certainly, many speakers without schizophrenia leave units of language incomplete. However, in the non-psychotic cases, there is an apparent reason (the speaker is interrupted, changes the wording, is thinking for a moment, etc). However, if the incompletions are rather too frequent or too close together, then these usual reasons, which may be supported by non-verbal contextual clues, are less likely. Similarly, if the language seems too inconsequential or meaningless, then there is a discontinuity with the context since the context seems to demand more information than we hear.

Flattening of affect

Flattening of affect is a negative symptom carried largely by the interpersonal metafunction. Affect conveys the speaker's attitude to interaction or to other elements of the environment. Individuals convey affect by facial expressions such as smiling, frowning, grinning, etc. However, language also conveys affect in two ways by language (see Table 7.7 for a summary). Firstly, speakers convey affect by affective statements that involve a mental process verb ('I *think* that is exciting') or an evaluative word ('an *exciting* trip'). Even intensifying a descriptive word can send an affective message ('a *very* red sweater'). Secondly, speakers convey commitment by a range of devices within the interpersonal metafunction: intonation, contrasts in meaning from speaker to speaker, attitudinal words, words of commitment and rate of speech. It is certainly easy to identify affect when it is expressed directly by affective statements. However, there are other linguistic means for expressing affect that require explanation. Intonation can convey surprise ('THEY came', with an unusually high rising tone), questioning or doubt ('They came on Tuesday!?' (falling-rising tone) 'but I was expecting them on Wednesday') and gentle chastisement of the hearer ('They came on Tuesday?!' (rising-falling tone) 'and you should have known that'). A speaker who does not use such intonation is not expressing an entire range of affect: the speaker's feelings about the expectedness of the information or what the hearer is thought to know.

Table 7.7	Kind of meaning	Language features	Examples
Schizophrenia: negative symptoms, flattening of affect – language features	Affective statements	Mental process verbs (think, hope …)	I *think* that is exciting
		Evaluative words	an *exciting* trip
		Intensifying words	a *very* red sweater
	Interpersonal Meta-function	Intonation	They came on Tuesday*!?*
		Contrast	Kim saw the *NEW* house
		Attitudinal words	some *fascinating*, suspenseful mystery novels
			Certainly I like chocolate ice cream
		Commitment	
		- modal verbs	I *may* like chocolate ice cream
		- modal adjuncts	*Possibly*, I like ice cream

Speakers also convey affect implicitly by the way they present new or unexpected information. As described in detail in Chapter 2, the placement of sentence stress indicates information coded for the hearer as given or new. In 'Kim SAW the new house', the speaker is encoding the 'seeing' as the new and unexpected information, in contrast to 'Kim saw the NEW house' or 'Kim saw the new HOUSE'. When information is marked as unexpectedly new, usually by sentence stress in the middle or beginning of the clause ('Kim SAW the new house', 'KIM saw the new house'), the implicit message to the hearer is 'I think you don't know this information'. Thus the speaker is displayed affect by relating to the information state attributed to the hearer. When the sentence stress is regularly and predictably at the end of the clause, then we hear the speaker as not adjusting the information flow for the hearer, as if the speaker has little affect to show the hearer. The language seems monotonous and possibly out of touch with the hearer.

Attitudinal words express affect and are found in a number of places in the clause. The people, places and objects of the world (functionally, 'things') may be modified by attitudinal words as well as by more neutral ideational information. In the following examples, the attitudinal words (attitudinal epithets) modify the nouns in combination with the ideational modifiers. We notice that the attitudinal modifiers usually come before the ideational modifiers: a *seemingly* bright student, a *terrific* long and interesting movie, the *amazing* wide desert, some *fascinating*, suspenseful mystery novels. As well as modifying people, places and objects, attitudinal words are used to modify entire propositions. These attitudinal words are often adverbs (attitudinal adjuncts) that can be placed in different places in the clause: '*Certainly* I like chocolate ice cream', 'I *certainly* like chocolate ice cream', 'I like chocolate ice cream, *certainly*'. Again, without such attitudinal words utterances sound affectively flat.

As well as attitudinal words, affect is also carried by expressing the speaker's commitment to his or her own utterances. There is a difference in the expression of affect between 'I like chocolate ice cream' and 'I may like chocolate ice cream'. The second expression is more tentative compared to the first. Commitment is expressed by certain modal verbs (may, might, can, could, would, should, ought to) that accompany ideational verbs (walk, throw, think, etc.) and by a wide range of adverbs (modal adjuncts) expressing commitment. The commitment can be expressed in terms of probability (possibly, probably, certainly), how usual (sometimes, usually, always), obligation (necessarily), or inclination (willingly) (see Halliday, 1994, Chapter 3, for many more details). As with the modal verbs, these modal adverbs convey the speaker's level of commitment and thus the affect of the speaker towards what he or she is saying and towards the hearer. The following passage from a speaker with schizophrenia (modified from Rochester and Martin, 1979: 97) is presented in two versions, the first with modal adjuncts and the second without. The second version explicitly expresses less commitment either strong or weak and so seems to convey less affect.

More modal adjuncts, more explicit signals of level of commitment:

> ...each life you know you can't *always* remember your past lives very few people *easily* remember their past lives in India there's *really* a lot of emphasis on reincarnation in India and Buddhism and Hinduism and that kind of thing but in western culture which we *usually* see variety and so forth there *necessarily* isn't very much emphasis there placed on reincarnation.

No modal adjuncts, few explicit signals of level of commitment, less expression of affect:

...each life you know you can't remember your past lives very few people remember their past lives in India there's a lot of emphasis on reincarnation in India and Buddhism and Hinduism and that kind of thing but in western culture which we see variety and so forth there isn't very much emphasis there placed on reincarnation.

Thus speakers use a range of words in different places in an utterance to express affect. Each linguistic device expresses a different kind of affect in terms of expectations, attitude and commitment in the interaction. These different kinds of affect must then be mapped onto the context. In general, we notice when a speaker expresses less affect. The flat language seems out of place.

CHANGED RATE OF SPEAKING

A final device for expressing affect, beyond the use of specific words or intonation, is change in the rate of speaking. Speeding up speech usually signals excitement, anger or irritability. Speeding up can also indicate that the information is less central to the issues being discussed (Auer, 1996), moving to a self-correction (Tarplee, 1996) or affective irritation (Gunthner, 1996). When the rate of speech is constant, then the affect is apparently even. Continuing the rate of speech of a prior speaker signals 'momentary speaker affiliation' (Couper-Kuhlen and Selting, 1996: 32) and so indicates perhaps an affective affiliation as well. The clinician must pay attention to the *change* in rate since speakers may have different base rates of speech depending on age, cultural background, personality, etc. Nevertheless, whatever the usual pace, variation in rate typically signals affect. When this variation is reduced, the language seems flat, monotonous and lacking in affect.

7.5   Summary

The positive and negative symptoms of schizophrenia thus draw on a large number of meanings and wordings in language. These meanings and word-ings articulate the individual diagnostic criteria and together combine to create the gestalt of schizophrenia that is heard in language. Although the descriptions are necessarily presented one by one and in rather obvious ways, the clinical picture can be a combination of parts of each criterion and various criteria at subclinical levels. In each case, the language makes the speaker sound detached from the context. The atypicality, though, is not random. Rather, the atypicalities of language found in schizophrenia implicate either the reality that the speaker seems to be living in or a dis-connection from the immediate ideational and interpersonal context. The schizophrenia will appear severe as a function of the number of linguistic factors that are atypical and how far the speaker departs from the expected meanings and wordings. The linguistic factors may be distributed in different ways as outlined in Chapter 1. The clinician must pay attention to both the kind of signal showing the disconnection and the distribution of the signals in terms of frequency and density. For example, one comment indicating a clear, bizarre hallucination forms an immediate impression of schizophrenia, whereas it may take ten to 15 per cent of nominals to be unclear to form an impression of disorganised speech. The clinician's intuitive judgements and the lay community's impression of bizarre behaviour use an unknown combination of these specific linguistic markers that are nevertheless quite reliable in identifying schizophrenia.

Chapter 8 contents

Chapter 8

Mood disorders

Overview of mood disorders 8.1

Both mania and depression have clear characterisations in language. As mood disorders, these features of language tend to appear in various contexts and in various social processes. There are three general areas of language that signal mood disorders for both depression and mania:

(1) affect in mood disorders is expressed by the interpersonal metafunction of language showing how the speaker is relating to the hearer;

(2) the changes in topics, such as flight of ideas in mania and negative thoughts in depression, are expressed by the ideational metafunction of language;

(3) the acoustics of language convey the clinical categories of pressure of speech in mania and slowed and decreased volume of speech in depression.

Sometimes a combination of these three general areas of language signals other clinical descriptions, such as irritability or depressed mood. Since the mood disorders are composed of episodes of depression and mania, we will describe these basic episodes in detail.

8.2	Depressive episode

8.2.1 Clinical features

There are two indicators of depressive disorder from a clinical perspective:

(1) depressed mood;

(2) diminished interest or pleasure with activities.

As with some other disorders, depressive disorder is present in language in two ways: as statements affected individuals make about the world and as observations by others of the signs of the disorder.

8.2.2 Language features

Depressed mood

An individual with depressed mood may make subjective reports about mood. These subjective reports include statements about being sad, empty, discouraged, hopeless, 'down in the dumps' or simply depressed. There are a number of classes of verbs that express feelings. These classes vary in how DIRECT REPORT   directly they express feeling. The most direct way to express a feeling is to use a verb that connects a characteristic to an individual (e.g., 'I am sad'). These verbs, such as the forms of the verb 'be' (am, is, are, was, etc.), seem ('I seem tired'), set up an individual as the 'carrier' ('I' in the above examples) of a characteristic that is often expressed as an adjective (sad, depressed). These verbs (technically, relational processes) state simply that the individual (e.g., 'I') has a characteristic (e.g., 'sad'). These verbs produce utterances such as: 'I'm sad', 'I'm angry', 'I'm in the dumps', 'I'm depressed', etc. Moods can be expressed less directly by using verbs of sensing ('I *feel* sad'). There are several subtypes of these verbs of sensing and each carries a slightly different force. These categories are:

(1) perception   I *see* / *hear* I'm sad;

(2) affect   I *feel* sad;

(3) cognition   I *think* / *know* / *understand* I'm sad.

The speaker can report the mood in these various ways, each with a different kind of meaning and a different strength of commitment. A speaker can also present the mood less directly by combining kinds of verbs, as in 'I *think* I'm sad', 'I *feel* I *am* sad', 'I *know* I *feel* sad', etc. More indirectly still, a speaker can use a verb of saying ('I *said* I am sad') rather than a verb of sensing. Again, these ways of stating a mood can be combined. For example, a verb of saying can be combined with a verb of affect ('I *said* I *feel* sad'), with a verb of cognition ('I *said* I *think* I am depressed') and so on. A speaker can thus express a large number of degrees of commitment to the subjective report of mood. Table 8.1 lists some of these ways of expressing commitment, but a larger number of combinations is possible.

Table 8.1

Mood disorders – language features: direct expression of mood from strongest to weakest

Type of verb (process)	Example
relational	I am sad.
perception + relational	I see I am sad.
cognition + relational	I know I am sad.
affection + relational	I fear I am sad.
sensing + relational	I feel I am sad.
saying + relational	I said I am sad.
perception + sensing	I see I feel sad.
cognition + sensing	I know I feel sad.
etc. with many possible combinations of these verb types	

As well as expressing mood directly, we can hear depressed mood even when the speaker is not talking directly about his or her mood. There are three verbal signs of depressed mood: negative sentences, intonation and choice of topics (see Table 8.2 for summary and examples). We produce negative sentences simply by using the small set of negative words in the language. These negative words ('not', or 'n't' in informal speech, is by far the most frequent) convey that some information in the sentence is not true. The negative words include: not, n't, no, never, neither, nothing, nor, nowhere, nothing. These words mark out different amounts of information as being negative. The general word 'not' signals that the proposition of the whole sentence is false ('They are not here'), The other negative words only make some of the sentence negative ('They are never to be seen' in which only the time is at stake). In the following part of an interview with a speaker with

INDIRECT SIGNS OF DEPRESSION

NEGATIVE SENTENCES

depression, there are frequent uses of 'n't' signalling that the entire state-ment is negative and one use of 'no'. Of course, such speech could easily be produced by a speaker without depression. However, these frequent negative markers help characterise the depressed mood and could occur with other verbal and non-verbal signs of depression.

I: was she willing to take care of the baby?

S: I wouldn't let her … no… you know… I just didn't feel like that um if I couldn't take care of her. I didn't want anybody else to

I: right

S: plus I didn't want to run into her… if I saw her I would keep her

I: right

S: I don't know… I don't know why she turned against me to tell you the truth … in fact that's one of the reasons … she doesn't like A (name), my husband

Table 8.2	Language feature	Examples
Depressive disorder, depressed mood – language features (also for diminished interests and activities with appropriate changes)	Negative words	The tables are *not* here. The tables *never* were here. *Nothing* is in the room.
	Intonation Infrequent stressed words Infrequent large rise or fall	Infrequent: The book is VERY expensive. They R E A L L Y are here.
	Choice of topic sad, funereal, hopelessness, suicidal, etc.	I saw a vision of the fire and thought it was the end of the world.

INTONATION

As well as these negative words, intonation signals depressed mood. We have two patterns of intonation to signal interest in the interaction and emotional involvement with the other speakers. One pattern is to stress a word (in capitals) that is not generally stressed: 'The book IS very expensive', 'The book is VERY expensive'. Such stress signals that the speaker is interested in the conversation and is expecting the hearer to be surprised by the word that is stressed. A second pattern that signals involvement between speaker and hearer is an unusually large rise or fall in pitch: 'They REALLY have their hands full with the new puppy', 'You THINK the stock market will go up?' A speaker who rarely uses these two patterns of intonation signalling involve-ment will sound uninterested in the interaction, detached and depressed.

The third signal of depressed mood in speech, in addition to negative words and intonation, is choice of topics. The topics of a speaker with depression may be sad, referring to death or suicide or show hopelessness. Though such topics do not necessarily indicate depression and can be found in any speaker's language, a speaker who uses them frequently in conversation can sound depressed. Obviously, then, the clinician must consider the frequency of these topics with respect to the age, role of the speaker and the cultural contexts the speaker is in. For example, initiating and sustaining a conversation on a sad topic with a clerk in a post office is atypical and more likely indicates a depressed mood than such a conversation with a friend (see, though, Segrin and Flora, 1998). In the following section of conversation with a woman with depression, relatives are the main topic for a number of turns. Notice the sustained negative approach to various relatives.

TOPIC CHOICE

1 I: what kind of person is she [your mother]?

2 S: she's nervous … she's worried … she worries a lot … about things (xxx) type um that's about it … generous? No … she's not very generous … nervous and worried

3 I: that's the main thing

4 S: that I can remember of her … yea … I don't know if she is still that way or not … she might be changed … but … I don't think so … I called her up a couple times and every time I phone she won't come to the phone … or she makes an excuse so that she can't come to the phone and talk to me … um … this kind of treatment … and you just get tired of it after a while … you just get so fed up and frustrated trying to talk to her … you just give up

5 I: what happens if you confront her with that and ask her directly … why don't you speak with me?

6 S: I have and she wouldn't give me an answer … I've asked her … I've phoned her once and I said look … why don't we talk I over with (xxx) bothering you … why don't you tell me what's bothering you instead of keeping it to yourself … tell me … but she wouldn't … she wouldn't even talk to me

7 I: what about your father?

8 S: my father is kind of under her thumb … sort of thing … he doesn't like (xxx xxx) either … he sticks on … he stays to her side mostly … I talked to him once … I talked to him the last time I called for a few minutes … not long at all … no he's mainly on her side (description of father continues)

9 I: do you have any other relatives that you are in contact with … like … uh

10	S:	(answer about cousin)
11	I:	what about your in-laws
12	S:	oh my mother-in-law … sorry … uh hum … I see her quite a bit (xxx)
13	I:	is she very different from your mother
14	S:	uh hum … uh hum … um … she won't …I don't know … I can't say that she's different … she's sort of the same as my mother … she's um … if she doesn't like something … or she doesn't like somebody … she let's you know about it … you know
15	I:	uh hum
16	S:	um … she's the nervous type too I imagine … yea … she's nervous … she's on some kind of medication right now too
17	I:	uh hum
18	S:	so … basically she's … the same as my mother … she worries too … basically she's the same but … she wouldn't turn her back on the kids … not like my mother's done to us … she's different that way

(concerning S's husband)

33	I:	what would he [your husband] do in a situation like that (during a conflict with S's mother-in-law)
34	S:	I don't know … I don't know … I don't think he would take sides I think he would try to stay neutral … and listen to both sides of it and then … come to his own conclusions … his mother did tell him what happened but … she exaggerates … to the point of lying almost … about things and … I don't know what A (S's husband) believes … whether he believes me or her … uh … what would A do? (the description of A continues)

In this passage, The speaker mentions the negative qualities of each relative. The mother worries, is nervous and not very generous. One gets frustrated talking to her. The father is under the mother's thumb, sticks to the mother and has only been spoken to once. The mother-in-law is the same as the mother, worries and exaggerates almost to the point of lying. Of course, there are positive statements and statements about happy topics. However, the speaker returns to the unhappy aspects of personalities beyond what is expected in the context. We thus get an impression of depressed mood.

Another speaker with depression described a dream with the following language: adjectives describing qualities: 'depressed', 'horrible', 'insecure', 'inadequate'; verbs describing events: 'turned against', 'fall off', 'battered', 'crying'; nouns describing things: 'only time', 'terrible dream', 'negative thinking'. We could, of course, find such a series of themes and wordings in any speaker's talk. However, when the balance is tilted towards such negative topics, crowding out more neutral or happier ones, then the impression of sad and depressed content is given.

Diminished interest or pleasure in activities

As with depressed mood, we can hear diminished interest or pleasure in activities either by a direct subjective report or by noticing how an individual speaks. The direct subjective reports may be similar to the reports of depressed mood. In particular, we heard diminished interest or pleasure in verbs that report affection (e.g., like, want, enjoy) and verbs and adjectives that report on a negative subjective state (bored, uninterested, fed up, tired of) (see Table 8.1). Of course, a speaker can negate a positive word to get the same effect (no fun, not interesting). The reports of lack of interest or pleasure may be concentrated in one area of activity or spread across many. If there was a particular area of interest, such as a hobby, that becomes uninteresting, the clinician must be prepared to notice the change. In fact, becoming bored with in one area of interest (the field, see Chapter 2) may be a sign of a more general reduction in interests and activities. Other individuals with depression can show the diminished interest or pleasure across many topics and interests. The clinician can explore the extent of the diminished interests by inquiring about a range of prior activities and the speaker's current interest in them. With more awareness, the speaker can speak about the mood and interests. With less awareness, the speaker may just speak in a way that indicates the diminished interests and activities.

Some speakers may not be aware or capable of directly expressing diminished interests. In these cases, as for the parallel cases of depressed mood, the clinician must listen for the range of topics or areas of interest that are both present and absent in spontaneous interaction (see Table 8.2 for depressed mood, with corresponding changes for 'interests and activities'). We can listen for which topics the speaker initiates and shows interest in as well as noting which topics the speaker responds to in detail or with interest and enthusiasm. The formula is straightforward: a change in levels of interests and pleasures is signalled by less enthusiasm, talk and initiation on once favoured topics. One simple marker of the lack of enthusiasm is the use of negative words, in particular, the use of 'not' and 'n't'. Another marker is the use of intensifiers that suggest interest and pleasure. Words such as 'very' and 'really' ('I really like to', 'I like it very much') as well as similar negative expressions ('not very much', 'not especially', 'not particularly') signal the positive or negative levels of interest. The clinician should ideally be able to compare premorbid and post morbid interests and pleasures to determine the changes in the specific speaker. As well, the clinician instinctively uses the community standards of interest in various activities.

Psychomotor retardation

Psychomotor agitation or retardation is another diagnostic criterion that is partly defined by language. The focus will be on the retardation, given that it is more typical and that the agitation is more or less merely overabundance in the dimensions we describe for retardation. Psychomotor retardation can be conceptualised as either slowed speech or the slowed thinking that we observe by the way someone speaks. We may hear speech that is simply slower with pauses in the typical places or there may be a range of other phenomena. If we notice that a speaker does not respond fast enough to the environment (other speakers, events), then this verbal behaviour may be interpreted as slowed thinking. We also notice psychomotor retardation in speech if there is reduction in:

(1) the amount of talk;

(2) variety of the content;

(3) variation in intonation.

To clarify this last dimension, a monotone may sound like a slow speech and a quiet voice may sound as if the speaker is devoting minimal energy to the interaction. The extreme of these three dimensions is muteness.

AMOUNT OF TALK

We now expand on these linguistic dimensions of psychomotor retardation (see Table 8.3 for a summary and examples). We can hear a reduction in the amount of talk (the first dimension) both within the clause and in how many clauses are combined together. Within the clause, a speaker can express more or less information that modifies the things of the world. Speakers with depression may express less information of a certain kind. Information describing the kind or type of something (classifiers, in Chapter 2) seems to be missing in the speech of speakers with depression. The same speakers, however, do describe the qualities of objects and people. For example, speakers without depression speak about kinds and types of objects, such as: 'this *rhyming* slang', 'the different things *that happened*', '*prisoner of war* camps' and 'a place *for them to stay*'. However, such information is missing in the speech of speakers with depression who restrict themselves to describing the qualities of things. Placing 'very' in front of the descriptive word can test for these qualities. Consider the following examples from the interactions of speakers with depression: '*truthful nasty* jokes', 'very *good* day', 'an *awful* difference', 'some *terrible* dreams', 'a *healthy* appetite'. All the descriptive words tell us about a quality of the object and can all be further modified by 'very'. There are no examples here of words that tell about the class of the objects (e.g., 'this *rhyming* slang', '*prisoner of war* camps').

Table 8.3

Language feature	Examples	
Slowed speech	each utterance spoken slowly	*Depressive disorder, psychomotor retardation – language features*
Reduction in amount of speech		
- within clauses	this (rhyming) slang (prisoner of war) camps	
- across clauses	(see extended examples in Section 8.2.2)	
Reduction in variety of content, expressed in restricted sets of	extended talk on one topic to exclusion of other topics	
- nominals encoding things, people, places	uninterrupted talk about the lake etc.	
- verbs encoding events	repeated talk about eating, sleeping etc.	
- adverbs, etc. encoding details of events	repeated talk about yesterday, here etc.	
Reduction in variation of intonation	utterances spoken with little change in pitch, loudness	

As well as a reduction in the amount of talk within a clause, the failure to expand on information from one clause to another indicates the reduction of amount of talk in depression. In the following interview with a speaker with depression, the answers are rather short and undeveloped.

LITTLE ADDED INFORMATION

> I: so we were talking about you and your present condition and that kind of thing
>
> S: right
>
> I: is there any way you are … all the time would you say I mean that's worse now and … other things are going on but would you say that by-and-large you always were a rather self-conscious person
>
> S: … yes I am
>
> I: do you know where it comes from … do you think that as a child you had experiences that made you ah … become self-conscious and kind of ashamed of some things about yourself
>
> S: … hmm … it could be

Of course, the personal nature of the topic could be shaping these short answers. When we find such short interactions in a number of contexts, we are more certain that it is the 'reduction in amount of talk' that is typical of speakers with depression.

REDUCED VARIETY OF
CONTENT

Related to a reduction in the amount of talk in depression is a reduction in the variety of content. We hear the restricted variety of content by listening to the nouns that express the objects, people and places of the world, the verbs that express the events in the world and the variety of words (adverbs, prepositions, clauses) that express the times and locations of those events. The speaker may talk about limited content because the speaker has a favourite or stereotyped topic that crowds out other topics. In any case, we hear a 'reduction' in variety of content in terms of our expectation for that particular social process. Furthermore, as there is a reduction in the variety of content, so there is a reduction in the variety of social processes that the speaker can contribute to. On the one hand, there are limited word meanings and on the other hand there are limited social processes. However, it is not clear what the causal relation is between the reduction in variety of content and the reduction in social processes.

DECREASED
INFLECTION

The third kind of decreased speech in depression, in addition to decreased amount of speech and decreased variety of speech, is a decrease in the inflection of speech. A narrower range in the ups and downs of sound (the pitch), leads to speech sounding monotonous. Changes in pitch, especially wider changes in pitch, express what is new in a message and what is emotionally important to the speaker. Without these specific meanings, a speaker certainly sounds less interested in the hearer and less interested in the content of the message.

Feelings of worthlessness or excessive guilt

As would be expected, feelings of worthlessness or excessive or inappropriate guilt are expressed directly through main content words (see Table 8.4).

In the following excerpts of conversation, some of the content words of worthlessness and guilt are emphasised.

I: why would people be so interested in you?

S: I don't know

I: What do you think they may be saying?

S: … about my *appearance* mainly

I: what … do they make derogatory remarks or?

S: yes

I: what would that be?

S: ah … you know some people *try* to *hide* their … acne

I: oh I see

S: you know … and you know … things like that you know wearing brown shoes with black pants

I: you have black now

S: yes … I *changed* them

S: it's a little *distressing* but it … it *will work out* … *start taking care of* myself and … *cut* my hair and stuff like that

S: I'm *afraid* to say something to somebody that *might hurt their feelings*

As a number of these utterances show, worthlessness and guilt are expressed in statements about events ('*try* to *hide*', 'I *changed* them', '*will work out*', '*start taking care of*', '*cut* my hair', '*afraid* to say', '*might hurt their feelings*') that imply that the current state is undesirable (worthless) and that a change of state would be an improvement. The judgement of 'excessive' feelings of guilt must, as usual, be made in the cultural and situational context of the interaction.

Clinical feature	Meaning in world at stake	Language features	Examples
Depressed mood	(See Table 8.2)		
Diminished interest or pleasure in activities	(See Table 8.2)		
Psychomotor retardation	(See Table 8.3)		
Feelings of worthlessness or excessive guilt	view of self-worth, guilt	content words (nominals, verbs, adjectives) of worth, guilt	I'm *afraid* to say something to somebody that *might hurt their feelings*
Diminished ability to think or concentrate, indecisiveness	subjective claims, mitigation of commitment to truth	modal verbs confirmation seeking level tone at end of clause	I can't think of the answer. I *would* take their advice. I left, *you know.* They should be here …
Recurrent thoughts of death, suicidal ideation		content words (nominals, verbs, adjectives) of death, suicide	I thought I should *go, end it all, be finished once and for all*

Table 8.4

Depressive disorder – language features

Diminished ability to think or concentrate, indecisiveness

The criterion of 'diminished ability to think or concentrate' is conceptualised in terms of thinking. The issue then is, what is the evidence for these particular kinds of thoughts. Naturally, the clinician will be listening for subjective claims that the speaker cannot concentrate or decide, e.g., 'I can't think of the answer', 'It's hard for me to make up my mind about that'. However, there are also indirect indications in language (see Table 8.4). Verbs that mitigate commitment to the truth of a statement (modal verbs, Chapter 2) are signals that the speaker is less than sure of what is being said. In the following examples, these verbs of mitigation are emphasised. As well, 'you know' is used frequently in this example to check the hearer's understanding. This frequent checking shows that the speaker is insecure about how the message is being understood.

MITIGATING VERBS

> I looked at my bosses… I looked at … people I *could* talk to you know people that *seem* friendly … you know … for a little bit of guidance well … at the time it didn't work out too well … you know … I *would* take their advice and sometimes it *would* backfire you know so …

> I *would* appreciate a doctor but at the moment I *can't* … *can't* even afford a a doctor's fees I *can't*

LEVEL TONE

Indecisiveness can also be signalled by a level tone at the end of clauses. A rising tone often indicates a question. A falling tone often indicates a statement, but a clause that could be a statement ('I think it's raining') with a level tone at the end sounds incomplete. It is unclear whether the speaker knows or does not know the truth of the statement. The impairment in concentration and thinking, we see, shows itself in the language of insecurity and indecisiveness through the use of certain verbs and intonation.

Recurrent thoughts of death and suicidal ideation

CONTENT WORDS

As with feelings of worthlessness, thoughts of death and suicide are features of depression that are conceptualised as thoughts but noticed mainly in language (see Table 8.4). As with other features implicating ideation, there will be the expected content words of the language that deal with death and suicide. The clinician must also be sensitive to the culturally based definition of what is 'recurrent' and therefore what is pathological. There is little need to list the words and social activities that express preoccupations with death or suicide.

Depression is conceptualised clinically as a number of largely ideational criteria (summarised in Table 8.4). These markers of depression are expressed mainly by nouns encoding the people and objects of the world and by verbs encoding the events of the world. The unusual expressions of loss of interest, worthlessness, guilt, death and suicide are the ideational content of depressive episodes. With increase in such expressions, there may be a corresponding decrease in other kinds of more typical ideation thus foregrounding the depressed ideation.

As well as the specific ideation, depression can be conveyed by the speaker's expressed attitude to the ideation. That is, the language carrying the speaker's enthusiasm, excitement and commitment is affected, further displaying the depressed mood. The interpersonal parts of language, such as modal verbs and aspects of stress and intonation carry these messages of enthusiasm and commitment. In all cases, the clinician must be aware of the usual language patterns that express ideation and interpersonal meanings to notice the atypical excesses and scarcities in the language of speakers with depression.

SPEAKER ATTITUDE

Manic episode   8.3

8.3.1 Clinical features

The main clinical categories of manic mood (see Table 8.5 for summary and examples) expressed in language are:

(1) euphoria;

(2) enthusiasm for interaction;

(3) inflated self-esteem;

(4) irritability;

(5) manic speech;

(6) flight of ideas;

(7) distractibility.

Of these clinical categories, euphoria or atypically good mood is a higher-level category. When the other more specific and more concrete clinical categories are present, then we hear euphoria.

Table 8.5

Manic disorder – language features

Clinical feature	Meaning in world at stake	Language features	Examples
Euphoria	Cheerfulness, well-being	Few negative words Positive attributes in relational clauses	n't, never, nothing I'm feeling *wonderful*
		Positive characteristics of nominals	The *delightful* movie
Enthusiasm for interaction	Interpersonal initiative	Initiating social processes Initiating speech functions for:	Let's play cards.
		• information • goods and services	It's time to swim. Would you like a drink?
Inflated self-esteem	Assuming important role in community	Speech functions and content words of giving advice, orders	I would see to that problem right away.
		Frequent specific, technical vocabulary	Release the dynamic pressure valve
Irritability	Angry exchanges Negative responses	Emotional vocabulary Contradiction and correction	I *hate* that behaviour. A: We will win tonight B: *No we won't.*
Manic speech	Pressured, loud, difficult to interpret	Fewer, shortened pauses Unusual loudness	
	Joking, punning, theatrical	Unusual people, things, places Unusual voice quality	This Martian came up to me . . . .
Flight of ideas	Ideas are fast and difficult to follow	Few pauses Increased rate of talk	
		Abrupt changes in topic	We watched TV. I have to go to the wedding night.
Distractibility	Stimuli external to the social process intrude	References to physical situation	*That* door over *there*.
		Changes in participants, processes, circumstances	The door opened. The *moon* is full.
		Changes in antecedents for reference	The door opened. It squeaked. The moon is full. *It* glowed.

We hear mania largely in the physical aspects of speech such as volume, rate and prosody. On the other hand, we notice the joking and theatrical speech in mania because they are special social processes that interrupt or compromise the main activity. The flight of ideas and distractibility in mania implicate more ideational jumping and, for flight of ideas, the rate of change of ideation. Vocabulary choice and reduced or strained linking in language (see cohesion, Chapter 2) create this ideational movement.

8.3.2 Language features

Euphoria

Our description then starts with this more general category of elevated mood. Euphoria is a general cheerfulness and feeling of well-being. Euphoria is created by language with positive statements of mood and mental state and by paralinguistic means such as laughs, smiles and accelerated rate of speech. The specific linguistic indicators will be:

(1) the relatively scarce use of the negative words found in depression (e.g., not, n't, no, never, neither, nothing, nor, nowhere), especially the use of 'n't' to make a whole statement negative;

(2) the frequent use of positive attributes of the people, places and things of the world expressed in sentences that characterise (relational sentences), such as 'I'm feeling *wonderful*', 'the trip was *exciting*', 'the sandwich was *delicious*'. We also find the positive characteristics of people, places and things expressed as descriptions before the nouns stating these things. The positive sounding descriptions may be either a class (classifier, see Chapter 2) of the things (the *automatic* machine) or a positive quality (epithet) of the thing (the *delightful* movie).

Enthusiasm for interaction

Enthusiasm for interaction means notably more participation than usual. Language conveys this enthusiasm by specific interpersonal and ideational meanings. Enthusiasm for interaction is created interpersonally in atypically high rates of initiating exchanges. These exchanges can be exchanges of information and perhaps even goods and services ('Would you like a drink?' 'Can I help you?' 'Please move over here.'). The initiations will be widespread, across contexts and across different topics of interaction (the 'fields' outlined in Chapter 2). If the initiations are only in a few favourite topics, then the speaker sounds more like someone with special interests, rather than a general enthusiasm for interaction.

INITIATING
EXCHANGES

To understand these interpersonal meanings, we must look at the abundance of initiating at a number of levels of analysis. At the most abstract level, the speaker will be heard as starting various social processes. For example, the speaker will be the one to start jokes, stories and introduce people to each other. A speaker who starts these interactions more than is expected gives the impression of wanting interaction. At a lower level of analysis, certain speech functions indicate enthusiasm for interaction. That is, statements, questions and imperatives all start local sequences of utterances signalling that the speaker is opening an interactional sequence and that the interlocutor is the one who is expected to respond. These interpersonal speech functions of conveying information (statements), seeking information (questions) and directing someone to give goods and services (imperatives) open up interactions that will be continued by other speakers. Of the two basic meanings of speech functions, initiating and responding, we see that the initiating speech functions and their expression in grammar by questions, statements and imperatives, show the enthusiasm of the speaker.

In extreme cases, this enthusiasm for interaction seems unceasing or indiscriminate. We notice these more severe cases by the rapid succession of turns at talk and by the speech functions in those turns. The speaker with enthusiasm for interaction will be initiating both social processes (the stories, the new activities, etc.) and use statements, questions and imperatives Other speakers, then, are not be able to take these roles. These other speakers may even find it difficult to fully respond to all the initiations by the affected speaker.

RANGE OF TOPICS

As indicated, we find much of the enthusiasm for interaction in a speaker's initiating. However, there are also aspects of ideational meaning that convey enthusiasm. A speaker who talks about a wide range of topics (the fields of Chapter 2) can create the unceasing flow of language that we hear as enthusiasm for interaction. That is, the speaker introduces a range of social processes involving many topics. It seems that there is nothing that the speaker does not talk about. In more typical interaction, a speaker sometimes takes on an initiating role and sometimes a responding role. This is particularly true as the interaction moves from one social process and topic to another. In some contexts, a speaker will typically initiate since the speaker may be more knowledgeable or interested in the social process at hand, whereas in other contexts the speaker will typically be more passive. If there is frequent initiating behaviour across various social processes and various contexts, then the interaction will be heard as forced, without regard to other speakers. To put this behaviour in clinical terms, the speaker is indiscriminately speaking about different things and indiscriminately initiating interaction. The initiating is sometimes inappropriate either in terms of the speaker (e.g., initiating a personal conversation with a distant superior at work), or in terms of the content (e.g, initiating a discussion of the importance of relativity theory).

In summary, for enthusiasm for interaction, the clinician will be attending to both the interpersonal aspects that signal enthusiasm and the ideational aspects of the interaction. If the enthusiasm seems constant across different social processes and different topics, then there may be the unceasing and indiscriminate use of language that is described in mania.

Inflated self-esteem or grandiosity

As with enthusiasm for interaction, it is ideational and interpersonal meanings that convey inflated self-esteem and grandiosity in mania. Interpersonally, the speaker takes on roles such as giving advice or talking about public figures in an intimate way. In general, these roles are higher than would be expected of the speaker's social roles in the community. For example, a speaker may mention 'my friend, the mayor' or 'the last time I spoke with the ambassador'.

There is an ideational aspect to inflated self-esteem as well. A speaker posing as an expert will sound as having inflated self-esteem. The specific linguistic markers of this inflated self-esteem are technical terms that are used out of place. We can usually recognise highly specific and technical language used by a speaker who does not really know the ideational material. In considering the actual wordings, the events that are mentioned (expressed by verbs), the people and things of the world (usually expressed by nouns) and the modifiers (worded as nouns and adjectives 'cool, light, Mosel wine') signal inappropriate technical language.

Irritability

Irritability is essentially a description of a reaction to people or to aspects of a situation. If the irritability is serious, then the social process itself may be interrupted. Irritability can be recognised by unexpected, short, angry exchanges. In particular, a speaker can show irritability by contradicting the prior utterance of another speaker. In the simplest case, responding negatively to a positive statement conveys irritability, as in the following example.

    A: the German team is much better this year
    B: no it isn't

Since contradiction and correction are a natural part of interaction, the clinician must pay attention to the frequency of these short contradictions. More broadly, irritability is displayed by responses that are confronting by expressing disagreement or non-compliance. For example, when goods and services are offered, a speaker may reject the offer ('I don't want any'); when a question is asked, a speaker may refuse to answer: 'What time is it?' 'I wouldn't tell you' (see Eggins and Slade, 1994: 180–213 for a detailed presentation of these confronting possibilities). Again, it is the rate of the confronting utterances with respect to the situation that indicates irritability. As well as by confronting speech functions, the irritability may also be expressed by short utterances and by exaggerated or loud intonation.

The rather negative quality of utterances that express irritability may be found in one ideational sphere (one field, to use the concept from Chapter 2) or cut across a number of ideational spheres, indicating a rather touchy personality in general. The clinician should then probe a number of ideational areas to explore whether the irritability is centred on one topic. In some cases of interaction, the irritability will be displayed when the speaker's wishes or statements are themselves contradicted. In the following example, the irritability is found in the third utterance in the sequence in reaction to the unexpected utterance of the second speaker that, in fact, interrupts the expected social process.

> A: I want a sandwich with mustard (request for goods and services)
> B: sorry we don't have any left (confronting response that denies the request)
> A: what's wrong with you (irritable follow-up to denial)

Manic speech

Manic speech is described clinically as:

(1) largely low-level phenomena in the delivery of speech: pressured, loud and difficult to interrupt;

(2) atypicalities at a higher level such as joking, punning and theatrical speech.

SHORTENED PAUSES

The low-level phenomena are rather evident to the hearer. We identify pressured speech by the fewer and shortened pauses and a rapid delivery of words. The hearer notices the absence and shortening of pauses particularly in locations that usually mark the transitions. These transitions may be from one social process to another or even from one part of a social process to another (for example, making introductions in a meeting and then turning to the agenda of the meeting itself).

Unusual loudness of speech is noticed especially on stressed syllables that normally are somewhat louder than other parts of the utterance. The exaggerated volume on these syllables may even interfere with the meaning of the message since loudness often expresses meanings of contrast, surprise, etc. These low-level phenomena in the delivery of speech collectively interfere with the larger social process, since other speakers may not be able to take turns in the usual way. For example, with pressure of speech, other speakers may not easily be able to take a turn to answer a question or even to ask for clarification when needed. That is, the pressure of speech and generally more rapid speech can change the social roles in the interaction and thus actually compromise the completion of the social process.

EXTRA LOUDNESS

The higher level atypicalities of manic speech include joking, punning, amusing irrelevancies and theatrical speech. All these characteristics express meanings atypical to the social context and the step-by-step development of the social process. Joking, punning and amusing irrelevancies intrude into the social processes when they are not expected. These intrusions all have a rather positive social dimension but are nevertheless out of place. If the intruding dimension were more neutral (such as asking for the time of day), the utterances would also be out of place but not indicate the positive, expansive, even comic, mood found in mania.

CHANGE IN SOCIAL PROCESSES

In contrast to the limited scope of jokes, puns and irrelevant comments, theatrical speech may continue beyond a few comments and may involve a number of departures from the social process. Theatrical speech involves playing an atypical role in the interaction. This theatrical social role may be used to attract attention. Within the theatrical role, there can be changes in voice quality, changes in facial expressions and body movements and mimicry. The result of all these changes in the use of language is to create a social role for the speaker that is markedly out of place in the context at hand.

Flight of ideas

Flight of ideas is, clinically, an unusually rapid flow of speech. It has few pauses and the actual rate of words is increased. Furthermore, there can be abrupt changes in topics (technically the fields and institutional foci of Chapter 2), similar to the derailment in schizophrenia (see Chapter 7). These changes in topic are signalled in language by changes in sets of vocabulary without the signals that a new topic is being introduced. The unsignalled changes in topic can sound incoherent and disorganised in their extreme forms. See the detailed linguistic descriptions of incoherence and disorganised speech in the description of schizophrenia (Chapter 7).

Distractibility

In a manic disorder, speakers may not be able to screen out irrelevant external stimuli. This characteristic is, in part, an inference from language behaviour. The external stimuli can appear in language either as:

(1) aspects of the physical situation;

(2) from outside the current social process.

PHYSICAL STIMULI   When the external stimuli are from the physical situation, then direct references (exophoric references) to this physical context will be found. The speaker will pay attention to and mention things such as '*this* table', '*that* phone', '*that* door over *there*', '*those* clouds in the sky', '*your* sun glasses'.

STIMULI FROM EXTERNAL SOCIAL PROCESSES   When the external stimuli are less connected to the physical situation, they may be tied to some social process, some activity, that does not appear to be connected to the on-going interaction. As with the abrupt changes in topic found in flight of ideas, distractibility is recognised by the unconnected sets of vocabulary. For example, part of an utterance can deal with automobiles or hobbies and then switch, unannounced, to the vocabulary of politics. As well as the changes in sets of vocabulary, a speaker may use references (endophoric reference) to the people, places and things of the world (through words such as 'he', 'she', 'it', 'they', 'them', 'their') atypically. As the topics change, the things that these words refer to also change. At one point, 'they' will refer to the television programmes being spoken about and soon afterwards 'they' will refer to the politicians who have just been elected.

A third type of distraction is a combination of an external stimulus and an external social process. That is, the speaker may enter into a social process that is overheard and switch between two activities. For example, while engaged in one interaction in a store (buying shoes), the speaker may be distracted and enter into an interaction with other individuals involved in a different social process (how to adjust the heating system so customers will be more comfortable in the store).

In all these cases of external stimuli, the language gives the impression that the speaker is attending to something outside the social process. The clinician will want to pay close attention to the nature of the linguistic signals mentioned above to form impressions of the kind of distraction involved. The feature of distractibility in a manic disorder should be compared to distractibility and inattention in attention deficit hyperactivity disorder (see Chapter 6).

We have seen that the detailed description of the characteristics of mania implicates many features of language. Some of these features overlap with features found in psychosis and even attention deficit hyperactivity disorder. In clinical diagnosis and description, it is important to consider the combination of features found in a speaker rather than be focused on what seems a clear feature of one or another disorder.

Chapter 9 contents

Personality disorders

Overview of personaility disorders 9.1

9.1.1 Patterns of meaning

Personalities are seen clinically as atypicalities in inner experience that interfere with normal social functioning. We will deal with four personality disorders in this chapter: schizotypal, histrionic, dependent and obsessive compulsive disorders. We will discover that since these disorders are related to inner experience, the linguistic descriptions that we will present for the four disorders do not have a strong common thread. Rather, the disorders show both an overlap of linguistic features and different combinations of linguistic features. The clinical approach is to say that personality disorders involve cognition, affect and impulse control. In this chapter we outline that linguistic appearance of these three categories. Along with the categories we describe the inflexibility and pervasive patterns of behaviour found in patients with personality disorders. To foreshadow the linguistic descriptions:

(1) cognition most clearly involves the ideational meanings of language;

(2) affect involves mainly the interpersonal meanings of language;

(3) impulse control involves interpersonal and interactional meanings (see Table 9.1).

Clinical features	Metafunctions of language at stake	Table 9.1
cognition	ideational	*Relation between clinical features for personality disorders and the metafunctions of language at stake*
affect	interpersonal	
impulse control	interpersonal	

In this chapter we show how excess or scarcity of specific interpersonal and ideational meanings are interpreted by the clinician as atypicalities of inner experience. Our approach is to conceptualise the disorders as observable characteristics of verbal behaviour rather than as the more traditional atypicalities of inner experience. The verbal characteristics are, though, linked to the underlying concepts of cognition, impulse control, etc. We must notice that the traditional concepts are of different kinds. Inner experience is a concept of the intraorganism state. It is accessible subjectively but can also be accessible objectively when a person describes an inner state. In contrast, cognition is a concept at the level of information processing that applies to both inner constructs and objective outer world constructs. It is how we process the information we deal with. The third concept, impulse control, is an abstract way of talking about one aspect of behaviour.

We use the details of the language phenomena to compare across individuals and across disorders. Although it requires patience to understand, we must give enough detail about the language so that individuals can be described at a phenomenological level. The disorders can then be understood in terms of language. More fundamentally, the goal is to use the language to describe the impairment in social functioning which is the core of the problem in personality disorders. We do not eliminate concepts such as inner experience or disturbance in affect. Rather, we identify such concepts through principled descriptions of the language behaviour that lead to the clinical identification of the concepts. In this way, commonalties across individuals are based on the language behaviour. The clinician can then use these commonalities to subgroup individuals according to behaviour. More importantly, we can use the behaviour subgroups as a starting point for exploring common underlying processes or emotional features. We can start to build new sets of concepts that may lie behind the disorders.

There are three kinds of patterning of behaviour in personality disorders. First, the behaviour is stable over time. Second, the behaviour is stable across social situations. Third, the behaviour includes at least two out of the three domains of: cognition, affectivity and interpersonal functioning, impulse control. This definition brings together the context of the interactions and the expected domain of the atypicalities (cognition, affectivity, interpersonal). From our perspective from language, the context of the social process interacts with the domain of atypicality. That is, the kinds of cognition, affectivity and interpersonal functioning that the clinician may see depend also on the context. For example, children learn early on to vary language behaviour to fit the situation in terms of ideational meanings and in terms of interpersonal meanings. They vary their language according to the addressee, the content that they are speaking about and the social process they are in. This variation is an important part of using language for social purposes. By varying language, speakers signal that they are aware of the social purposes of the interaction and signal that they know the social roles that they and others are taking. When there is less of this variation, due to personality traits or other reasons, then the social functioning is itself at risk. If we heard someone speaking the same way all the time it would sound odd indeed. Sometimes the speaker would be too formal, sometimes too relaxed, sometimes giving too much detail, sometimes sounding like a person avoiding certain issues. That is, variation, both in meanings and in how those meanings are worded, is expected and part of the patterning of social interaction across social contexts and across speakers. The description of personality disorders will be organised according to the domains of cognition, affectivity and interpersonal interaction since these are the clinical categories that are most apparent when interacting with an individual with a personality disorder.

9.1.2 Language signalling cognition

Cognition is taken as underlying the inflexible traits in a personality disorder. What is important in cognition is how the individual perceives the world and the self. Of course, it is largely in language that we find the evidence for these perceptions and for the difficulty in cognition. We then study the language to draw inferences about the cognition. The atypicalities in language then lead us simultaneously to a description of:

(1) atypical language;

(2) the evidence that is used to infer atypical cognition;

(3) the evidence for the key clinical requirement of maladaptive social and occupational behaviour.

Our description and understanding of personality disorders is from:

(1) a description of language, to

(2) the atypical ways of perceiving the self and outside people and events, to

(3) the atypicalities in cognition that lead to the odd perceptions in (2).

However, the construction of the concepts is not so linear. For example, the concept of perceiving the self may be more established than either the description of language which reflects those perceptions or the specific cognitive processes underlying the perceptions. Depending on our interests, we can start the different clinical and research tasks (diagnosis, classification, evaluation, etc.) at different levels of the description.

Table 9.2

Relation between clinical features for personality disorders and language features

Clinical features	Language features at stake	Examples
Cognition	Participants expressed by: • nominals (especially encoding of self)	Repetitions of I, the boss
	Descriptions of participants expressed by: • qualifier	The play *they were late for*
	Events expressed by: • verbs	Repetitions of running, fighting
	Circumstances (time, place, causes, etc.) expressed by: • adverbs • prepositional phrases	 She did it *quickly*. They ate *at home*.
Affect	Determined polarity (positive or negative) expressed by: • falling or rising pitch	It is raining. **(falling pitch)** It is raining? **(rising pitch)**
	Unexpected information expressed by: • extra stress	The FURNITURE arrived.
	Degree of commitment expressed by: • modal adjuncts • modal verbs	 It is *probably* raining. It *might* be raining.
	Kinds and range of emotions expressed by: • adjectives • verbs of emotion • verbs of behaviour	 I was *frustrated*. I *felt* terrible. I *cried* all day.
	Intensity of emotions as expressed by: • intonational stress • change in emotions (lability)	 I LAUGHED through supper.
Impulse control, interpersonal functioning	Wrong social process	Profession criticism taken for personal attack
(see also Table 6.3)	Inappropriate language for social process	Swearing or shouting in a post office

First and very clearly for personality disorders, there are major atypicalities of ideational meanings (see Table 9.2). These ideational meanings include the people, places and objects of the world (participants in linguistic terms), the events of the world and information of times, locations and causes of these things and events. In listening to speakers with personality disorders, we hear unusual expression of the self as well as other things and the events they are involved in. That is, these expressions of things and events are not what we usually hear in the language community. In particular, we hear an inflexibility in the ideational content. A speaker will talk about the same people, places, things and events despite changes in the context. The speaker seems to be talking about the same things no matter what.

IDEATIONAL MEANINGS

To take a wider perspective, speakers try to accomplish different social goals in different contexts: sometimes to convince a neighbour to lend a cup of sugar, sometimes to invite a friend for a cup of coffee, sometimes to make an appointment with the dentist. However, if the speaker returns to the same ideational content, then there will be difficulty in attaining a variety of social goals. Usually, we achieve specific social goals by a certain combination of ideational information, interpersonal meanings and the meanings imposed by the constraints of the channel of communication (letter, email, telephone conversation, shouting over loud music, etc.). When the ideational meanings are relatively constant (e.g., a certain expressed view of oneself, a repeated concern over the health of others), then these meanings will intrude into contexts where they are usually not found and the social processes themselves will be at risk. To take an example that occurred in a clinical interview, one stage of the interview concerned taking a history and speaking about family relations. However, the patient repeatedly talked about another clinician eventually compromising the on-going social process: the interview. Clinically, the concern about the other health professional sounded like inflexible and inappropriate cognition.

In practice, the clinician must identify the specific components (things, people, events, time periods, etc.) that intrude into the social process in order to recognise the nature of the inflexibility. With this added detail, the clinician can characterise and compare different speakers and build more detailed hypotheses about the kind of cognitive inflexibility involved. Similarly, if a speaker characterises individuals, things and events too consistently, then hearers will think that the speaker is inflexible in describing the world. These descriptions of the outside world can appear as details (technically a qualifier, see Chapter 2) after a noun naming a person, place or object ('The monster *that I wish I hadn't seen*', 'The play *that they were late for*'). The speaker with a personality disorder may also repeated descriptions of time, place or the manner of the action ('*Three years ago*, they really had a hard time', '*In our neighbourhood*, there is always something interesting happening', 'She did it *as fast as lightening*'). Focusing on the descriptions relating to the self, whether in modification ('my *poor* dog', 'my *steaming* apartment'), attributing qualities or actions to the self ('I am *worried* again', 'I *beat* them at their own game'), or describing when or where events happened ('*For the fourth time*, I found myself *in the castle*'), may be particularly helpful in identifying the ideational inflexibility within a personality disorder. Furthermore, the self, in particular, may be introduced into the interaction rather more than is expected. The most explicit linguistic signals of the self are the first person pronouns (I, me, my, mine, myself, we, us, our, ours, ourselves). A speaker who returns to these pronouns more often than usual, across various contexts and especially with set descriptions of the self, will be heard as having a personality disorder.

9.1.3   Language signalling affect

The usual approach is to attribute these atypical expressions of the self and others to perceptual and other processes that are taken as central to personality disorders. Another central characteristic of personality disorders is atypical emotional response (affectivity). This characteristic is like the perceptual processes in identifying a source for various observable, largely verbal, phenomena. We now develop a linguistic interpretation of affectivity. Language expresses emotional response through a specific, limited number of devices in the interpersonal metafunction. Emotional response is also encoded in a minor and obvious way in the ideational meanings of language. These points will be outlined after discussing the important interpersonal resources for conveying emotional response.

INTONATION

Language gives us a rich set of resources for signalling emotional responses. Firstly, the rise and fall of intonation (the intonation contour) encodes whether the speaker thinks that the positive or negative meaning of the sentence is known. Rising intonation ('They are here?') indicates that the speaker is not sure whether the sentence is positive or negative, true or false. In contrast, falling intonation ('It is raining', 'It is not raining') signals that the speaker's message has a known truth-value (positive or negative). At the simplest level, unusual rising intonation indicates ideational and emotional uncertainty, whereas falling intonation indicates certainty. At a more sophisticated level, combinations of rising and falling intonations carry meanings of being first sure and then unsure (falling then rising intonation) or first unsure and then sure (rising then falling intonation). These complex combinations of rises and falls in intonation express the emotional state of the speaker with respect to the ideation of the utterance.

We have seen that the direction of intonation carries emotional meaning. In addition, the stress or loudness on certain parts of an utterance express surprise by indicating that a certain part of the utterance is unexpected or is just encoded as unexpected for the hearer (see Chapter 2 and the discussion of intonational prominence). A speaker who rarely indicates surprise by intonational prominence conveys a message of uninvolvement, apathy or indifference to the interaction and to other speakers.

To express a full range of emotional involvement we express the degree of commitment to our messages. The main kinds of meaning that express commitment are: probability ('It is *possibly* snowing'), usuality ('It *usually* snows at this time of year') and inclination ('They *must* come now'). These meanings and how they are expressed (see Chapter 2 for a more detailed outline of the meanings), tell us how the speaker is reacting to the utterances of others and how committed the speaker is to the current utterance. The changes in affectivity found in personality disorders can be either little qualification of commitment, suggesting unusually strong commitment, or unusually frequent qualification of commitment, suggesting self-doubt or extreme caution.

COMMITMENT

The emotional responses in personality disorders can be specified further. Clinically, the emotional responses in personality disorder are atypical in terms of:

(1) the kinds of emotions expressed;

(2) the intensity of the emotions;

(3) the change in emotions over time (lability).

The clinician should be aware of the language of each of these dimensions. The emotions can be expressed as adjectives that attribute qualities to the speaker ('I am *mad/happy/frustrated*'), verbs that express emotions ('I *feel* terrible') or verbs that express the actions of the speaker ('I *laughed/cried* all day'). In personality disorders, we will hear an unusual variety of emotions (the specific adjectives, verbs of emotion, verbs of action) as well as unusual ways of expressing these emotions. In particular there can be a narrowing of the usual range and perhaps a focus on a very limited number of emotions.

The intensity of the emotions also departs from the typical in a personality disorder. As described earlier, we hear the intensity of emotions through intonation and the level of commitment to the ideational material. The change in emotional reactions over time, lability, is heard in terms of both the on-going interaction and the pattern of change usually found in the speech community for similar contexts. The clinician must monitor both the changes in meaning as the interaction develops and the ways those meanings are expressed. We always track the three dimensions of range, intensity and lability in context and instinctively compare them to the emotional reactions we expect in the social process. If a social process is accomplished with little problem, then any difference in emotional reaction is below a threshold for being noticed and below a threshold for compromising social activity.

9.1.4   Language signalling: interpersonal functioning

The third main clinical description of personality disorder, in addition to disturbances in cognition and affectivity, is a disturbance in interpersonal functioning. The clinical approach suggests that the problem in cognition is a problem of thinking. Here we are interested in the linguistic evidence for the construct of atypical cognition. Similarly, the odd affect is a difficulty conceptualised at an emotional level that is then expressed verbally and non-verbally. The third aspect of personality disorder, interpersonal functioning, is not a conceptualisation of a cause (either cognition or emotions) and identified from observable verbal and non-verbal data. Rather, interpersonal functioning is itself, a description of largely verbal behaviour (see Table 9.2). In the most general sense, the individual is not mutually building a social process with one or more people.

The disturbances in interpersonal functioning cover a large range of verbal behaviour and a range of possible underlying causes. As indicated earlier, the speaker may not understand what the current social process is (for example, mistaking mild criticism of performance at work for a vicious personal attack, or mistaking a neighbourly comment for an expression of romantic interest). At a lower level of abstraction, the individual may play an inappropriate social role in terms of the role of another individual (for example, to become an aggressive customer demanding personal attention when the government clerk is in fact trying to be helpful in solving a problem). At a still lower level, the disturbance in interpersonal functioning may appear as inappropriate use of language (swearing or shouting when inappropriate) that interferes with the social process. The root of the inappropriate use of language may be a separate disturbance at the level of production (for example, a complex verbal tic) or a misunderstanding of what language is appropriate when. In all these cases, the social process is at risk and the individual is seen as having an identifiable disturbance in interpersonal functioning. Clinically, it is important to identify the sources of the disturbance. The speaker may either:

(1) misunderstand the social processes and social roles themselves or

(2) use language inappropriately for constructing the social interaction; that is, the mapping between language and social processes is odd.

Impulse control is an especially important part of interpersonal functioning. A fuller description of impulse control is presented in Chapter 6 where
impulsivity is discussed as a characteristic of attention deficit – hyperactivity
disorder. Impulsivity involves a verbal or a non-verbal behaviour that occurs
somewhat ahead of its time in interaction or that seems to be out of place.
Such behaviours should have been suppressed in the on-going context (see
Table 6.3 reproduced here again). The behaviours that are ahead of their
time are associated with the interpersonal meanings and the behaviours
that seem out of place are usually associated with ideational meanings. The
speaker is talking about things and events that are out of the context. In the
mutual construction of interaction, the speakers take roles in terms of both
turns at talk and the information that is contributed in these turns (see the
discussion of exchange structure and speech functions in Chapters 2 and 3).
When speakers enter into interaction too quickly, creating overlapping talk
or when they take a speech role that is out of sequence (answering a question
before it is asked), then the verbal behaviour seems impulsive. These kinds of
impulsivity are largely carried by the interpersonal resources of language such
as turn-taking and functions of speech. The impulsivity affects the organisation of talk and ultimately the social processes that depend on organised talk.
Impulsivity has this deleterious effect by breaking the patterns of turns and
creating new patterns, including starting new sequences of: question – answer
and statement – response to statement when they are out of place.

Clinical feature	Language features	
Overlapping speech	interactants speak at same time	*Table 6.3 (Reproduced)*
Changing topics	infrequent repetition of vocabulary infrequent pronouns signalling same things, people, place	*Attention deficit hyperactivity disorder: impulsivity – language features*
Initiating interaction	frequent first pair partners in adjacency turns often expressed as question or imperative	

As well as this interpersonal turn-taking, we can see impulsivity in the
ideational aspects of language. Usually, a speaker who knows the social
process suppresses ideas and topics that are not relevant to what is happening. If material from another social process does intrude, then we hear
a discontinuity of ideational meaning and perhaps the social process itself
is compromised. The exception happens when the unconnected material
is signalled as different ('Hold on, just let me tell you about …'). Speakers
with schizophrenia in particular introduce such unconnected material and

in the extreme produce disorganised speech (see Chapter 7 for a detailed development of the language features of disorganised speech).

Each of the specific personality disorders involves different combinations of the clinical and language features outlined above. We describe four personality disorders in terms of their linguistic characteristics and how those characteristics both define the disorders and also are important for the clinical recognition of specific diagnostic criteria.

9.2   Schizotypal personality disorder

9.2.1   Clinical features

Broadly, schizotypal personality disorder involves pervasive social and interpersonal deficits with few close personal relationships. More specifically, the disorder involves a number of atypicalities of language (see Table 9.3). These atypicalities are similar to those found in schizophrenia (see Chapter 7) and include:

(1) idiosyncratic speech;

(2) loose, digressive and vague language;

(3) concrete or abstract responses;

(4) word level atypicalities.

In addition to these atypicalities in language, there can be:

(5) a narrowing in the expression of affect that is conveyed by language.

	Clinical feature	Language features	Examples
Table 9.3 *Schizotypal personality disorder – language features*	Idiosyncratic speech	Unusual word order	Today, in the morning, at the table, he sneezed.
		Low frequency structures	What I wanted to do was eat cake.
		Highly marked structures	Tomorrow, in the cupboard, it is the GREEN sweater you will want.

Table 9.3 (Continued)

Loose, digressive, vague language (see derailment and incoherence, Table 7.5)	Change in lexical sets	They answered the *phone*, but he's a real *phoney*.
	Little description of people, objects within nominals	The (round) hill (over there).
	Reference to entire class of objects	*Insects* are repulsive.
	Events with little meaning expressed by:	
	verbs with minimal semantics	You should *do* it.
	Little detail of time, location, manner, etc. in circumstances expressed by:	
	• adverbs	(Yesterday,) they swam
	• prepositional phrases	(in the pool) (to stay cool).
Concrete or abstract responses	Concrete ideation expressed by nominals	The *floor* is dusty.
	Abstract ideation expressed by:	
	• abstract nominals	Love, hate, justice
	• verbs of mental activity	She *thought* it was a good idea.
	• verbs of relating	The idea *seemed* wonderful.
Word level atypicalities	Archaic or rare words, neologisms	behove, notwithoutstanding redly
Narrow affect	stiff presentation as expressed by:	
	• few back-channel markers	um hmm
	• few requests for confirmation	The train leaves at ten. (At ten?)
	Uncontracted forms	I did not think so.
	Few hesitation markers	ah, um, well, you know
	Little overlap of speech	

9.2.2 Language features

Idiosyncratic speech

The first atypicality is idiosyncratic speech and is constructed by:

(1) unusual word order ('*Yesterday, if you don't mind me saying so and I know you may disagree*, my cousins had the best day of the summer' compared to the more usual 'My cousins had the best day of the summer yesterday if you don't mind me saying so and I know you may disagree'),

(2) by low frequency structures ('What I wanted to do was go swimming');

(3) by highly marked structures that are both infrequent and are appropriate only in very restricted structures ('Tomorrow, in the cupboard, it is the GREEN sweater that you will want' – an utterance appropriate when the speaker assumes that the hearer does not expect (a) the time, 'tomorrow', (b) the location, 'in the cupboard' and (c) a feature of a thing, 'green'.

Loose, digressive or vague language

The second atypicality in language is loose, digressive or vague language. This atypicality resembles the derailment and incoherence found in schizophrenia (see Chapter 7) but is not as extreme. In schizotypal personality disorder, the language departs from the social processes at hand. Ideationally, the content words are first from one set of related items, for example, cooking and then from a different set of items, say, astronomy, without sufficient warning of the change. This change in the semantic direction of the interaction is sometimes based on the sound characteristics of words (from 'tele*phone*' to '*phoney*') or on mainly irrelevant semantic features (from 'My *glasses* are fogged up' to 'The *champagne glasses* are really delicate and may break'). The vagueness in language is largely conveyed by little ideational information about the things and events in the world. In language, this scarcity of information happens because there is relatively little modification of the nouns that convey information about people, places and objects ('the (round) hill (over there)'), by the specification of whole classes of things ('*desks* are fine if you need to write', '*insects* are repulsive', 'never climb *a tree*') rather than specific things ('*my/the desk* is brown', '*that bug* went under the carpet', '*the tree in the yard* is ten years old').

As we have seen sometimes the vagueness in language stems from little information about the things of the world. A speaker can also be vague by saying little about the time, location and manner of events. This information (the 'circumstances' discussed in Chapter 2) is largely expressed by prepositional phrases ('in the city', 'around the corner', 'in fifteen minutes', 'at ten o'clock') and by adverbials (quickly, suddenly, unexpectedly). The events themselves (largely expressed by verbs) may have unusually little ideational information. For example, 'think' expresses less information than 'want', 'know' or 'wish'. Similarly, the verb 'do' can replace many verbs of physical action but does not carry much ideational meaning. The more different forms of vagueness a speaker uses and the more the speaker uses them, the more the speaker is noticed as giving less information than expected. The deficit is even more apparent if it extends from one context to another.

Concrete or abstract responses

The language of schizotypal personality disorder involves a third atypicality of language: responses that are unusually concrete or unusually abstract. Concrete language is tied to the physical situation of the speech events (e.g., 'The objects in the room', 'The speakers themselves') or picks out the physical characteristics of what is said ('That idea floored me' leading to the more concrete statement 'The floor sure is dusty'). Abstract language, on the other hand, involves the things of the world that do not have material form (love, hate, injustice, acupuncture). Verbs of mental activity ('She *thought* it was a good idea') or verbs of relating ('The idea *seemed* wonderful') also sound rather abstract. These are, respectively, the mental and relational processes outlined in Chapter 2.

Word level atypicalities

A speaker with schizotypal personality disorder may also use language that is atypical at the level of the word. We readily notice unusual word choices, such as archaic or rare words (behove, notwithoutstanding) and odd constructions that follow the word patterns of the language (redly). These word choices may not specifically interrupt the social process but do still mark the speaker as unusual in context.

Narrow range of affect

A final characteristic of schizotypal personality disorder is narrowing of the range of affect. As described for personality disorders in general, there are many ways to express affect. A stiff presentation is conveyed by not following up one's own comments and by not interacting fully with others. Typically, personal and emotional commitment to interaction is signalled by using back-channel information such as head nods, expressions such as 'uh hmm' to signal that one is following the other speaker and requesting confirmation of information ('At ten?'). When these markers are not used, the interaction sounds stiff or self-centred. Other markers of stiff communication are using the full form of words instead of contractions ('did not' instead of 'didn't', 'it is' instead of 'it's') and little overlap with the speech of others. These ways of expression make the speech sound overly formal. Even using few of hesitation markers such as 'uh', 'well', 'okay', 'um' makes the speaker sound stiff. In summary, using fewer signals of affect than the expected reduces the range of interpersonal meanings. Without these meanings, the interaction sounds overly concerned with the ideational meanings, rather than the interpersonal meanings that lubricate communication.

In schizotypal personality disorder we hear a number of ideational and interpersonal atypicalities in language that mark the interaction as not quite as clear as we expect and as missing the usual amount of affect. That is, there is an unusual configuration of meanings for the contexts we hear. The interactions are not as disruptive as in schizophrenia and the social processes may generally succeed. However, hearers notice the pervasive nature of the atypicalities and the interactions are compromised to some extent.

9.3   Histrionic personality disorder

9.3.1   Clinical features

Histrionic personality disorder essentially includes 'pervasive and excessive emotionality and attention-seeking behavior' (American Psychiatric Association, 1994, 655). First we discuss the features of emotionality and attention-seeking behaviour (see Table 9.4) and then turn to the pervasive and excessive nature of these features.

Table 9.4	Clinical feature	Language features	Examples
Histrionic personality disorder – language features	Emotionality	Verbs of mental processes	I *love/hate/enjoy* those things.
		Verbs of relation + attribute of emotion	They *were annoying.*
		Stressed intonation	Such *REVOLTING* ideas.
		Unusually slow or fast tempo	
	Attention-seeking	Unusual topics of discourse (field) as expressed by: • verbs • nominals	

Table 9.4 (Continued)

• unusual formality/friendliness (tenor) as if unusual channel (mode)	Now all pay attention as I tell you …
Speaking about self by:	
• first person pronouns	*I* want to tell you what *I* did.
• statements about self	*I* have three new umbrellas.
• questions about self	What do you think of *my* new coat?
• startling statements about self	*I've* just won three prizes!

9.3.2   Language features

Emotionality

Emotionality is expressed in language by both ideational and interactional meanings (the ideational and interpersonal metafunctions). Emotionality is expressed ideationally by the choice of words that focus on emotions. In particular, verbs that express the mental processes of thinking and feeling (e.g., like, love, hate) convey emotionality. Furthermore, there are verbs such as 'am', 'seem' that combine with words of emotion; e.g., 'I *seem angry*', 'I *am aghast* with the situation', 'I *was happy* to see them'. As is clear, references to the self ('I', 'my', 'mine', etc.) are a natural part of expressing emotionality and are used more than usual. Emotionality is also expressed interpersonally by add commitment and surprise to the ideational meanings. The commitment is expressed by intensifiers such as 'really' and 'very' ('He was *really* angry'. 'They were *very* annoying'), by loud and pronounced intonation or by unusually slow or fast tempo that adds emotion to the utterance. Interactionally, a speaker with histrionic personality disorder may respond less than usual to what others say or may not respond at all to some topics. The clinician must listen closely to hear if a speaker varies in responding according to the situation or topic.

IDEATION

INTERPERSONAL

Attention-seeking

Attention-seeking behaviour is the second major feature of histrionic personality disorder, in addition to emotionality. In a general sense, attention-seeking behaviour can just be the attempt to be different and in the difference get attention. More specifically, an individual can be dramatic in language and non-verbal behaviour. This dramatic behaviour is conveyed by taking on the role of another person such as by speaking about unusual topics (the field or institutional focus, see Chapter 2), setting up an unusual interpersonal relationship such as unusual formality or friendliness (tenor) or interacting as if there is an unusual channel of communication, for example, as if acting on stage, or speaking for a television camera (mode).

A speaker can also directly seek attention by asking about the self ('What do you think about my new umbrella?') and by making statements about the self ('In fact, I have three new umbrellas'). More explicitly still, a speaker can seek attention by initiating exchanges: by asking questions (demanding information), giving commands (demanding goods and services) and by making startling or unusual statements (giving information). These exchanges tend to start social processes and require a response from others. Merely starting such an exchange and having others respond seeks attention. If this pattern repeats, then there is reason to consider a diagnosis of histrionic behaviour.

Pervasiveness and excessiveness

As well as emotionality and attention-seeking behaviour, an individual with histrionic personality disorder exhibits pervasive and excessive behaviours that make the speaker stand out in context. If even common behaviours occur too frequently or too close together, then they are noticed since our intuitions are well tuned to pick up differences. The features of the interaction that are unusual can in principle be quantified and unusual frequencies and thresholds determined. However, lay and clinical listeners readily, regularly and accurately identify atypical frequencies in interaction.

9.4   Dependent personality disorder

9.4.1 Clinical features

Dependent personality disorder is defined in part by a difficulty expressing disagreement with others, especially with someone whom the speaker is dependent on. This characteristic is clearly based on verbal behaviour. The linguistic description of difficulty expressing disagreement mainly involves the interpersonal meanings of language and especially the sequencing of moves in interaction (see Chapter 2).

9.4.2 Language features

As outlined in Chapter 2, exchanges in interaction are usually composed of two utterances adjacent to each other in specific patterns. For example, the following patterns are quite common (examples repeated from Chapter 2):

Offer	Acknowledge offer	A piece of home-made pie? – Sure
Command	Response offer to command	Get me two painkillers – Will do
Statement	Acknowledge statement	Hottest day of the summer – Guess so
Question	Response statement to question	When will I see you? – At eleven

If a speaker uses the typical sequence too often, that is, without the second utterance contradicting or questioning the first utterance even occasionally, then we have evidence for difficulty expressing disagreement (see Table 9.5). To express disagreement, the second utterance will usually have a negative word such as 'not', 'n't', 'never', 'no'. A speaker can also express disagreement by challenging the right of the first speaker to make the utterance, whether it is a statement, question or command. Disagreements may take the form of a question responded to with a challenge ('When do you want supper?' 'Why even ask?') or a statement responded to with a denial of the speaker's right to make the statement ('It's raining in Spain.' 'You have no idea about anything' 'How do you know?' 'Who would believe you?'). Although such challenges strongly express disagreement, they are atypically used occasionally. Their complete absence gives the impression that the individual cannot disagree.

Language features	Examples	Table 9.5
Infrequent disagreement with other speakers, as expressed by:		*Dependent personality disorder – language features*
• positive (rather than negative responses)	It is hot in here.	
	Yes it is. (*No, I'm cold*)	
	Would you like some?	
	Sure. (No thank you / not a chance)	
Infrequent challenges to right of other speaker	It's going to be a bad summer.	
	I guess. (How would you know?)	

In summary, the feature of not being able to disagree with another is largely expressed by the failure to construct negative and challenging utterances to the utterances of other speakers. That is, the clinician should be attuned to pairs of utterances from different speakers and especially to the positive or negative status of the second utterance in the pair. It is to be expected that an individual may express agreement and disagreement with some speakers but only agreement with other speakers. In a case of dependent personality disorder, the interlocutor who is not disagreed with is the person that the affected individual is dependent on.

9.5   Obsessive-compulsive personality disorder

9.5.1   Clinical features

Obsessive-compulsive personality disorder implicates language in a number of ways. It should be noted that these features are not directly part of the diagnostic criteria for the disorder. We will outline two major features of the disorder in terms of their expression in language:

(1) being wrapped up in one's own perspective;

(2) affective atypicalities.

9.5.2   Language features

Wrapped up in own perspective

Someone who both speaks about the self and ignores the positions of others seems wrapped in his or her own perspective. The simple markers of speaking about oneself are using first person pronouns (I, me, my, myself, etc.) that refer to the speaker rather than using pronouns that refer to either the hearer in the situation (expressed as: you, your, yourself, etc.) or to things that are spoken about (he, she, they, his, hers, etc.). It is the imbalance of speaking too much about oneself that marks the disorder, rather than the complete exclusion of other people or things.

Ignoring the ideas and interactions of others is also expressed through the interpersonal metafunction of language. As outlined for dependent personality disorders above (and in greater detail in Chapter 2), we expect certain pairs of utterances to be next to each other and dependent on each other. In not giving an appropriate response to the first speaker's utterance (e.g., not supplying an answer in response to a question, not acknowledging that a statement has been made), a speaker seems out of touch with the other individual. Rather, by continuing one's own topic of interaction and one's own role in the social process, the cooperative nature of the social process is not developed and the social process is jeopardised. For example, by continuing to tell a story and not responding to offers for food ('Would you like a bite?') or change of location ('Let's stand over there'), a speaker may find that others will not listen and may eventually move away from the interaction. More specifically, a speaker shows continuity with the self and little connection with others by using pronouns such as it, they, she, he to refer to entities that he or she has mentioned, rather than to pick up on things that the other speaker has said. Similarly, a speaker who repeats only his or her own words rather than the words of others is heard as ignoring those other speakers. That is, the speaker is sending the message: 'I am continuing to talk about what I just talked about rather than what you just talked about'. Such concentration on the meaning and wordings of the speaker does not seriously imperil the social process, but does skew the interaction away from its usual balance.

A second consequence of being wrapped up in one's own perspective is not being able to acknowledge the perspectives of others. This feature of obsessive-compulsive personality disorder is also largely conveyed by the interpersonal metafunction of language. In the utterance-by-utterance construction of interaction, utterances frequently begin with an acknowledgement that the previous utterance has been heard. Remarks such as 'okay', 'yes', 'ya', 'um hum' often indicate that the speaker has heard what the other has said and will continue building the interaction from this acknowledged common ground. When these seemingly minor markers are absent, it appears that the speaker is not attending to the other speaker and is perhaps skipping over what the other speaker is contributing.

Affect

A second aspect of the obsessive-compulsive personality disorder, in addition to being wrapped up in one's own perspective, is controlled, formal or stilted affect. Clinically, the description is in terms of the speaker's internal state: the speaker feels uncomfortable. The language that expresses uncomfortable feelings is similar to the language expressing affect (see Table 9.6). The controlled expression of affect is noticed by the use of frequent words. Frequent words such as 'good', 'nice', 'awful' make a speaker sound predictable, understated and controlled. Using of more infrequent words (such as 'super', 'fantastic', 'disastrous') makes affect sound less controlled, less predictable, more spontaneous. In addition, the use of expressive intonation by varying the loudness of speech, the tempo and the pitch contours (the ups and downs of the tone) also adds spontaneity to the affect. However, consistently slow speech is likely to sound lacking in affect. This happens since the speech sounds as if it is being controlled to monitor and moderate the direct expression of emotion.

CONTROLLED AFFECT

Clinical feature	Language features	Examples
Table 9.6 *Obsessive-compulsive personality disorder – language features*		
Wrapped up in own perspective	Speaking about self, expressed by:	
	• first person pronouns	*My* garden is better than ever.
	Ignoring others, expressed by:	
	• few third person pronouns	
	• few responses to other's initiatives	A: What do you think of that book? B: I am still wondering how they saw me.
	Few links to other's speech, expressed by:	
	• third person pronouns	A: I saw the book and the flower. B: I saw Kim (*them*).
	• substitution/ellipsis	A: I saw the book and the flower. B: I saw them *too*.
	Acknowledgement of previous utterance	A: I saw the book and the flower. B: *Yes/ya/um hum* I saw them too
Affect	Controlled affect, expressed by: • frequent words • slow speech • even intonation	nice, good, bad, awful
	Failure to express compliments	
	Discomfort with other's emotions, expressed by:	
	• changing topics (content words)	A: I really feel hurt by his anger. B: *But the whole day was good*.
	• short answers	A: I'm fed up with this place. B: *So.*
	• negative responses	A: It's the best beer in town. B: *No it isn't*.

Table 9.4 (Continued)

Formal, serious relationships	Interpersonal meanings of social distance, expressed by:	
	• topic of interaction not personal or emotional expressed by nominals, verbs, adjectives	Do you think the economy will improve? (You seem *down* today)
	• few contractions	I *do not* (don't) think so.
	• formal vocabulary (rare words)	I'll *consider* (think about) it.
	• even intonation	
	• little modulation of commitment	They ate the supper I made (They *may* have eaten at home)
	Preoccupation with intellect and logic, expressed by: • few emotion words	
	• more conjunctions of cause, time	*Since* they came, it has rained
Holding back	Pauses before starting turn Fewer corrections as a result of: • planned speech • slower speech	

A specific example of not expressing affect is not expressing compliments. Compliments are specific social processes that express positive affect about another person. Compliments thus combine an expression of an emotion and a personal relationship with another person. Both these specific tasks seem particularly difficult for an individual with obsessive-compulsive disorder so it is not surprising that compliments are not expressed often.

As well as controlled affect, a speaker with obsessive-compulsive disorder may be uncomfortable when others are expressing emotions. We know that an individual is uncomfortable in these cases from several aspects of the individual's interaction. The speaker may:

DISCOMFORT EXPRESSING EMOTIONS

(1) change topics (by changing the content words, by not using pronouns such as they, it, she to follow up what others are saying);

(2) give short answers without adding relevant information;

(3) make negative comments about what others are saying ('That's not right').

These linguistic markers of discomfort will vary depending on the emotional content in the speech of others. The more the other speaker talks of emotions, the more the speaker with obsessive-compulsive disorder will produce these markers of discomfort.

FORMAL, SERIOUS
RELATIONSHIPS

A further clinical characteristic of obsessive-compulsive disorder is that these individuals have formal and serious relationships. Again, we come to this conclusion largely from language data (see again Table 9.6). It is the interpersonal meanings that express social distance and relationships between individuals (the personal tenor of language) that express the formal and serious relationships. One aspect of the social distance is the restriction of interaction to topics (the field of interaction) that do not touch on emotions, personal matters and affect. For example, talk that largely centres on occupations, public discourse such as politics or weather and abstract philosophy, rather than the speakers themselves, sounds formal and serious.

Specifically, formal and serious relationships are expressed by:

(1) fewer contractions ('cannot' instead of 'can't', 'will not' instead of 'won't');

(2) slower speech that sounds more monitored and deliberate;

(3) less frequent vocabulary that sounds more formal ('considered it'/'pondered it' instead of 'thought about it', 'the car halted' instead of 'the car stopped');

(4) monotonous intonation that expresses little affect or involvement in the context;

(5) little modulation of commitment to the content of utterances by terms such a possibly, possibly, sometimes, likely (see the discussion of modality in Chapter 2).

The presence of formal and serious relationships is most obvious in contexts where we usually find lighter, happier relationships evident by smiling, jokes and personal comments.

Most of the atypicalities we have discussed in obsessive-compulsive disorders have to do with affect and emotions. However, there are elements of language that involve more ideational meanings. Preoccupation with the logic and the intellect can push out the expression of emotions. Speakers express logical and intellect by vocabulary that avoids emotions and by connectors (largely conjunctions) that encode causal and temporal relations. Even in talking about the events of the world, verbs expressing saying and thinking (say, mention, think, considered, 'He *said* he was fine') will be favoured over those encoding feelings ('He *felt* fine'). In interaction, the speaker may ignore utterances that involve emotions and respond mainly to those utterances that express abstract or concrete ideation. In particular, the speaker avoids expressing personal feelings (e.g., '*my* anger', '*I felt* terrible', '*I* seemed *happy* then').

There is a general characteristic of the language of speakers with obsessive-compulsive personality disorder that applies to the expression of both affective and ideational meaning. Clinically, this characteristic is described as holding back to fashion a perfect utterance. In language, this characteristic is found in:

(1) the delay of contributions beyond the usual slight delay we use to plan utterances;

(2) less correction, repetition and hesitation markers in spontaneous speech;

(3) slower speech, with perhaps some pauses, as the the speaker plans what to say.

In summary, speakers with obsessive-compulsive personality disorder use atypical expressions of affective meaning in certain contexts and restrictions in the expression of some ideational meanings. Each of these kinds of meaning is carried by a number of specific linguistic features and are heard as unusual interaction or unusual emotional or cognitive states. To identify obsessive-compulsive disorder more clearly and accurately, the clinician can deliberately attend to this set of language features. To consider the clinical problem the other way round, when a specific clinical feature is suspected, the clinician can specifically attend to the linguistic features that often encode the clinical features.

Chapter 10 contents

The partnership of language and psychiatry

This volume has considered psychiatric disorders and their criteria from the perspective of language. This approach raises a number of important conceptual issues that will be discussed in this chapter. These conceptual issues interact with:

(1) the methods of studying psychiatric disorders;

(2) the problems that must still be investigated both clinically and in terms of research.

This chapter is therefore divided into three sections: Section 10.1 where we are in terms of conceptualising psychiatric categories in terms of language; Section 10.2 which explores the conceptual problems and research issues that are raised by considering psychiatric categories in terms of language used in context and Section10.3, the new areas that are opened up for investigation and the new goals that can be set for research on language and psychiatric disorders.

Conceptualising psychiatric categories in terms of language 10.1

There is a necessary relationship between language and psychiatric disorders. These disorders are largely characterised by the way individuals speak, both in the community where some atypicality is first noticed and in the clinical setting where the clinician probes atypicalities and considers diagnoses. The clinical approach to disorders is generally through the categories of:

disorders, symptoms, signs and diagnostic criteria. These entities tend to take on the qualities of pure Aristotelian categories that are either present or not present. The temptation is to also regard linguistic categories as pure entities. However, specific linguistic characteristics (for example, unclear pronominal referencing or rising intonation to create questions) are related only indirectly to the meanings they send (the specific functions they accomplish). These characteristics are themselves graded since they occur with various frequencies and co-occur with other linguistic characteristics. That is, we should not see the linguistic categories as pure entities mapped directly onto functions or simply combined in various ways to create or express the psychiatric categories. Any set of defining language features for psychiatric categories must be treated very cautiously. Arriving at such possibly defining features depends on the kinds of individuals considered (for example, with mild, moderate or severe symptomatology, as will be discussed below) and whether the purpose is to describe the phenomenology of the disorder or to hunt for underlying causes and mechanisms. Of course, each different model of language and each model of psychiatric categories (Freud, DSM-III, or DSM-IV) leads to different descriptions and eventually to different empirical studies.

It is useful to think of the linguistic categories as highly specific, reliable and function-based categories. Being specific, these categories can be easily identified on the basis of observable characteristics of language and each characteristic can be independently identified. Such properties also make the categories reliable across observers and across those being observed. As functional categories, the linguistic descriptions account for how speakers sound unusual and why listeners notice the atypical language and interactions. These functional categories can describe language from many kinds of speakers both with and without psychiatric diagnoses.

There are a large number of disorders and an even larger number of diagnostic criteria that are directly and indirectly dependent on language. Most of the detailed empirical work in linking the disorders and their diagnostic criteria to specific features of language has not been attempted let alone completed. What has been presented in the preceding chapters is a detailed mapping of clinical features onto specific linguistic features. Much work remains to empirically establish the connections and to establish the relative contributions of the various linguistic features to the diagnostic categories. Empirical work may also show that some diagnostic criteria that could be potentially definable in terms of specific linguistic features first need further clinical refinement or specification.

Conceptual problems and research issues   10.2

The thesis that has been presented is that functional linguistic categories can capture just those aspects of language that characterise psychiatric categories. Functional linguistic categories give us tools for conceptualising the psychiatric categories and lead to clarifying the phenomena of the disorders. More particularly, we see disorders as failures to build social processes. Essentially, this is just a specific way of talking about the failure in social or occupational functioning that is used in clinical contexts. The failure to build social processes is then traced to the language that is usually used to build those social processes and whose atypicality is noticed in the speech community. These categories of language thus directly map onto to the clinical categories. The language categories then represent a way of studying the aetiology, trajectory and effects of treatment. Simultaneously, we take language as the means that largely builds social processes and also take the language categories as evidence for the cognitive and emotional systems that are affected in psychiatric disorders. The proposal is that the language categories both represent the phenomena that are noticed clinically and also index the underlying cognitive and emotional systems. The research problem is to build specific connections between functional linguistic categories and psychiatric categories that inform us both about the ability to build social interaction and about the underlying cognitive and emotions systems that are compromised in the disorders.

SOCIAL PROCESSES

10.2.1 Conceptualising disorders from language on up to the social processes

The approach to the necessary relationship between language and psychiatric categories is to describe verbal behaviour 'bottom-up', from the observable characteristics of language to the psychiatric concepts. At the most apparent, observable level, the speech community notices that some individuals are not following the typical and expected patterns of verbal behaviour. As a consequence, the expected social norms are not met and the expected social goals are not attained. This approach does not deny the role of cognitive or organic factors, but rather, in a manner following Kandel (1998), the atypical behaviour is seen as a product of the neurobiology and vice versa.

Disorders

The features and diagnostic criteria of psychiatric disorders necessarily involve impaired social functioning. These features and diagnostic criteria are grouped into disorders with at least a family resemblance across individuals with a specific disorder even if there is no common aetiology or even a single common characteristic across all the individuals. The phenomenological entities may, though, have a common trajectory or a common response to medication.

Certainly, it would be too strict a criterion to expect that individuals with a specific disorder have a common pattern of communication. Rather, we could expect a few common patterns that then have a 'family resemblance' to each other. For example, in schizophrenia, there may be tangentiality, loose associations and even delusions that all implicate detachment from the context (as discussed in detail in Chapter 7). In language, then, we expect that specific language characteristics will be typically associated with a disorder or a diagnostic criterion but may not be defining of either kind of category.

Middle-level categories

Considering middle-level categories is one approach to finding common characteristics across speakers with a disorder. The diagnostic criteria of a disorder can often be grouped into these 'middle-level' categories (middle between the diagnostic criteria and the disorder). Examples of these middle-level categories are hyperactivity in attention-deficit hyperactivity disorder or social interaction impairments in pervasive developmental disorders. These middle-level categories may be more characteristic of the disorders than specific diagnostic criteria. Furthermore, the middle-level categories may reflect more general underlying cognitive or neurobiological functions. From the perspective of language, the middle-level categories may be more stable and characteristic of the disorders than specific diagnostic criteria. The difficulty is that the diagnostic criteria cut across various disorders. For example, rambling thoughts and speech are found in mania, schizophrenia and caffeine intoxication. Just looking at individual linguistic characteristics may then be misleading. The middle-level categories cover a wider spectrum of behaviour and can be more characteristic of the disorders. Rather than describing the language features of individual diagnostic criteria, it may ultimately be more fruitful to describe the language of these middle-level categories. Such descriptions are likely to involve combinations of linguistic features that tend to co-occur to create the 'family resemblance' of how a certain disorder sounds (see Lott et al., 2002).

Kinds of disorders

Moving up from the level of the disorder to broad kinds of disorders (e.g., mood disorders, psychoses), we may find common linguistic characteristics that reflect a common impairment in attaining social processes within these groups of disorders. More likely, broad categories of language use are systematically related to these broad categories of psychiatric disorders. For example, the linguistic characteristics that convey being out of touch with reality may be found across the spectrum of psychoses. The categories in psychiatry can be conceived of atomically from bottom up (from features to diagnostic criteria, to middle-level categories, to disorders and to complexes of disorders). In this sequence, the linguistic descriptions can establish the reliability and validity of the features and diagnostic criteria. The categories in psychiatry can also be conceived of from top down: complexes of disorders, to disorders, to middle-level categories, to diagnostic criteria to features. These categories often involve fuzzy concepts that can be sharpened by linguistic description of individual cases of language use. Working from abstract psychiatric concepts, such as a complex of disorders, challenges the linguistic approach to identify the types of meaning that are at risk throughout the category. For example, even the category of schizophrenia is broad and includes various subtypes of schizophrenias. If the category is valid in describing a common set of phenomena, then there is likely a set of related meanings that are atypical across cases. The proposal that has been presented in Chapter 7 is that meaning is disconnected from the context in schizophrenia. Once a basic meaning is identified, then we can start to describe how affected individuals express that meaning at the levels of vocabulary, grammar and intonation (the wordings).

Language

As we have recounted, psychiatric categories exist at different levels of abstraction. Similarly, language is also viewed as a series of categories at different levels of abstraction. However, the levels of language, as explained in Chapters 2 and 3, are regarded as 'actualisations' or 'realisations' of each other. At the lowest levels, for example, a word is actualised or expressed by its sounds. At a higher level, we can say that the interpersonal meanings of language are expressed in terms of the grammatical structures and intonations that are used to convey statements, questions and commands. As indicated above, we can conceptualise a psychiatric category such as a disorder or a diagnostic criterion as atypicality in meaning that the lay and clinical communities detect and describe. However, the linguistic approach also suggests that sometimes the difficulty may not be in the meaning itself, but rather in terms of how a meaning is expressed. That is, in a given disorder, or for a given diagnostic criterion, a speaker may have a restricted, stereotyped or idiosyncratic way of saying things. This manner of expressing meaning itself then suggests that the speaker is autistic, depressed, agitated, etc. If so, the linguistic approach asks what area of the linguistic system (vocabulary, grammar, intonation, etc.) is affected and how does that specification of the atypicality suggest an underlying cognitive, emotional or other impairment. The atypicality in realisations may just be in the sequence of realisations, for example, an unending series of questions or short monotone phrases even though the speaker may have been intending more variegated meanings. At the highest levels of abstraction, the linguistic approach asks which social processes a speaker fails to achieve. That is, we see language as actualising and expressing social processes. By specifying the social processes at risk, the linguistic approach aims to describe the particular social impairment of the speaker and how that impairment is perceivable in the language used.

REALISATIONS

MEANING IS DISPERSED

As indicated in Chapters 2 and 3, meaning is seen as dispersed at several levels. For example, social processes have specific sequences of activities (such as requesting a paper, tendering money, accepting change, departing, in buying a newspaper), to patterns of interpersonal meaning (formal or informal), to selection of vocabulary. Each of these levels of meaning may be independently affected, reflecting a specific compromise in the ability to accomplish social processes. Again, the linguistic approach then asks: at what level is the impairment in a specific disorder and why is that the problem?

To review the elements of the linguistic approach:

(1) meaning is seen as dispersed across the several levels that have been mentioned and the meanings are conceived of as different options that may be expressed (rude or polite, question or statement, positive or negative statement);

(2) language is then a vast repertoire of meanings, i.e., a set of semantic resources, some of which are used frequently and some of which are almost never used;

(3) these meanings must also be expressed or worded by the grammar, vocabulary and sounds of the language.

NO 'ONE-TO-ONE' MAPPING OF MEANING AND WORDING

It is important to realise that there is not a one-to-one mapping between meanings and that a speaker chooses how to 'word' a message. The atypicalities found in psychiatric disorders may then be either at the level of which meanings are expressed or in terms of how those meanings are put into language for the hearer. The fact that there is not a one-to-one mapping between meanings and how they are worded creates variety in language use but also allows for a rather loose connection between meanings and expressions. This connection is too loose in cases of pathology: individuals seem to be using inappropriate vocabulary, grammar and intonation to express their meanings.

Sounds

We will now consider the meanings as they are built bottom-up from the sounds and wordings of language towards the social processes that they should accomplish. At the lowest level of language, there is some 'substance' that the hearer or reader confronts or produces: the sounds or written symbols of the language. This discussion confines itself to sounds since there is very little research on the writing of psychiatric patients and very little clinical use of writing samples. The sounds of a language carry the words and meanings of the speaker but can also be atypical in themselves sending unusual meanings. Speech that is particularly loud or quiet, fast or slow, filled with pauses or slurred together may itself indicate one or more diagnostic criteria or disorders. Even then, at this most concrete level, patients with psychiatric disorders sound different from others.

Vocabulary and grammar (lexicogrammar)

From the sounds, now we move upwards to the vocabulary and grammar of language. The vocabulary of language encodes the people, places, objects, events and circumstances of the world (ideational meanings). These ideational meanings are specifically at risk in some disorders, e.g., the expression of delusions in psychosis or depressed mood in depression. The vocabulary is assembled together by the grammar of language and thus a great number of additional meanings can be expressed. For example, the grammar can take essentially the same content words and express:

IDEATIONAL MEANING

(a) a statement ('The table is wet'),

(b) a yes-no question ('Is the table wet?')

(c) a wh- question ('Why is the table wet?'), or

(d) a command ('Wet the table!').

Many of these different meanings are interpersonal in nature since they set up different interpersonal relationships between speaker and hearer. As well as ideational meanings and interpersonal meanings, the vocabulary and grammar convey meanings that connect the language to the verbal and non-verbal context. This is textual meaning. Words such as 'they', 'it', 'this', 'you', 'afterwards', 'however', 'then' connect what is said ('it') to something else that was said earlier ('the table') or connect a word ('you') to the environmental context (the addressee). This connection is also meaning since it signals to the hearer that speaker and hearer share the same world. Thus the vocabulary and grammar of language enable ideational, interpersonal and textual meanings to be conveyed. Within each of these broad categories of meaning, there are many specific meanings each of which may be at stake in some disorder. The meanings at stake may be rather specific (e.g., a particular ideational focus on playing cards) or rather general (not responding in interpersonal interactions). In psychiatric disorders, the question is what particular meanings are atypical and characteristic of a disorder or indexical of a diagnostic criterion.

INTERPERSONAL MEANING

TEXTUAL MEANING

Social processes

Moving up yet further from the sounds, the vocabulary and grammar bring about or actualising the social processes of a society. That is, the problem for patients with psychiatric disorders is not one of sound, vocabulary or grammar, but how social processes are not effectively accomplished. These social processes have several facets. First, social processes are composed of ordered steps or stages of activity. An individual must attempt and accomplish these stages:

STAGED ACTIVITY

(1) in the right order (first decide if the sweater fits and then pay for it; first say 'hello' and then ask how the family is doing);

(2) with the usual frequency (not speaking about football scores, one's latest medical problems, or a voice from heaven 70 per cent of the time).

Human language is very creative partly because it enables social processes to be accomplished by many different wordings. However, there are still loose limits to the variation. Beyond these limits, hearers start to react to a speaker as if that speaker has a disorder.

SETS OF MEANING IN
SOCIAL PROCESSES

As well as stages of activity, social processes are characterised by typical sets of meanings and how they are accomplished. For example, buying a newspaper or attempting a seduction are usually not done in loud, shouting voices. Swearing is usually not the way to introduce strangers to each other. Discussing which package of cheese to buy is usually done with simple, frequently occurring words rather than multisyllabic, scientific sounding vocabulary. A speaker may use atypical sets of meanings at this level of abstraction by:

(1) speaking about atypical things (a disturbance in subject matter or institutional focus);

(2) assuming an unusual channel of communication, implied by shouting, whispering, telegraphic speech, clipped words (a disturbance in mode of communication);

(3) using language associated with an inappropriate personal relationship, e.g., formal, informal, angry (a disturbance in tenor of communication).

In each case, the usual social process will be compromised or destroyed by these atypical meanings. Again, the challenge in the study of psychiatric disorders is to determine which meanings are associated with which disorders and with each particular diagnostic criterion or middle-level category.

COGNITIVE AND
NEUROBIOLOGICAL
IMPAIRMENT

Beyond the of kinds of meanings and how they are worded by individuals with psychiatric disorders, a careful examination of these kinds of meanings starts to provide hypotheses about the kinds of underlying cognitive and neurobiological impairments involved in psychiatric disorders (see, for example, the approaches in Cloninger, 2002; Szatmari, 2003). That is, a pattern of atypical language use either in one individual or across a class of individuals suggests an impairment in the mechanism responsible for that level of language processing. Clinically, it is important to relate the atypicality in the functional use of language to the underlying mechanism so that the appropriate management can be instituted.

Mapping between language and clinical categories

As we have outlined, functional linguistics provides a series of levels of analysis for meanings and for wordings that then be connect to psychiatric disorders and their specific features. A close reading of earlier chapters shows that there are many overlaps across the disorders. One atypical characteristic of language may be found in a number of disorders. Finding linguistic characteristic L does not unambiguously suggest disorder D or even diagnostic criterion R. The approach is to relate linguistic characteristics to diagnostic criteria and, where possible, to middle-level clinical categories that include a number of specific diagnostic criteria. We will now explore the relationship of language features to these psychiatrically defined categories.

At a simple level, the linguistic descriptions may just be specific descriptions of behaviour common to more than one disorder. For example, pressure of speech may be found in mania and attention deficit hyperactivity disorder. The linguistic description provides a more objective, principled description of the phenomenon than the clinical feature. The more difficult challenge is to relate a common phenomenon to deeper characteristics of the disorders. The close description of the linguistic phenomena can suggest underlying causes of the disorder (an impairment in an inhibitory mechanism, or in a monitoring mechanism) or perhaps to a fundamental principle of the disorder (an impairment in information processing or an impairment in relating to social reality in schizophrenia). A single atypical language characteristic can be produced by different underlying causes or even some combination of causes. In these cases, perhaps, in fact, this is the default case, it is the combination of language features that must be studied in order to hypothesise reasonable underlying mechanisms. These mechanisms then account for both the set of language features that are atypical and the co-variation of those atypicalities across individuals and across time in a single individual.

The use of middle-level categories (e.g., hyperactivity in attention-deficit hyperactivity disorder, or one-sided social interactions in pervasive developmental disorders) provides a level of conceptualisation that is more stable than individual diagnostic criteria. That is, as the notion of the disorder evolves, the middle-level categories will tend to remain, although their definitions may change in terms of diagnostic criteria. It is unclear whether these middle-level categories or more specific language features are the right level of abstraction for exploring the neurological basis of the disorders or their disruptive effect on social processes. The more specific language features may serve these purposes better. Language is organised both functionally and in terms of wordings to create social interaction. This organisation is both a phylogenic and ontogenic reality. Languages all have the same general principles, including a vast set of resources of meanings and the means for expressing those meanings so others can understand

MIDDLE-LEVEL
CATEGORIES

them. These characteristics of language are then the bases for building and sustaining social realities. Ontogenically, children are able to learn languages organised according to these principles. Without entering into the debate as to whether the mechanisms that underlie language are specific to language or not, it is clear that some of the neurophysiological processes that enable language to be used are impaired in psychiatric disorders. In these disorders, the specific atypicalities in using language can thus be a way of exploring the neuropsychological mechanisms. For example, is unclear pronoun use a function of an attention mechanism, a memory mechanism or some other mechanism? Does the occurrence of unclear pronouns in different disorders imply the same underlying mechanism? Is it reasonable to postulate such an impaired mechanism for that disorder given other behavioural (both verbal and non-verbal) or neurobiological characteristics of the disorder? This is the line of reasoning suggested by the close description of the language of psychiatric disorders.

It is important not to reify the psychiatric categories. Neither disorders nor diagnostic criteria are pure essences. The linguistic descriptions are not descriptions of clear, homogeneous, psychiatrically defined categories. Rather, the linguistic approach can clarify some of these categories. For example, pedantic speech in pervasive developmental disorders could be sharpened by much linguistic description of actual speech that is clinically regarded as 'pedantic'. As the clinical categories are redefined from one edition of the clinical manuals to another, the concepts that language must describe and explain are themselves evolving. In fact, the mapping of linguistic categories and psychiatric categories onto each other is bi-directional. The task is not the linguistic description of psychiatric categories, but the development of psychiatric categories and their linguistic characteristics at the same time. This is a very difficult enterprise with many stages of clinical clarification, linguistic development and the empirical study of much discourse from many speakers.

This section dealt with how functional linguistic categories specify psychiatric categories and explain how the impairments in academic and occupational functioning come about through the impairment in building social processes. In turn, social processes are seen as the outcome of interacting with language. By considering the various levels of linguistic analysis, we specify the impairments in various psychiatric disorders. The linguistic and psychiatric categories, though, exist only in relation to individuals with the disorders. The discussion now turns to how we classify and group these individuals to learn more about the disorders and to treat the individuals more effectively.

10.2.2 Which individuals to study

In the study and linguistic definition of psychiatric disorders, we must care-fully consider which individuals to study and how to study their language. For both the subjects and the language, the discussion is in terms of how to set up studies. More importantly, though, is how the research must reflect fundamental issues in psychiatry and language. We start with considering which subjects to study. There are three dimensions in considering which subjects to study in order to map language onto psychiatric categories of diagnostic criteria, disorders and complexes of disorders. One dimension is the severity of the disorder in terms of mild or severe symptomatolgy. A second dimension is the relative absence or presence of co-morbidities, a pure-mixed dimension. A third dimension is the typicality of the case along a continuum of common – uncommon. These three dimensions are conceptually independent, though in practice they are related since pure cases of many disorders are uncommon and extremely severe cases are also uncommon. Selecting subjects along each of these dimensions involves both advantages and disadvantages. Two of the dimensions are plotted against each other in Table 10.1. Although the dimensions are portrayed as having two poles they should be considered as continua.

	Pure case	Mixed case	Table 10.1
Severe symptomatology	Linguistic characteristics are very evident. Generalisation to large numbers of patients is indirect and difficult.	Linguistic characteristics are hard to identify since they are present with atypicalities in language derived from other disorders. In some cases, the language features will become very salient despite the co-morbidities and so mask the co-morbidities. Generalisation should be easy since many cases of disorders involve co-morbidity.	*Dimensions of subjects (severity of symptomatology / amount of co-morbidity) mapped against each other*
Mild symptomatology	Linguistic characteristics are hard to identify. There will be considerable overlap across disorders.	Linguistic characteristics may be masked by the linguistic characteristics of the co-morbidities.	

Mild or severe symptomatology

Individuals with severe symtomatology certainly demonstrate the relevant language characteristics clearly. These tend to be good cases to exemplify and describe the phenomenon and to teach from. However, relatively few individuals will have such extreme features and the future clinician will have to notice the phenomenon when it occurs in much less severe forms. Furthermore, if the linguistic characteristics are severe, they may make other features harder to identify. More fundamentally, the individuals with severe characteristics may differ in some other way from those with less severe characteristics. From the perspective of scientific explanation, an assumption has to be made that the severe case is produced by the same mechanisms that underlie the less severe and more common cases. This assumption must be examined anew for each language characteristic and for each putative mechanism. It is possible, for example, that the severe cases involve interactions of mechanisms that are not present in the more frequent, less severe cases. Extrapolation about mechanism from the severe cases may thus be inappropriate.

In contrast to severe symptomatology, mild symptomatology is harder to detect. The clinician will wonder whether the language really indicates depression or whether the talk really is tangential. Using these cases to build a description and definition of the disorder has questionable reliability and validity. Further, when the speaker displays only mild symptomatology, the language itself may not be clearly atypical in some specific feature. For example, if there is mild pressure of speech, it may not be clear if there is also tangentiality; if there is mildly pedantic speech it may not be clear if there is also tangentiality or one-sided social interaction. On the other hand, these mixtures of mildly atypical linguistic features are clinically frequent.

Pure or co-morbid cases

In order to understand a disorder or to map a diagnostic criterion onto an underlying mechanism, it is desirable to examine an individual with only a single disorder or a single, clear diagnostic criterion. In these cases, there is less difficulty separating the concept of interest from other phenomena. Interactions among phenomena are also minimised. However, it may not be justifiable to generalise from these cases to the more frequent cases with their considerable co-morbidity. The interactions of underlying mechanisms found in the frequent cases of co-morbidity may be important in themselves to understand how the disorders arise and are manifested. The few 'pure' cases may not involve such interactions. Valid generalisability is then again jeopardised. Clinically, the 'pure' cases are initially appealing but using them for defining the disorders or the diagnostic criteria may result in overly narrow concepts that can rarely be applied in a clinical population.

Common or uncommon cases

This dimension overlaps with the first two dimensions of severity of symptomatology and amount of co-morbidity. As we study the common cases, so the ability to generalise about the use of language increases. Certainly, the challenge is to be able to describe and understand the frequently occurring cases so that diagnosis and treatment can be optimised for the greatest number of people. However, the clinical approach of describing clear (but likely unusual) cases and the research approach of studying relatively rare pure or extreme cases both have their place and are necessary at early stages of understanding the relation between psychiatric categories and the use of language.

Purposes

The purposes of inquiry also have an important role in determining which individuals to study. If the purpose is the definition of disorders and their diagnostic features, then pure and extreme cases are best. The goal is to deal with individuals who 'really have' the disorder or criterion. From these cases, then, the milder forms can be derived. Similarly, if the purpose is to uncover mechanisms underlying the psychiatric categories, then the pure and severe cases may be of interest first. As noted above, though, such an approach requires an assumption that the mechanisms in the mixed and less severe cases are similar to the pure and severe cases. This is often a good working assumption. At some stage of research, though, this assumption must be challenged so that interactions of the mechanisms with severity and co-morbidity are investigated.

If the major purposes are diagnosis and treatment, then the more common cases with co-morbidity and less severe symptomatology are the ones to start with. These are the kinds of people that are seen frequently and for whom treatment must work, even if there are many complicating factors due to the co-morbidities. Ultimately, these are the individuals who need treatment in order to be able to accomplish the social processes that they are unable to effect.

The clinical perspective and the research perspective are not mutually exclusive or based on non-overlapping goals. For both, there is a set of profound issues to be faced. Are there pure essences in the categories they each deal with? Whether these categories are disorders, behavioural features, underlying neurobiological processes, or models of neurological systems, there may be assumptions of certainty or assumptions of fuzzy categories. Some of these assumptions can be working assumptions that are then modified when the phenomena turn out to be discrete when they were assumed to be fuzzy or fuzzy and interacting when they were assumed to be discrete and independent. On the face of it, many connections between language and psychiatric disorders seem based on interactions and graded phenomena. We find more or less of a language characteristic that is associated more or less frequently with other language features and with psychiatric categories at different levels of abstraction, from features to diagnostic criteria, to disorders.

INDIVIDUAL OR
GROUP STUDIES

Taking all the conceptual and research issues together leads to the question of whether it is optimal to study single cases, series of cases or to study groups of individuals. This question deserves an extended treatment on its own. It is just raised here since it derives from the issues just discussed. By studying individual cases in depth, we can see more clearly the interactions among the linguistic characteristics and relate them to the psychiatric and treatment status of the individual. When individuals are grouped, the grouping itself may be questionable and then phenomena found in one subset of individuals may be balanced out by phenomena in another subset. Some of these phenomena can be regarded as noise that makes an understanding of the disorder difficult. However, the variation itself is important to consider and could be lost in a quantitative group study. Unfortunately, the close study of several simultaneous language factors is often too time-consuming to permit multivariate statistical treatment of large amounts of data from numbers of individuals. Both the study of individual cases and of properly defined groups with various control groups are needed at various stages in the investigation and theorising about the connection between psychiatric categories and their linguistic characteristics.

10.2.3 Functional model of language

As well as considering which subjects serve as the basis for learning about language in psychiatry, there is an important issue of how to analyse the language itself. The reasons for using a functional approach were given in Chapter 1. Briefly, the functional approach is used so that the linguistic characteristics of each disorder will account for the specific impairment in social processes attributed to the disorder. The goal is to find the linguistic characteristics that are responsible for the disorder sounding the way it does and impairing the individual's social behaviour in the particular way it does.

Social interaction usually takes place as each speaker takes a turn at talk in a real social context. In analysing data or formulating a clinical picture, we tend to see the conversation as a completed whole, recorded or transcribed on the page. To be true to the data, we should see conversation as unfolding as two or more speakers contribute to building interaction that constitutes a social process. This is a dynamic view of interaction that looks at verbal interaction as if it were unfolding step by step. At each step in the conversa- tion, we can ask: why was the conversation continued in one way and not in another? That is, at each point in the situation or the actual construction of the interaction, we can consider the options available to the speaker and assess the option taken in terms of the options that were not taken. For example, do some speakers typically expand on their responses to ques- tions whereas other speakers do not? In this case, the latter speakers may seem laconic or withdrawn or the former speakers may seem loquacious, depending on which pattern is more typical in the context. One strategy that is equally important in the clinical setting and for opening up new research questions is to listen for and notice atypicalities in language use and then identify the immediately preceding context. This context (that can be called a micro-context) can suggest clues for why the speaker used an unusual language option; for example, perhaps a sensitive emotional issue was introduced, or the interlocutor spoke quickly, or demanded too much attention or information.

DYNAMIC UNFOLDING

MICRO-CONTEXT

Distribution of language features

We hear the atypicalities of language that signal psychiatric disorders both in these micro-contexts and in the wider contexts of social processes. The atypicalities may be distributed in a number of ways and so impinge on the hearer differently, entailing different research strategies and clinical attention. Table 10.2 presents these distributions schematically. Firstly, some linguistic feature may be distributed ('average frequency' (1)) in the speech of an affected individual with a frequency that is heard as greater or less than is typical. For example, a speaker may have relatively more hesitation markers (e.g., 'ah', 'uhm') than is expected. Secondly, certain features of language may clump together in an uncharacteristic way ('density or clumps' (2)). For example, a speaker may ask two or three questions in a row and sound atypical, even though the overall frequency of questions is not strikingly atypical. Thirdly, linguistic features may be atypically juxtaposed (3), such that feature C is used after feature B instead of after feature A where it is usually used. For example, a simple 'yes' answer typically follows a question and then afterwards there may be some further explanation. Placing the explanation before the simple 'yes' answer sounds rather peculiar.

Typically we find:

A: Do you want to go for a hike this afternoon? (question)

B: Yes. (direct answer) I have nothing else to do except call Kim, rearrange the books and get to the library. (further explanation)

Atypically we could hear the following. This sequence does not indicate pathology in itself but if the pattern is repeated would sound unusual:

A: Do you want to go for a hike this afternoon? (question)

B: I have nothing else to do except call Kim, rearrange the books and get to the library. (explanation) Yes. (direct answer)

A fourth distribution is the use of even a few rare instances of highly atypical features (4). For example, just one convincing statement of a delusion ('I AM Napoleon whether you think so or not') is sufficient to suggest psychosis.

Table 10.2

Distributions of atypicalities of language in affected speakers compared to typical distributions

(1) Average frequency

Typical: A A B A A B A A B A A B; A:B = 2:1

Affected: A B A B A B A B A B A B; A:B = 1:1

(2) Density or clumps

Typical: A A B A A B A A B A A B

Affected: A *BB* A A B A A A *BB* A A A

(3) Atypical juxtaposition

Typical: A C A B A C A B A A C B A A B

Affected: A A *BC* A B A B A *BC* A B B A

(4) Rare instances of highly atypical language characteristics

Typical: A A B A A B A A B A A B

Affected: A A B *C* A A B A A B A *C* A B

It is easy to think of examples and speakers who say unusual things in terms of word order, sequencing of statements, or word choices. However, we can use a much wider view of the distribution of atypicalities to notice other phenomena that are important in psychiatric diagnosis and formulations. For example, in considering the roles individuals take in social processes, are there individuals who take initiatives so frequently that it is noticeable and disruptive of social activities? Are there individuals who rarely take the initiative or perhaps rarely respond to the initiatives of others? In considering the sets of interpersonal and ideational meanings, a speaker who uses language that is formal or informal, sad or enthusiastic, with atypical frequency can sound socially inappropriate and even pathological. The overall point is that language must always be heard in terms of successive levels of context, from the social processes sanctioned by the culture to the micro-contexts of preceding sentences, words and intonations.

All four of the atypical distributions of language features presented in Table 10.2 must be considered in listening to and analysing the language of speakers who may have psychiatric disorders. The clinician is probably clearer about the importance of all four kinds of atypicalities than the academic researcher who is inclined to study only the first type: differences in average frequency of a given feature distributed over a sample of talk.

New areas and new goals for language and psychiatric disorders   10.3

The aim of this work has been to describe the phenomena of psychiatry in functional linguistic terms. The results have shown that there remain a number of serious problems. Two sets of these problems have just been outlined:

(1) the difficulty in capturing how the language is atypical and is mapped onto the psychiatric categories;

(2) the difficulty in deciding which speakers to study.

The results of the detailed descriptions of disorders show that there is considerable overlapping of linguistic characteristics across disorders. For example, entering into an interaction too early may be characteristic both of a personality disorder and of attention-deficit hyperactivity disorder. To give another example, disorganised speech may derive from both impulsivity in a personality disorder or tangential thinking in schizophrenia. A simple atomic examination of language and psychiatric disorders is not sufficient. Consistent overall patterns of features in language and psychiatric disorders are needed to understand the complex gestalt of psychiatric disorders and their relationship to the language that so largely conveys the disorder. These patternings of features must be found for both language and for psychiatric categories at different levels. Coherent pictures of the disorders and of diagnostic criteria may be found at various levels of the organisation of language from the sounds, up to the words, clauses, types of meaning and to the genres, social processes and culture. Similarly, the psychiatric levels of features, diagnostic criteria, middle-level categories, disorders, complexes of disorders constitute the concepts onto which language must be mapped. Theory and understanding of both language and psychiatric concepts may change the levels we now have. These levels are not necessarily the most informative ones for mapping language onto psychiatric disorders. They are the ones that are now available and that have been used to start exploring the connections between language and psychiatric disorder.

Although the purpose in this study has been to account for a wide range of phenomena, there are very large issues that have scarcely been mentioned. Much work remains to be done to properly deal with emotional issues and how they are expressed in language. Furthermore, non--verbal communication is a feature of both typical interaction and social processes and of psychiatric pathologies. The patterns of non-verbal communication would generally be expected to parallel verbal communication in both the typical and pathological cases. However, this is only a rough guess that needs empirical research. On a more abstract level, we must learn much more about the range of typical interaction and language use and the range of the atypical and noticeable uses. At what point does the use of language or non-verbal communication become so atypical that it interrupts the social process or calls attention to the individual? Certainly, different societies, different individuals and even different clinicians have a variety of thresholds for both noticing atypicality and for labelling it pathological. These issues are critical for defining the notion of mental health and for defining the concept of society that is the setting for the definition of mental health.

References

Alverson, H. and Rosenberg, S. (1990) Discourse analysis of schizo-phrenic speech: a critique and proposal. *Applied Psycholinguistics*, 11, 167–84.

American Psychiatric Association (1994) *Diagnostic and Statistical Manual of Mental Disorders*. 4th edn. Washington, D. C. : American Psychiatric Association Press.

Andreasen, N. C. (1979a) Thought, language, and communication dis-orders: I Definition of terms and their reliability. *Archives of General Psychiatry*, 36, 1315–21.

Andreasen, N. C. (1979b) Thought, language, and communication dis-orders: II Diagnostic significance. *Archives of General Psychiatry*, 36, 1325–30.

Auer, P. (1996) On the prosody and syntax of turn-continuations. In E. Couper-Kuhlen and M. Selting (eds) *Prosody in Conversation: inter-actional studies*. 57–100. Cambridge: Cambridge University Press.

Baltaxe, C. A. M. and Simmons, J. Q. (1995) Speech and language disor-ders in children and adolescents with schizophrenia. *Schizophrenia Bulletin*, 21, 677–92.

Beitchman, J. H., Cohen, N. J., Konstantareas, M. M. and Tannock, R. (1996) (ed.) *Language, learning, and behavior disorders: develop-mental, biological, and clinical perspectives*. Cambridge: Cambridge University Press.

Butt, D., Fahay, R., Feez, S., Spinks, S. and Yallop, C. (2000) *Using Functional Grammar: an explorer's guide*. 2nd edn. Sidney: National Centre for English Language Teaching and Research, Macquarie University.

Caplan, R. (1996) Discourse deficits in childhood schizophrenia. In J. H. Beitchman, N. J. Cohen, M. M. Konstantareas and R. Tannock (eds) *Language, Learning, and Behavior Disorders: developmental, biological, and clinical perspectives.* 156–77. Cambridge: Cambridge University Press.

Caplan, R., Guthrie, D., Tang, B., Komo, S. and Asarnow, R. F. (2000) Thought disorder in childhood schizophrenia: replication and update of concept. *Journal of the American Academy of Child and Adolescent Psychiatry*, 39, 771–8.

Caramazza, A. (1986) On drawing inferences about the structure of normal cognitive systems from the analysis of patterns of impaired performance: the case for single patient studies. *Brain and Cognition*, 5, 41–66.

Caramazza, A. and McCloskey, M. (1988) The case for single patient studies. *Cognitive Neuropsychology*, 5, 517–58.

Chaika, E. (1974) A linguist looks at 'schizophrenic' language. *Brain and Language*, 1, 257–76.

Chaika, E. (1990) *Understanding Psychotic Speech: beyond Freud and Chomsky.* Springfield Il. : Charles Thomas.

Chaika, E. and Lambe, R. (1985) The locus of dysfunction in schizophrenic speech. *Schizophrenia Bulletin*, 11, 8–15.

Cloninger, C. R. (2002) The discovery of susceptibility genes for mental disorders. *Proceedings of the National Academy of Science*, 99, 13365–7.

Couper-Kuhlen, E. and Selting, M. (1996) Towards an interactional perspective on prosody and a prosodic perspective on interaction. In E. Couper-Kuhlen and M. Selting (eds) *Prosody in Conversation: interactional studies.* 11–56. Cambridge: Cambridge University Press.

Eggins, S. (1994) *An Introduction to Systemic Functional Linguistics.* London: Pinter.

Eggins, S. and Slade, D. (1994) *Analysing Casual Conversation.* London: Cassell.

Fawcett, R. (2000) *A Theory of Syntax for Systemic Functional Linguistics.* Amsterdam/Philadelphia: Benjamins.

Fine, J. (1991) The static and dynamic choices of responding: toward the process of building social reality by the developmentally disordered. In E. Ventola (ed.) *Functional and Systemic Linguistics.* 213–34. The Hague: Mouton DeGruyter.

Fine, J. (1994) *How Language Works: cohesion in normal and non-standard communication*. Norwood, N. J. : Ablex.

Fine, J. (1995) Towards understanding and studying cohesion in schizophrenic speech. *Applied Psycholinguistics*, 16, 25–41.

Fine, J. and Knizhnik, A. (1993) *Exchange Structures and Realizations Across Languages: what must be learned*. Paper given to Twentieth International Systemic-Functional Congress, Victoria, July 1993.

Fries, P. H. (2001) Issues in modelling the textual metafunction. In M. Scott and G. Thompson (eds) *Patterns of Text: in honour of Michael Hoey*. 83–107. Amsterdam/Philadelphia: Benjamins.

Gentner, D. (1982) Why nouns are learned before verbs: linguistic relativity versus natural partitioning. In S. A. Kuczaj *Language Development. Vol. 2: Language, thought and culture*. Hillsdale, N. J. : Erlbaum, 301–34.

Goren, A. R., Fine, J., Manaim, H. and Apter, A. (1995) Verbal and nonverbal expressions of central deficits in schizophrenia. *Journal of Nervous and Mental Disease*, 183, 715–9.

Gunthner, S. (1996) The prosodic contextualization of moral work: an analysis of reproaches in 'why'-formats. In E. Couper-Kuhlen and M. Selting (eds) *Prosody in Conversation: interactional studies*. 271–302. Cambridge: Cambridge University Press.

Halliday, M. A. K. (1984) Language as code and language as behaviour: a systemic-functional interpretation of the nature and ontogenesis of dialogue. In R. Fawcett, M. A. K. Halliday, S. M. Lamb and A. Makkai (eds) *The Semiotics of Language and Culture. Vol. 1: Language as social semiotic*. 3–35. London: Pinter.

Halliday, M. A. K. (2004) *An Introduction to Functional Grammar*. 3rd edn. Revised by C. M. I. M. Matthiessen. London: Arnold.

Hamaguchi, P. A. (2001) *Childhood Speech, Language and Listening Problems*. 2nd edn. New York: Wiley.

Hoffman, R. E., Stopek, S. and Andreasen, N. (1986) A comparative study of manic vs. schizophrenic speech disorganization. *Archives of General Psychiatry*, 43, 831–8.

Kandel, E. R. (1998) A new intellectual framework for psychiatry. *American Journal of Psychiatry*, 155, 457–69.

Lanin-Kettering, I. and Harrow, M. (1985) The thought behind the words: a view of schizophrenic speech and thinking disorders. *Schizophrenia Bulletin*, 11, 1–7.

Leonard, L. (1998) *Children with Special Language Impairment.* Cambridge, MA: MIT Press.

Levinson, S. C. (1983) *Pragmatics.* London: Cambridge University Press.

Lott, P. R., Guggenbühl, S., Schneeberger, A., Pulver, A. E., Stassen, H. H. (2002) Linguistic analysis of the speech output of schizophrenic, bipolar, and depressive patients. *Psychopathology*, 35, 220–7.

Malcolm, K. (1985) Communication linguistics: A sample analysis. In J. D. Benson and W. S. Greaves (eds) *Systemic Perspectives on discourse. Vol. 1: Selected theoretical papers from the 9th International Systemic Workshop.* 136–51. Norwood, N. J. : Ablex.

Martin, J. R. (1992) *English Text: system and structure.* Philadelphia: Benjamins.

Matthiessen, C. (1995) *Lexicogrammatical Cartography.* Tokyo: International Language Sciences.

Owens, R. E., Metz, D. E. and Haas, A. (2002) *Introduction to Communication Disorders: a life span perspective.* 2nd edn. Boston: Allyn & Bacon.

Rochester, S. and Martin, J. (1977) The art of referring: The speaker's use of noun phrases to instruct the listener. In R. Freedle (ed.) *New Directions in Discourse Processing.* 245–70. Norwood, N. J. : Ablex.

Rochester, S. and Martin, J. (1979) *Crazy Talk: a study of discourse of schizophrenic speakers.* New York: Plenum.

Rutter, M. (2002) The interplay of nature, nurture, and developmental influences. *Archives of General Psychiatry*, 59, 996–1000.

Segrin, C. and Flora, J. (1998) Depression and verbal behavior in conversations with friends and strangers. *Journal of Language and Social Psychology*, 17, 492–503.

Shames, G., Anderson, N. (2002) *Human Communication Disorders: an introduction.* 6th edn. Boston: Allyn and Bacon.

Szatmari, P. (2003) The causes of autism spectrum disorders. *British Medical Journal*, 326, 173–4.

Tarplee, C. (1996) Working on young children's utterances: prosodic aspects of repetition during picture labelling. In E. Couper-Kuhlen and M. Selting (eds) *Prosody in Conversation: interactional studies.* 406–35. Cambridge: Cambridge University Press.

Ventola, E. (1987) *The Structure of Social Interaction: a systemic approach to the semiotics of service encounters.* London: Pinter.

Zurif, E., Gardner, H. and Brownell, H. (1989) The case against the case against group studies. *Brain and Cognition*, 10, 237–55.

Glossary

adjacency pair
    Pairs of turns in conversation (first pair partner, second pair partner) that are typically adjacent to each other. The utterance of the first partner in the pair controls the interpretation of the next turn as being the second partner in the pair; for example, greeting-greeting ('Hi' – 'Hi'), invitation-acceptance or decline ('Want to come for lunch?' – 'No, I'm too busy'). Chapter 2, p. 53.

attitudinal epithet
    Epithets in the nominal group that express a quality of the thing being described ('the *disgusting* weather'). Attitudinal epithets differ from other epithets in that they describe the speaker's opinion about the thing rather than some more objective quality. Non-attitudinal epithets (the predicate adjectives) include examples such as 'the *warm* weather', 'the *record-breaking* weather', 'the *unusual* weather', whereas attitudinal epithets convey more opinion: 'the *lovely* weather', 'the *fantastic* weather', 'the *beastly* weather'. Chapter 2, p. 45, 65.

circumstances
    The surroundings of events in the world (one of the basic categories of reality, along with things and events) that fill in details of events. Also, the functional grammatical category that encodes these details of events. Circumstances are worded mainly by adverbials (quickly) and prepositional phrases ('in the sitting room'). Chapter 2, p. 42.

classifier
    Information (in the nominal group) about which subclass of the thing is being mentioned. As well as adjectives ('the *private* party',

'a *manual* transmission'), classifiers can be expressed by nouns ('the *office* building', 'the *computer* table'), and verbs ('a *running* dispute', 'the *shined* shoes'). Chapter 2, p. 46.

clause
A grammatical unit that more or less conforms to the patterns of the language. Participants, processes and circumstances are organised into clauses. The central or defining feature of a clause is the process usually expressed by a verb. There can be several clauses in one utterance. Chapter 2, p. 49.

conjunctive adjunct
Category of adjuncts (largely worded by adverbs) that relates the clause to an earlier clause. ('The sky is shimmering yellow. *Actually*, it looks warming and soothing to tired eyes.') Chapter 2, p. 71.

deictics
Pointing information (in the nominal group) that helps to identify the thing to the hearer. These deictics include words that indicate which subset of the things is intended and sometimes how much of the subset. The most frequent deictics are the demonstratives (the, this, that, these, those) and possessives (my, our, his, her, their, her brother's, etc.). Chapter 2, p. 45.

discourse structure
The arrangement of clauses into a socially acceptable pattern to convey typical meanings with the typical arrangement of words and grammatical structures. Language (e.g., a story, conversation) that is completely and uncompromisingly in the passive would sound strange. The telling of a story or the development of a conversation requires, among other things, the use of the right amount of repeated words, the use of conjunctions (but, then, because, however, etc.) and an appropriate use of pronouns and other referring expressions (he, it, theirs, *the* house). Chapter 2, p. 31.

epithet
Information (in the nominal group) about a quality of the things. Adjectives usually fill this role of epithet; e.g., 'a *large, blue* pen'. Chapter 2, p. 45.

events

The 'goings-on' in the world that things are involved with (one of the basic categories of reality, along with things and circumstances). Some events are not perceptually accessible but are nevertheless much more like perceptual events than they are like things. Chapter 2, p. 22, 24, 36.

field

Language that reflects the institutional focus of what is happening (a contextual variable, along with tenor and mode). This institutional focus then leads to the 'content' or subject matter of the talk. For example, a focus on the social activity of sowing grass seeds leads to the selection of certain kinds of vocabulary that is different from a focus on bicycle repairs. Institutions within the society are the focus of activity and that focus is reflected in the language. Chapter 2, p. 35.

finite verbal element

Part of the verbal group that carries meaning about the time and probability of the process. It takes the negative 'not' or 'n't'. The function of the finite element is to make the proposition definite enough to be 'at stake' in the conversation. This finite element may be included with the main verb ('They ate lunch', in which *ate* includes information about the material process of eating and involves the past tense 'the action happened in a time passed') or the finite element may be separated from the main verb and placed before it in an auxiliary verb ('They had (hadn't) gone home' in which the auxiliary verb *had* encodes the time (and can carry the negative *n't*) and the main verb *gone* encodes the lexical meaning 'to leave a place' as well as a signal that it is to be combined with an auxiliary: the use of *gone* instead of *go*). Chapter 2, p. 61.

genre

The way language is organised to achieve social processes (staged goal-oriented activities). Just as the genre of a mystery story has components of introduction of characters, inciting event, search for clues and the villain, discovery of villain, denouement, etc., so the genre that accomplishes a social process (e.g., a casual conversation that continues and solidifies a friendship) may have elements such as Greeting, Approach to neutral topic like weather, Approach to a substantive topic (why we are having this meeting),

Leave taking. Such elements establish a schematic structure that speakers are expected to be familiar with. Chapter 2, p. 32.

ideational meaning
The meanings expressed in language that reflect the reality external to ourselves and our experience of this reality. In the most general way, our experience of reality is experience of things, events and circumstances. These things, events and circumstances are then expressed by language. Chapter 1, p. 23–4.

interpersonal meaning
The meanings expressed in language that encode how the speaker relates to the ideational meaning of the utterance. These meanings concern the role relationships with others and the speaker's attitude to the ideational meaning and to other individuals. Chapter 1, p. 25.

lexicogrammar
The words and the grammatical structures that carry much of the meaning of language. Intonation carries additional meaning. Chapter 2, p. 31.

material processes
Processes (expressing the events of the world) that largely express experience of the world outside of the individual. These processes are most clearly processes of doing (e.g., 'She *opened* the box') and typically have an actor as the participant. Chapter 2, p. 41.

mental processes
Processes (expressing the events of the world) that involve experience of the individual's inner world. Mental processes include perception (e.g., 'They *heard* the music'), affection (e.g., 'They *enjoyed* the music'), and cognition (e.g., 'They *understood* the music'). Chapter 2, p. 41.

metafunctions
The three major categories of meanings in language (ideational, interpersonal, textual) and how language conveys those meanings. Chapter 1, p. 23.

modal adjunct
Category of adjuncts that expresses how relevant the speaker

thinks the message is (Halliday, 1994: 49). The subcategories are: a comment on the whole proposition ('*Unfortunately*, we have not resolved the issues yet'), a signal about the time ('*Soon*, there will be no more left'), polarity ('*No*, they haven't seen the movie') or other aspect of the mood of the clause ('*Probably*, that is not the way to do it'. '*Certainly*, I'll help out'. '*In fact*, it's an ace'). Chapter 2, p. 64.

mode

Language that reflects the role that language itself is playing in the situation (a contextual variable, along with field and tenor). For example, language may be spoken, written, spoken as if it were written (a newscast), spoken as if it was not written (a play). The channel of communication (e.g., face-to-face, telephone, via windows facing each other over a roadway) can substantially affect which messages are sent and how they are formulated. As with tenor and field, though, the mode itself is an organization of meanings. There is a meaning to interacting spontaneously that is different to the meaning of a written text. For example, in organizations one sometimes hears 'Will you put that in writing?' or 'Come say that in person.' That is, the same words with the same sender and receiver mean something different when they are in a different mode. Chapter 3, p. 99.

move

A functional structural unit in interaction that fills a slot in conversational exchanges. Moves are combined into different kinds of exchanges. The basic functional distinctions of moves are: information or action as the basis of the social activity, primary knower or actor (the one who knows the information or does the action) or secondary knower or actor (the one who does not know the information or does not do the action) and identification of the contribution as follow up to some other part of the interaction or not. The scope of the move is the 'clause selecting independently for mood' (Martin, 1992: 59). Chapter 2, p. 54.

nominal group

A group of adjacent words in which the primary word is a noun. The whole nominal group can be replaced by a pronoun; e.g., '*a house*', '*a tall house*', '*the delightful old house I saw yesterday morning*', all replaceable by '*it*'. Chapter 2, p. 44.

numerative
   Information (in the nominal group) about how many of the thing
   is being considered ('*three* pens') or the order of the thing ('the
   third pen'). Chapter 2, p. 45.

participant
   A functional linguistic category that expresses the things in the
   world. Participants in discourse are largely worded by nouns for
   the objects of the speaker's experience. The kinds of participants
   are: actor, goal, senser, phenomenon, behaver, sayer, receiver
   verbiage and target. Chapter 2, p. 40.

process
   A functional linguistic category that expresses the events, the
   goings-on, of the world. Processes are mainly worded by verbs
   (see the subcategories of processes: material, mental, relational
   and further detail in Halliday, 1994, Chapter 5). Chapter 2, p. 41.

qualifier
   Information (in the nominal group) that is placed after the thing.
   This information characterizes the thing but does so by a phrase
   or a clause that can itself be quite complex; e.g., 'The pen *in the
   penholder that my sister made for me*'. Chapter 2, p. 46.

register
   Aspects of meaning related to three standard contextual variables:
   field (meanings reflecting the institutional focus of the interaction,
   loosely, subject matter), tenor (meanings reflecting the social roles
   of speakers) and mode (meanings reflecting the role of language
   itself). Speakers are expected to combine meanings from field,
   tenor and mode to sound like other speakers in parallel situations. This combination of field, tenor and mode is called register.
   Register is thus a combination of values that represent meanings
   and that go together to 'achieve a text's goals' (Martin, 1992:
   502–3). Chapter 2, p. 36.

relational processes
   Processes (expressing the events of the world) that enable speakers
   to generalize by relating one kind of experience to another, as in:
   'John *is* short', 'The butler *is* the culprit'. Chapter 2, p. 31.

rheme
> The non-initial element in a thematic structure that expresses the development of the theme. The initial element in thematic structure is the theme (the point of departure of the clause as a message or what the message is about). Chapter 2, p. 67.

situation
> The relevant physical circumstances of each interaction. In any given interaction, there are physical aspects of the world that impinge on the interaction. The people involved in the interaction are the most obvious components that are relevant to the interaction. Other factors may be the objects around the interaction, the location of the interaction, the medium of the interaction (by face-to-face oral language, by telephone, letter, electronic mail, voice mail, etc.) and the ambient sounds. Speakers, to the best of their ability, perceive and analyse the physical attributes of the communication event (the situation) in terms of the relevant factors. Situations, then, as the specific physical circumstances of an interaction, must be perceived and parsed in terms of what is culturally and interactionally relevant. Chapter 2, p. 33.

social processes
> Staged and goal-oriented activities are formed and present in a culture. Established collections of meanings are typically combined into an overall activity in the society. Examples of social processes in common activities are buying stamps, introducing strangers to each other, saying good morning to a neighbour, or engaging in a psychiatric interview. The social processes in turn are structured in terms of sequences of elements and the dependencies among them. Simple social processes with few elements are, for example, asking for a telephone number from an information service or buying a newspaper. More complex social processes have many elements, for example, buying a home or negotiating a management labour union agreement. Chapter 1, 2, p. 23, 33.

speech function
> The semantic roles that are taken by speakers in interaction defined by the dimension of 'giving' or 'demanding' and the dimension of 'information' or 'goods and services'. Chapter 2, p. 57, 59.

tenor

Language that reflects the structuring of the social roles of speakers in interaction (a contextual variable, along with field and mode). Speakers may have formally defined roles, such as judge and prosecutor, or less formally defined roles, such as current resident of an apartment building and incoming resident or roles related to age, sex or family relationship. These roles, in turn, have a range in status, rules of formality, and rules of interaction attached to them. The tenor is the configuration of meanings associated with the social roles. For example, there are things that a teacher can say to a fourth grade pupil ('sit down now right away') that are not generally said by speakers in other roles in other interactions. Chapter 2, p. 35.

text

An instance of language that is operative in context. A stretch of language which is not text is citational. Chapter 1, p. 9, 14.

textual meaning

The meanings created when fitting an utterance into its context. The specific textual meanings are: cohesion (lexical, reference, conjunction, substitution, ellipsis), information structure (information coded as given or new) and thematic structure (information coded as theme (the starting point) or rheme). Chapter 1, 10, p. 26, 289.

theme

The first element in a thematic structure that expresses 'the point of departure of the clause as a message' or 'what the message is about'. The theme ties down the text by showing how the speaker looks at things (Martin, 1992: 489). What is not theme is called rheme and has the meaning of 'the development of the theme'. Chapter 2, p. 67.

theme-marking

Theme-marking (i.e., placing as theme some element that is usually not theme) highlights certain kinds of meaning for the hearer (e.g., '*In the middle of the night*, they discovered the parcel'). Chapter 2, p. 72.

things

The objects, people and concepts that are talked about, however abstract, fictional, or whimsical (one of the basic categories of reality, along with events and circumstances). 'A unicorn', 'Big Bang' or 'material socialism' are all things in the real world that are talked about, even though we cannot point to an exemplar of them. Chapter 1, 2, p. 24, 40.

turn

A turn is the talk of one speaker that is bounded by the talk of other speakers. What one person manages to say before someone else speaks. Turns may be very long, since in some situations other speakers do not interrupt or they may be very short, as in an animated conversation where a simple 'yes' or 'ya' or even 'y-' may constitute a turn. Chapter 2, p. 53.

utterance

A stretch of language that is used in oral interaction. Most utterances are spontaneous, although they may be planned. Utterances may be relatively long or short. Chapter 2, p. 49.

verbal group

A group of words in which the primary word is a lexical verb and the other words come before this verb; e.g., 'could have come', 'whispered', 'was eating'. Chapter 2, p. 46–7.

wordings

The particular language resources that are used to express the meaning in a given instance. The wordings of language are said to 'realise' or actualise the meanings by exploiting the linguistic patterns available in the particular language. Chapter 2, p. 49, 87.

Appendix A

Language systems grouped by the metafunctions of ideational, interpersonal, textual

---

Ideational meaning

In the world

Things	objects, people, things that are talked about
Events	goings-on, activities of the world
Circumstances	fill in details of events

In language

Participants: encoding things (following Halliday, 1994):

Actor	the one that does something
Goal	the one to which the process is extended
Senser	the conscious being that feels, thinks or sees
Phenomenon	what is being felt, thought or sensed
Behaver	a conscious being, acting physiologically or psychologically
Sayer	an entity that puts out a message
Receiver	one who is to receive the saying
Verbiage	what is said
Target	that which is targeted or the subject of the saying

Processes: encoding events:

Material	doing something in the external world
Mental	experience of the inner world
• *Perception*	
• *Affection*	
• *Cognition*	
Relational	relate one experience to another

Circumstances: encoding details of events:

Extent:	distance	They travelled *for three miles*
	duration	They travelled *for three days*
Location:	place	They ate *in the lunchroom*
	time	They ate *at noon*
Manner:	means	They built it *with scrap metal*
	quality	They built it *carefully*
	comparison	They built it *unlike any other*
Cause:	reason	They considered it *because it was important*
	purpose	They considered it *in order to help the poor*
	behalf	They considered it *for the relatives*
Contingency:	condition	She studied in case there would be no time later
	concession	She studied in spite of the noise
	default	She studied in the absence of an incentive
Accompaniment:	comitative	The couple departed with/without the children
	additive	The couple departed as well as/instead of the children
Role:	guise	They behaved as wild animals
	product	They were transformed into angels
Matter		She spoke of shoes and ships and sealing wax and cabbages and kings
Angle		Oh my papa, to me you are so wonderful

Interpersonal meaning

Speaker roles:

	Giving	Demanding
Goods and services	offer	command
Information	statement	question

Adjacency pairs of turns (Martin, 1992: 45):

Call	Response to call	John – Yes
Greeting	Response to greeting	Hi – Hi
Exclamation	Response to exclamation	Disgusting – You bet
Offer	Acknowledge offer	A piece of home-made pie? – Sure
Command	Response offer to command	Get me two painkillers – Will do
Statement	Acknowledge statement	Hottest day of the summer – Guess so
Question	Response statement to question	When will I see you? – At eleven

Moves:
Information or goods and services
       Information
        Goods and services

Speaker or hearer oriented
        Speaker primary knower
        Speaker secondary knower
        hearer primary knower
        hearer secondary knower
        speaker primary actor
        speaker secondary actor
        hearer primary actor
        hearer secondary actor

Follow up to another contribution or independent contribution
        Follow up
        Non-follow up

Speech functions:

Initiating
Responding
Attending
        Call
        Greeting

Exchanging
        Giving
        Demanding
        Goods and services
        Information

Textual meaning

Thematic organisation:

Theme	the point of departure of the clause as a message
Rheme	how the message is developed

Information structure:

New	information as new to the hearer
Given	information as know to the hearer

Cohesion:

Reference   (continuity of participants – people, places, things)

personal	he, she, it
demonstrative	this, that
comparatives	*more* drivers

Conjunction   (continuity and development of message)

additive
temporal
causal
internal
external

Lexical   (continuity of institutional focus – subject matter of talk)

repetition
synonym
co-occurrence

Substitution and ellipsis   (direct copying of information)

nominal
verbal
clausal

Contextual variables

Field:	meanings and wordings reflecting focus of activity, institution (content)
Tenor:	meanings and wordings reflecting social roles of speakers
Mode:	meanings and wordings reflecting role of language in communication, channel of communication

Appendix B

DSM-IV diagnostic categories with language systems that are at risk.

Psychiatric categories – disorders and diagnostic criteria are <u>underlined.</u>

The linguistic categories listed are those that are at risk and may be used atypically. The linguistic categories are labelled as ideational, interpersonal and textual where possible.

Communication Disorders (Chapter 4)

<u>Expressive language disorder</u>

<u>Limitations</u>
Amount of speech
> Short responses (interpersonal)

Range of vocabulary (ideational)
> Nouns expressing things
> Verbs expressing events
> Adverbs expressing circumstances
> Adjectives giving details about things

Range of grammatical structures (ideational)
> Time expressions, gender, number
> Speech functions (interpersonal)
> Intonation (interpersonal)

Simplified grammatical structures, omitted elements, shortened sentences
> Word level
> Group level (expressing things, events, circumstances)
> Clause level
> New information omitted at ends of clauses
> (especially, goals, phenomena, verbiage, circumstances)

Unusual word order
> Group level

Clause level

Mixed expressive-receptive language disorder

Expressive language disorder as outlined above
Speaker roles (especially giving) affected by anxiety in social context
Adjacency pairs
Second turn in pair not given: response to call, response to greeting, response to exclamation, acknowledge offer, response offer to command, acknowledge statement, response statement to question

Speech functions – responding
Ideational meaning (shifting topics)
Participants
Processes
Circumstances

Textual meaning
Reference – pronouns tracking different participants

Phonological disorder

Sounds affected

Stuttering

Sounds affected
Information structure (new – given) as location of stuttering (textual)
Repetitions heard as clarifications (interpersonal)
Circumlocutions heard as unexpected meaning (ideational)

Pervasive development disorders (Chapter 5)

Autistic disorder

Impaired social interaction
Failure to develop peer relationships
Frequency of typical social activities
Frequency of ideation about peers
Reactions of peers
• *Moves: follow up*
• *Speech functions: responding to affected speaker*

Lack of spontaneous seeking to share
Speech function: lack of initiations
• *Lack of giving: information; giving: goods & services*
• *Lack of attending: call; attending: greeting*

Lack of social or emotional reciprocity
>
> Speech roles: imbalance in giving and demanding
>
> • *Especially information about emotions; emotion descriptions of participants, events; intonation encoding emotion*
>
> Moves: lack of follow up moves to signal continuing interaction
>
> • *Especially about topics (participants, events) introduced by interlocutor*
>
> Cohesion: lack of cohesion (reference, conjunction, lexis, substitution, ellipsis) linking to language of interlocutor
>
> Information structure of given and new by intonation, theme-rheme structure; inappropriately encoding what is known or unknown to the interlocutor
>
> Speech function: lack of responses
>
> • *Lack of typical mixture of responses and initiations*

Impaired communication

Delay or lack of development of spoken language
>
> Sounds, vocabulary and grammar below developmental level

Impairment in initiating and sustaining conversation
>
> Impairment in initiating conversation
>
> • *Speech roles: demanding information, goods and services*
>
> • *Speech functions: initiating attending, exchanging*
>
> • *Ideational meaning: new things, events*
>
> Impairment in sustaining conversation
>
> • *Vocabulary reflecting institutional focus (ideational)*
>
> • *Adjacency pairs – failure to supply second turn (interpersonal)*
>
> • *Speech functions – failure to respond (interpersonal)*
>
> • *Information structure – failure to use new, given meanings as appropriate (textual meaning)*
>
> • *Cohesion (textual meaning)*
>> *Reference (continuity of participants – people, places, things)*
>> *Conjunction (continuity and development of message)*
>> *Lexical (continuity of institutional focus – subject matter of talk)*
>> *Substitution & ellipsis (direct copying of information)*

Stereotyped, repetitive, idiosyncratic language
>
> Stereotyped
>
> • *Fixed participants (expressed by nominals), events (expressed by verbs), circumstances (expressed by adverbs, prepositional phrases) (ideational)*
>
> • *Fixed speech functions (interpersonal)*
>
> • *Language from another context, social process, genre*
>
> Repetitive
>
> • *Cohesion*
>> *Lexical (continuity of institutional focus)*
>
> Idiosyncratic
>
> • *Restricted use of moves, speech functions, vocabulary*

<u>Lack of varied, spontaneous make-believe play, social imitative play</u>
    <u>Make-believe play</u>
      • *Social processes atypical for the speaker's role in society*
    <u>Social imitative play</u>
      • *Using language from another context, social process*
        Vocabulary (ideational meaning)
        Speech roles (interpersonal meaning)

Restricted repetitive, stereotyped behaviour, activity, interests
    Fixed participants (expressed by nominals), events (expressed by verbs), circumstances (expressed by adverbs, prepositional phrases) (ideational)
    Fixed speech functions (interpersonal)
    Fixed intonation patterns
    Language from another context, social process, genre
    <u>Repetitive</u>
    • *Cohesion*
      Lexical (continuity of institutional focus)

Asperger's disorder

Impaired social interaction
<u>Failure to develop peer relationships</u>
    Frequency of typical social activities
    Frequency of ideation about peers
    Reactions of peers
    • *Moves: follow up*
    • *Speech functions: responding to affected speaker*
<u>Lack of spontaneous seeking to share</u>
    Speech function: lack of initiations
    • *Lack of giving: information; giving: goods & services*
    • *Lack of attending: call; attending: greeting*
<u>Lack of social or emotional reciprocity</u>
    Speech roles: imbalance in giving and demanding
    • *Especially information about emotions; emotion descriptions of participants, events; intonation encoding emotion*
    Moves: lack of follow up moves to signal continuing interaction
    • *Especially about topics (participants, events) introduced by interlocutor*
    Cohesion: lack of cohesion (reference, conjunction, lexis, substitution, ellipsis) linking to language of interlocutor
    Information structure of given and new by intonation, theme-rheme structure; inappropriately encoding what is known or unknown to the interlocutor
    Speech function: lack of responses
    • *Lack of typical mixture of responses and initiations*

Restricted repetitive, stereotyped behaviour, activity, interests

> Fixed participants (expressed by nominals), events (expressed by verbs), circumstances (expressed by adverbs, prepositional phrases) (ideational)
>
> Fixed speech functions (interpersonal)
>
> Fixed intonation patterns
>
> Language from another context, social process, genre
>
> Repetitive
>
> • *Cohesion*

Attention Deficit Hyperactivity Disorder (Chapter 6)

Inattention

Difficulty sustaining attention in tasks or play

> Lack of consistency in social process and stages of social processes
>
> • *Jumps (within a speaker) in participants (ideation)*
>> *Actor – the one that does something*
>> *Goal – the one to which the process is extended*
>> *Senser – the conscious being that feels, thinks or see*
>> *Phenomenon – what is being felt, thought or sensed*
>> *Behaver – a conscious being who is acting physiologically or psychologically*
>> *Sayer – an entity that puts out a message*
>> *Receiver – one who is to receive the saying*
>> *Verbiage – what is said*
>> *Target – that which is targeted or the subject of the saying*
>
> • *Jumps (within a speaker) in processes (ideation)*
>> *Material – doing something in the external world*
>> *Mental – experience of the inner world (Perception / Affection / Cognition)*
>> *Relational – relate one experience to another*
>
> • *Jumps (within a speaker) in circumstances (ideation)*

Extent:	*distance*	They travelled *for three miles*
	duration	They travelled *for three days*
Location:	*place*	They ate *in the lunchroom*
	time	They ate *at noon*
Manner:	*means*	They built it *with scrap metal*
	quality	They built it *carefully*
	comparison	They built it *unlike any other*
Cause:	*reason*	They considered it *because it was important*
	purpose	They considered it *in order to help the poor*
	behalf	They considered it *for the relatives*
Contingency:	*condition*	She studied *in case there would be no time later*
	concession	She studied *in spite of the noise*
	default	She studied *in the absence of an incentive*
Accompaniment:	*comitative*	The couple departed *with/without the children*
	additive	The couple departed as *well as/instead of the children*

Role:	guise	They behaved *as wild animals*
	product	They were transformed *into angels*
Matter		She spoke of *shoes and ships and sealing wax and cabbages and kings*
Angle		Oh my papa, *to me* you are so wonderful

Does not seem to listen when spoken to

- *Jumps (across speakers) in participants (ideation), especially across adjacency turns and in responding speech functions (interpersonal)*

 Actor – the one that does something
 Goal – the one to which the process is extended
 Senser – the conscious being that feels, thinks or see
 Phenomenon – what is being felt, thought or sensed
 Behaver – a conscious being who is acting physiologically or psychologically
 Sayer – an entity that puts out a message
 Receiver – one who is to receive the saying
 Verbiage – what is said
 Target – that which is targeted or the subject of the saying

- *Jumps (across speakers) in processes (ideation), especially across adjacency turns and in responding speech functions (interpersonal)*

 Material – doing something in the external world
 Mental – experience of the inner world (Perception / Affection / Cognition)
 Relational – relate one experience to another

- *Jumps (across speakers) in circumstances (ideation), especially across adjacency turns and in responding speech functions (interpersonal)*

Extent:	distance	They travelled *for three miles*
	duration	They travelled *for three days*
Location:	place	They ate *in the lunchroom*
	time	They ate *at noon*
Manner:	means	They built it *with scrap metal*
	quality	They built it *carefully*
	comparison	They built it *unlike any other*
Cause:	reason	They considered it *because it was important*
	purpose	They considered it *in order to help the poor*
	behalf	They considered it *for the relatives*
Contingency:	condition	She studied *in case there would be no time later*
	concession	She studied *in spite of the noise*
	default	She studied *in the absence of an incentive*
Accompaniment:	comitative	The couple departed *with/without the children*
	additive	The couple departed as *well as/instead of the children*
Role:	guise	They behaved *as wild animals*
	product	They were transformed *into angels*
Matter		She spoke of *shoes and ships and sealing wax and cabbages and kings*
Angle		Oh my papa, *to me* you are so wonderful

• *Incompatible level of certainty across speakers (interpersonal)*

  Modal verbs should, would, *etc.*
  Modal adjuncts possibly, probably

• *Repeated questions, commands by interlocutor (interpersonal)*
• *Attention getting devices, calling, raising voice by interlocutor (interpersonal)*
• *Information structure of given and new by intonation, theme-rheme structure – inappropriately encoding what is known or unknown to the interlocutor (textual)*

  Inappropriate intonation marking new information (textual)
  Inappropriate word order

• *Cohesion jumps across speakers (textual)*

  Reference (continuity of participants – people, places, things);
  - *personal* he, she it, *etc.;*
  - *demonstrative* (this, that, *etc;*
  - *comparatives* more drivers
  Conjunction (continuity and development of message)
  - *additive*
  - *temporal*
  - *causal*
  - *internal*
  - *external*
  Lexical (continuity of institutional focus – subject matter of talk)
  - *repetition*
  - *synonym*
  - *co-occurrence*
  Substitution & ellipsis (direct copying of information)
  - *nominal*
  - *verbal*
  - *clausal*

Does not follow through on instructions, fails to finish activities

  • *Direct expressions of not wanting to finish activities*
  • *Interlocutor notes that activities are not complete*
  • *Inappropriate responses (speech function) to exchanging goods and services (interpersonal)*

Difficulty organising tasks, dislike for tasks with sustained mental effort, easily distractible

  • *Direct expressions of difficulty*
  • *Reference to physical aspects of the environment* that desk

Hyperactivity

Rate of speaking
  Fewer pauses, shorter pauses
More talk than usual
  Conjunction (continuity and development of message)
  • *Additive*
  • *Temporal*
  • *Causal*
  • *Internal*
  • *External*
  Lexical (continuity of institutional focus – subject matter of talk)

- *Repetition*
- *Synonym*
- *Co-occurrence*

Talks excessively, often 'on the go'

Domination of ideational meaning – participants, processes, circumstances

Difficult for interlocutor to contribute responding speech function (interpersonal)

Impulsivity

Interrupts and intrudes on others

Overlapping with speech of previous speaker

Changing topics (ideational)

- *Change topics without notification of the change*
- *Less cohesion, lexical*

   (continuity of institutional focus – subject matter of talk)
   repetition
   synonym
   co-occurrence

Excess of initiating speech functions (interpersonal)

Blurting out answers before questions have been completed, difficulty waiting a turn

Starting too early the second turn in pairs of turns

- *Adjacency pairs of turns:*

Call	Response to call	John – Yes
Greeting	Response to greeting	Hi – Hi
Exclamation	Response to exclamation	Disgusting – You bet
Offer	Acknowledge offer	A piece of home-made pie? – Sure
Command	Response offer to command	Get me two painkillers – Will do
Statement	Acknowledge statement	Hottest day of the summer – Guess so
Question	Response statement to question	When will I see you? – At eleven

---

Psychotic disorders (Chapter 7)

Delusions

Mismatch of objects, people, things, events and information surrounding events of the world with those mentioned by the speaker in participants, processes, circumstances in language (ideational)

In the world

Things – objects, people, things that are talked about, especially in identity of speaker (I, etc.) and interlocutor (you, etc.)

Events – goings-on, activities of the world

Circumstances – fill in details of events

In language – participants

> *Actor – the one that does something*
> *Goal – the one to which the process is extended*
> *Senser – the conscious being that feels, thinks or see*
> *Phenomenon – what is being felt, thought or sensed*
> *Behaver – a conscious being who is acting physiologically or psychologically*
> *Sayer – an entity that puts out a message*
> *Receiver – one who is to receive the saying*
> *Verbiage – what is said*
> *Target – that which is targeted or the subject of the saying*

In language – processes

> *Material – doing something in the external world*
> *Mental – experience of the inner world (Perception / Affection / Cognition)*
> *Relational – relate one experience to another*

In language – circumstances

Extent:	distance	They travelled *for three miles*
	duration	They travelled *for three days*
Location:	place	They ate *in the lunchroom*
	time	They ate *at noon*
Manner:	means	They built it *with scrap metal*
	quality	They built it *carefully*
	comparison	They built it *unlike any other*
Cause:	reason	They considered it *because it was important*
	purpose	They considered it *in order to help the poor*
	behalf	They considered it *for the relatives*
Contingency:	condition	She studied *in case there would be no time later*
	concession	She studied *in spite of the noise*
	default	She studied *in the absence of an incentive*
Accompaniment:	comitative	The couple departed *with/without the children*
	additive	The couple departed as *well as/instead of the children*
Role:	guise	They behaved *as wild animals*
	product	They were transformed *into angels*
Matter		She spoke of *shoes and ships and sealing wax and cabbages and kings*
Angle		Oh my papa, *to me* you are so wonderful

In language – circumstances

Intonation indicating conviction
Adverbs of certainty (attitudinal adjuncts)
Moves, follow up that contradicts interlocutor

Hallucinations

Restricted ideational focus (aural, tactile, etc.) that does not match reality
Participants:

> *Actor – the one that does something*
> *Goal – the one to which the process is extended*

Senser – the conscious being that feels, thinks or see
Phenomenon – what is being felt, thought or sensed
Behaver – a conscious being who is acting physiologically or psychologically
Sayer – an entity that puts out a message
Receiver – one who is to receive the saying
Verbiage – what is said
Target – that which is targeted or the subject of the saying

Processes:

Mental – experience of the inner world (in particular)
- perception
- affection
- cognition

Material – doing something in the external world

Information structure

Assuming information as known to the hearer
- unusual sentence stress, word order

Disorganised speech

Derailment (between clauses)
Lack of ideational consistency in objects, people, things, events and information surrounding events of the world with those mentioned by the speaker in participants, processes, circumstances in language from one sentence to another (ideational).
In the world

Things – objects, people, things that are talked about,
especially in identity of speaker (I, etc.) and interlocutor (you, etc.)
Events – goings-on, activities of the world
Circumstances – fill in details of events

In language
Participants: consistency in objects, people, things that are talked about

Actor – the one that does something
Goal – the one to which the process is extended
Senser – the conscious being that feels, thinks or see
Phenomenon – what is being felt, thought or sensed
Behaver – a conscious being who is acting physiologically or psychologically
Sayer – an entity that puts out a message
Receiver – one who is to receive the saying
Verbiage – what is said
Target – that which is targeted or the subject of the saying

Cohesion (textual)

Reference	(continuity of participants – people, places, things) incorrect or absent
personal	he, she, it
demonstrative	this, that
comparatives	*more* drivers

Processes, consistency in goings-on, activities of the world

Material   doing something in the external world
Mental   experience of the inner world
• *Perception*
• *Affection*
• *Cognition*
Relational   relate one part of external world to another

Circumstances, consistency in time, place, details of events

Extent:	distance	They travelled *for three miles*
	duration	They travelled *for three days*
Location:	place	They ate *in the lunchroom*
	time	They ate *at noon*
Manner:	means	They built it *with scrap metal*
	quality	They built it *carefully*
	comparison	They built it *unlike any other*
Cause:	reason	They considered it *because it was important*
	purpose	They considered it *in order to help the poor*
	behalf	They considered it *for the relatives*
Contingency:	condition	She studied *in case there would be no time later*
	concession	She studied *in spite of the noise*
	default	She studied *in the absence of an incentive*
Accompaniment:	comitative	The couple departed *with/without the children*
	additive	The couple departed as *well as/instead of the children*
Role:	guise	They behaved *as wild animals*
	product	They were transformed *into angels*
Matter		She spoke of *shoes and ships and sealing wax and cabbages and kings*
Angle		Oh my papa, *to me* you are so wonderful

Lack of signals that the ideation is changing from sentence to sentence
<u>Topic shifting</u>
Atypical pattern of ideation changing from sentence to sentence (as for derailment)
<u>Incoherence</u> (within clauses)
<u>Word salad</u>

 Almost random and inconsistent selection of participants, processes, circumstances
 Disturbances in word order
Disconnection from social reality

 Inconsistent or disordered stages in social processes (ideational)
 • *Adjacency pairs of turns*:

Call	Response to call	John – Yes
Greeting	Response to greeting	Hi – Hi
Exclamation	Response to exclamation	Disgusting – You bet
Offer	Acknowledge offer	A piece of home-made pie? – Sure
Command	Response offer to command	Get me two painkillers – Will do
Statement	Acknowledge statement	Hottest day of the summer – Guess so
Question	Response statement to question	When will I see you? – At eleven

Disconnection interpersonally
- *Addressing interlocutors not present*
- *Speaking in third person* he, she
- *Speaking in plural* we
- *Unusual terms of address* Sir, comrade, butler
- *Atypical intimacy or distance*
  Formal intonation, low frequency, technical vocabulary
- *Atypical social roles*
  Authoritative, passive
  Atypical frequency of imperatives
- *Changing social roles without adequate signals*

Disconnection in channel of communication
- *Overly loud or quiet*
- *Speaking over other speakers*

Negative symptoms
Blocking
Pausing, stopping – within words, phrases, clauses
Poverty of speech
Less than expected talk, especially in second turns of adjacency pairs
- *Adjacency pairs of turns:*

Command	Response offer to command	Get me two painkillers – Will do
Statement	Acknowledge statement	Hottest day of the summer – Guess so
Question	Response statement to question	When will I see you? – At eleven

Poverty of content of speech
Less than expected content of talk (objects, people, things, events, circumstances), especially in second turns of adjacency pairs (ideation, interpersonal)
- *Adjacency pairs of turns:*

Command	Response offer to command	Get me two painkillers – Will do
Statement	Acknowledge statement	Hottest day of the summer – Guess so
Question	Response statement to question	When will I see you? – At eleven

Flattening of affect
Speaker's attitude to interaction expressed less than expected (interpersonal)
- *Mental process verbs*
- *Evaluative words*
- *Intensifying words*
- *Intonation*
  Contrary to expectation
  Contrast
  Attitudinal words
  Commitment to statements
  - modal verbs
  - modal adjuncts

Mood disorders (Chapter 8)

<u>Depressive episode</u>
Depressed mood (ideational)
In the world

> **Relational verb with adjective** I'm sad, depressed
> **Verb of sensing**
> • *Perception* I see I'm sad
> • *Affect* I feel sad
> • *Cognition* I think I'm sad
> **Negative sentences – negative words** not, never, no, nothing, etc.
> **Intonation – little contrastive stress or pitch changes**
> **Topics – refer to death, suicide, hopelessness**
> • *Participants, processes of death, suicide, hopelessness*

<u>Diminished interest or pleasure in activities</u>

> **Verb of affection** like, don't like, want, enjoy
> **Verb or adjective of negative subjective state** bored, uninterested, fed up, tired of
> **Negate positive process, adjective** no playing, not interesting
> **Lack of intensifiers** really, very
> **Negation of intensifiers** not really, not very, not especially, not particularly
> **Above linguistic markers found across different topics**

<u>Psychomotor retardation</u>

> Slower speech
> Longer than usual pauses
> Reduced amount of talk
> • *Fewer classifiers* a *carving* knife
> • *Less expansion for one clause to another, by conjunctions*
> • *Conjunction (continuity and development of message)*
>   *additive*
>   *temporal*
>   *causal*
>   *- internal*
>   *- external*
> Reduction in variety of content
> • *Participants, fewer or stereotyped objects, people, things that are talked about*
>> *Actor – the one that does something*
>> *Goal – the one to which the process is extended*
>> *Senser – the conscious being that feels, thinks or see*
>> *Phenomenon – what is being felt, thought or sensed*
>> *Behaver – a conscious being who is acting physiologically or psychologically*
>> *Sayer – an entity that puts out a message*
>> *Receiver – one who is to receive the saying*
>> *Verbiage – what is said*
>> *Target – that which is targeted or the subject of the saying*

- *Processes, fewer or stereotyped goings-on, activities of the world*
  - *Material – doing something in the external world*
  - *Mental – experience of the inner world*
  - *Perception – seeing, hearing*
  - *Affection – liking, fearing*
  - *Cognition – thinking, knowing*
  - *Relational – relate one experience to another*
- *Circumstances, less information of time, place, details of events*

Extent:	*distance*	They travelled *for three miles*
	duration	They travelled *for three days*
Location:	*place*	They ate *in the lunchroom*
	time	They ate *at noon*
Manner:	*means*	They built it *with scrap metal*
	quality	They built it *carefully*
	comparison	They built it *unlike any other*
Cause:	*reason*	They considered it *because it was important*
	purpose	They considered it *in order to help the poor*
	behalf	They considered it *for the relatives*
Contingency:	*condition*	She studied *in case there would be no time later*
	concession	She studied *in spite of the noise*
	default	She studied *in the absence of an incentive*
Accompaniment:	*comitative*	The couple departed *with/without the children*
	additive	The couple departed as *well as/instead of the children*
Role:	*guise*	They behaved *as wild animals*
	product	They were transformed *into angels*
Matter		She spoke of *shoes and ships and sealing wax and cabbages and kings*
Angle		Oh my papa, *to me* you are so wonderful

Decrease in inflection of speech
- *Narrow pitch range*

Feelings of worthlessness or excessive guilt

Content words of 'worthlessness' 'guilt'

Diminished ability to think or concentrate, indecisiveness

Subjective claims of inability to think, concentrate, decide
- *First person pronoun* I *with verb of cognition* think
Modal verbs would, could
Modal adverbs possibly, probably
Level final intonation (neither rising nor falling sentence intonation)

Recurrent thoughts of death and suicidal ideation

Participants, processes of death

Manic episode

Increased volume, rate of talk, pitch changes

Euphoria

Few negative words not, n't, never, nothing
Increase in positive attributes in relational sentences the trip was exciting
Positive characteristics of participants
• *Classifers* the automatic machine
• *Epithets* the delightful movie

Enthusiasm for interaction

Initiating social processes
• *Frequent initiation in speech function, for information, for goods and services, in different contexts (interpersonal)*
• *Statements*
• *Questions*
• *Imperatives*
Wide range of social processes, topics (ideational)

Inflated self-esteem

Social roles of giving information (advice), relating to public figures (interpersonal)
• *Technical and specific vocabulary (ideational)*

Irritability

Frequent contradiction, correction of prior utterance (ideation)
Rejection of offers, commands (interpersonal), with exaggerated intonation

Manic speech

Pressured, loud, difficult to interpret
• *Fewer, shortened pauses, loud stressed syllables*
Joking, punning, theatrical speech
• *Intrusion into step-by-step stages of social process*
    Unusual participants, processes, circumstances (ideation)
    Changes in voice quality

Flight of ideas

Few pauses
Increases rate of talk
Abrupt changes in topic (ideational)
• *Changes in participants, processes, circumstances*

Distractibility

Direct references to physical situation (textual)
Changes in participants, processes, circumstances to different social process (ideational)
Changes in referents for cohesion, reference (textual)

Personality disorders (Chapter 9)

<u>Schizotypal personality disorder</u>
<u>Idiosyncratic speech</u>

>> Unusual word order
>> Low frequency grammatical structures
>> Contextually restricted structures (interpersonal)
>> • *Information structure, given-new*

<u>Loose, digressive, vague language</u>

>> (see <u>psychotic disorders</u> (Chapter 7) <u>derailment, incoherence</u>)
>> participants, processes, circumstances from different social processes
>> lack of ideation information in participants, processes, circumstances
>> • *Little modification of nominals by classifiers, epithets, qualifiers*
>> • *Little use of prepositional phrases, adverbials to express circumstances*

<u>Concrete or abstract responses</u>

>> Cohesion, reference to physical speech event *that* desk
>> Participants without material form
>> Processes
>> • *Mental*
>> • *Relational*

<u>Word level atypicalities</u>

>> Archaic words
>> Low frequency words
>> Morphological errors redly

<u>Narrow range of affect</u>

>> <u>Stiff presentation (interpersonal)</u>
>> • *lack of follow up moves to interlocutor turns*
>> • *lack of confirming or requesting confirmations*
>> • *lack of contractions*
>> • *lack of overlapped speech*

<u>Histrionic personality disorder</u>
<u>Emotionality</u>

>> Mental process verbs like, love, hate (ideational)
>> • *relational process verbs with attribute of emotion* I was aghast *(ideational)*
>> intensifiers really, very (interpersonal)
>> loud, pronounced intonation
>> slow or rapid rate of speaking

<u>Attention-seeking behaviour</u>

>> Take on unusual social role in unusual social process (interpersonal)
>> Unusual topics, by unusual participants, processes, circumstances (ideational)
>> Speaking about self (interpersonal, ideational)
>> • *Speech function, giving information about self, statements*

Dependent personality disorder

Attention-seeking behaviour

Responding to speaker roles without contradicting or questioning
(interpersonal)
• *Speaker roles:*

	Giving	Demanding
Goods and services	offer	command
Information	statement	question

Giving second pair in pairs of adjacent turns without contradicting or questioning
Adjacency pairs of turns: (interpersonal)

Call	*Response to call*	John – Yes
Greeting	*Response to greeting*	Hi – Hi
Exclamation	*Response to exclamation*	Disgusting – You bet
Offer	*Acknowledge offer*	A piece of home-made pie? – Sure
Command	*Response offer to command*	Get me two painkillers – Will do
Statement	*Acknowledge statement*	Hottest day of the summer – Guess so
Question	*Response statement to question*	When will I see you? – At eleven

Obsessive-compulsive personality disorder

Wrapped up in one's own perspective

Speech about self, first person participant (ideational)
• *Expressed by first person pronouns*
Less talk about other participants or interlocutors (ideational)
• *Expressed by second* you, *third* it, they *person pronouns*
Ignore ideas and interactions of others (interpersonal)
• *Giving second pair in pairs of adjacent turns that ignore the first turn*
  – adjacency pairs of turns: (interpersonal)

Call	*Response to call*	John – Yes
Greeting	*Response to greeting*	Hi – Hi
Exclamation	*Response to exclamation*	Disgusting – You bet
Offer	*Acknowledge offer*	A piece of home-made pie? – Sure
Command	*Response offer to command*	Get me two painkillers – Will do
Statement	*Acknowledge statement*	Hottest day of the summer – Guess so
Question	*Response statement to question*	When will I see you? – At eleven

Cohesion, lack of continuing language of others, by: (textual)
• *Reference (continuity of participants – people, places, things)*

personal	he, she, it
demonstrative	this, that
comparatives	more drivers

• *Conjunction (continuity and development of message)*

additive
temporal
causal
- internal
- external

• *Lexical (continuity of institutional focus – subject matter of talk)*
> repetition
> synonym
> co-occurrence

• *Substitution & ellipsis (direct copying of information)*
> nominal
> verbal
> clausal

Affective atypicalities
Controlled, formal, stilted
• *Overuse of high frequency words* good nice awful
• *Slow, unvarying rate of speech*
• *Level volume*
• *Relatively level pitch, small changes in pitch*
Failure to express compliments (interpersonal)
Discomfort when others express emotions
• *Changing topics, by changing participants, processes after interlocutor expresses emotion (ideational, interpersonal)*
• *Short second turn after interlocutor expresses emotion (interpersonal)*
• *Negative comments after interlocutor expresses emotion (ideational, interpersonal)*
Formal, serious relationships
• *Topics (field of discourse) that are not personal (ideational)*
• *Few contractions*
• *Low frequency vocabulary, formal vocabulary*
• *Monotonous intonation, limited pitch and loudness changes*
• *Limited modulation of commitment, by*

> attitudinal adjuncts
> modal verbs

Preoccupation with logic and intellect
• *Increased use of vocabulary that avoids emotions (ideational)*
• *Increased use of conjunctions of cause and temporal relations (interpersonal)*
• *Infrequent assigning of emotions to self, first person carrier of emotional attribute* I seemed happy
Holding back to fashion a perfect utterance
• *Delay in starting turn or clause*
• *Infrequent self-correction, repetition, hesitation markers*
• *More frequent and longer pauses*

Index